AF678820

Early Brain Damage

Volume 1
Research Orientations and Clinical Observations

BEHAVIORAL BIOLOGY

AN INTERNATIONAL SERIES

Series editors

James L. McGaugh
Department of Psychobiology
University of California
Irvine, California

John C. Fentress
Department of Psychology
Dalhousie University
Halifax, Canada

Joseph P. Hegmann
Department of Zoology
The University of Iowa
Iowa City, Iowa

Holger Ursin, Eivind Baade, and Seymour Levine (Editors), Psychobiology of Stress: A Study of Coping Men

William W. Grings and Michael E. Dawson, Emotions and Bodily Responses: A Psychophysiological Approach

Enoch Callaway, Patricia Tueting, and Stephen H. Koslow (Editors), Event Related Brain Potentials in Man

Larry L. Butcher (Editor), Cholinergic–Monoaminergic Interactions in the Brain

Aryeh Routtenberg (Editor), Biology of Reinforcement: Facets of Brain-Stimulation Reward

Richard N. Aslin, Jeffrey R. Alberts, and Michael R. Petersen (Editors), Development of Perception: Psychobiological Perspectives. Vol. 1: Audition, Somatic Perception, and the Chemical Senses; Vol. 2: The Visual System

Joe L. Martinez, Jr., Robert A. Jensen, Rita B. Messing, Henk Rigter, and James L. McGaugh (Editors), Endogenous Peptides and Learning and Memory Processes

James W. Maas (Editor), MHPG: Basic Mechanisms and Psychopathology

Harman V. S. Peeke and Lewis Petrinovich (Editors), Habituation, Sensitization, and Behavior

C. Robert Almli and Stanley Finger (Editors), Early Brain Damage, Volume 1: Research Orientations and Clinical Observations

Stanley Finger and C. Robert Almli (Editors), Early Brain Damage, Volume 2: Neurobiology and Behavior

In preparation

Martin Reite and Tiffany Field (Editors), The Psychobiology of Attachment

Stanley D. Glick (Editor), Cerebral Lateralization in Nonhuman Species

Early Brain Damage

Volume 1
Research Orientations and Clinical Observations

EDITED BY

C. ROBERT ALMLI
Programs in Occupational Therapy and Neural Sciences
Departments of Anatomy and Neurobiology,
Preventive Medicine, and Psychology
Washington University School of Medicine
St. Louis, Missouri

STANLEY FINGER
Department of Psychology and Neurobiology Program
Washington University
St. Louis, Missouri

1984

ACADEMIC PRESS, INC.
(Harcourt Brace Jovanovich, Publishers)
Orlando San Diego San Francisco New York London
Toronto Montreal Sydney Tokyo

To our families:
Sheila, Todd, and Lynn
Wendy, Robbie, and Brad

COPYRIGHT © 1984, BY ACADEMIC PRESS, INC.
ALL RIGHTS RESERVED.
NO PART OF THIS PUBLICATION MAY BE REPRODUCED OR TRANSMITTED IN ANY FORM OR BY ANY MEANS, ELECTRONIC OR MECHANICAL, INCLUDING PHOTOCOPY, RECORDING, OR ANY INFORMATION STORAGE AND RETRIEVAL SYSTEM, WITHOUT PERMISSION IN WRITING FROM THE PUBLISHER.

ACADEMIC PRESS, INC.
Orlando, Florida 32887

United Kingdom Edition published by
ACADEMIC PRESS, INC. (LONDON) LTD.
24/28 Oval Road, London NW1 7DX

Library of Congress Cataloging in Publication Data

Main entry under title.

Early brain damage.

(Behavioral biology)
Order of editors' names reversed on v. 2.
Includes bibliographical references and index.
Contents: v. 1. Research orientations and clinical observations -- v. 2. Neurobiology and behavior.
1. Brain damaged children. 2. Developmental neurobiology. 3. Developmental psychobiology. I. Almli, C. Robert. II. Finger, Stanley. III. Series: Behavioral biology (New York, N.Y. : 1978) [DNLM: 1. Brain damage, Chronic--In infancy and childhood. 2. Brain injuries--In infancy and childhood. WS 340 E12]
RJ496.B7E27 1984 618.92'8 83-25833
ISBN 0-12-052901-7 (v. 1 : alk. paper)
ISBN 0-12-052902-5 (v. 2 : alk. paper)

PRINTED IN THE UNITED STATES OF AMERICA

84 85 86 87 9 8 7 6 5 4 3 2 1

Contents

Contributors

Numbers in parentheses indicate the pages on which the authors' contributions begin.

George M. Anderson (111), Department of Laboratory Medicine and the Child Study Center, Yale University School of Medicine, New Haven, Connecticut 06510

Thomas J. Boll (215), Department of Psychology, University of Alabama, Birmingham, Alabama 35294

Thomas H. Burnstine (3), Rush Medical College, Chicago, Illinois 60612

Donald J. Cohen (111), Pediatric Neurology, Yale University School of Medicine, New Haven, Connecticut 06510

Constance J. D'Amato (127), Department of Pathology, University of Michigan Medical School, Ann Arbor, Michigan 48109

Jack M. Fletcher (189), Developmental Neuropsychology Section, Texas Research Institute of Mental Sciences, Texas Medical Center, Houston, Texas 77030

Robert B. Glassman (35), Department of Psychology, Lake Forest College, Lake Forest, Illinois 60045

Roy A. Glover (127), Department of Anatomy and Cell Biology, University of Michigan Medical School, Ann Arbor, Michigan 48109

William T. Greenough (3), Department of Psychology, University of Illinois, Urbana-Champaign, Illinois 61820

Henri Hécaen[1] (277), Unité 111 — INSERM, 75014 Paris, France

Thomas G. Heffner (93), Department of Pharmacology, Warner-Lambert/Parke Davis, Ann Arbor, Michigan 48105

Alfred Heller (93), Department of Pharmacological and Physiological Sciences, University of Chicago, Chicago, Illinois 60637

Rolando R. Henry (253), Department of Psychiatry, Neuropsychiatric Institute, University of California, Los Angeles, School of Medicine, Los Angeles, California 90024

Samuel P. Hicks (127), Department of Pathology, University of Michigan Medical School, Ann Arbor, Michigan 48109

Hendrik J. Huisjes (169), University Hospital Groningen, Department of Obstetrics, 9713 EZ Groningen, The Netherlands

Marc Jeannerod (277), Laboratoire de Neuropsychologie Expérimentale, Unité 94 — INSERM, 69500 Bron, France

Malcolm A. Jeeves (233), Psychological Laboratory, University of St. Andrews, St. Andrews, Fife, Scotland, KY16 9JU

Katherine L. Kreusser (151), Department of Pediatrics, St. Louis Children's Hospital, St. Louis, Missouri 63110

Susan H. Landry (189), Developmental Neuropsychology Section, Texas Research Institute of Mental Sciences, Texas Medical Center, Houston, Texas 77030

Harvey S. Levin (189), Division of Neurosurgery, Department of Surgery, University of Texas Medical Center, Galveston, Texas 77550

Daniel S. O'Leary (215), Department of Psychology, University of Health Sciences, The Chicago Medical School, North Chicago, Illinois 60064

M. T. Perenin (277), Laboratoire de Neuropsychologie Expérimentale, Unité 94 — INSERM, 69500 Bron, France

Lisa A. Raskin (111), Department of Psychology, Amherst College, Amherst, Massachusetts 01002

Eric Saslow (253), Division of Pediatric Neurology, Department of Pediatrics, University of California, Los Angeles, School of Medicine, Los Angeles, California 90024

Paul Satz (253), Department of Psychiatry, Neuropsychiatric Institute, University of California, Los Angeles, School of Medicine, Los Angeles, California 90024

Lewis S. Seiden (93), Department of Pharmacological and Physiological Sciences, University of Chicago, Chicago, Illinois 60637

[1]Deceased.

Bennett A. Shaywitz (111), Pediatric Neurology, Yale University School of Medicine, New Haven, Connecticut 06510

Sally E. Shaywitz (111), Department of Pediatrics, Yale University School of Medicine, New Haven, Connecticut 06510

Aaron Smith (299), Neuropsychological Laboratory, The University of Michigan, Ann Arbor, Michigan 48109

Oswald Steward (59), Department of Neurological Surgery and Department of Physiology, University of Virginia, Charlottesville, Virginia 22908

H. Gerry Taylor (325), Child Development Unit, Department of Pediatrics, Children's Hospital of Pittsburgh, Pittsburgh, Pennsylvania 15213

Richard C. Tees (3), Department of Psychology, University of British Columbia, Vancouver, British Columbia V6T 1W5, Canada

Bert C. L. Touwen (169), Department of Developmental Neurology, Institute for Developmental Neurology, University Hospital Groningen, 9713 EZ Groningen, The Netherlands

Marcus W. van Hof (81), Department of Developmental Neurology, Institute for Developmental Neurology, University Hospital Groningen, 9713 EZ Groningen, The Netherlands

Joseph J. Volpe (151), Department of Pediatrics, St. Louis Children's Hospital, St. Louis, Missouri 63110

E. M. W. Wildervanck de Blécourt (81), Department of Physiology, Erasmus Universiteit Rotterdam, Rotterdam, The Netherlands

William C. Wimsatt (35), Committee on Conceptual Foundations of Science, University of Chicago, Chicago, Illinois 60637

Preface

One of the more intriguing and perplexing questions in the brain-damage literature on human patients and laboratory animals concerns the nature of the relationship between the organism's developmental status at the time of brain damage and the capacity for sparing or recovery of function. Almost 50 years ago, Margaret Kennard suggested that early brain damage may not be as deleterious as later brain damage, and hypothesized that this reflected a greater capacity for reorganization in the immature nervous system. But is there always greater sparing and recovery following early brain damage? And what evidence is there for neural reorganization on an anatomical or a physiological level? Indeed, even today the associations between age at the time of brain damage, performance, and developmental biology are far from being completely understood. It is in this context that the present two volumes were assembled. We asked noted workers to summarize and integrate their experiments and observations pertaining to early brain damage, and compiled a series of chapters into two volumes that emphasized the most salient new findings and developments in the field.

Early Brain Damage (Volumes 1 and *2)* presents a broad-based coverage of the many facets of current research being conducted on the topic of brain damage sustained early in life. Both volumes are oriented toward researchers and professional personnel interested in the topic of brain damage, and especially toward those interested in the many developmental brain-damage issues emanating from laboratory animal studies and human case reports. The collection of topics covered in the two volumes are representative of the multiple levels of analysis currently being used to assess the effects of early brain damage both experimentally and in neurological patients.

Volume 1, Research Orientations and Clinical Observations, is a collection of chapters oriented toward early brain damage in human clinical populations. This volume is divided into four basic parts. Part I presents research strategies and theoretical issues, such as intermodal compensation and evolutionary considerations, relating to early brain-damage phenomena. Part II presents research on animal models of infant neuropathological conditions such as hypoxia, fetal radiation, locomotor hyperactivity, and attentional disorders. Part III is concerned with short-term and long-term neurological effects of brain damage in children, including chapters on perinatal asphyxia, behavioral consequences of cerebral insult sustained during infancy, and correlates of early generalized brain dysfunction in children. Part IV presents chapters on cerebral lateralization and higher-order functions as they are altered by early brain damage.

The companion volume, *Early Brain Damage (Volume 2, Neurobiology and Behavior),* is a collection of chapters dealing with controlled experimentation on laboratory animals. The three parts of Volume 2 deal with recent advances in the anatomy and physiology of early brain damage, behavioral biology, and variables interacting with early brain damage.

While the principal thrust of both volumes of *Early Brain Damage* is to provide state-of-the-art information on the topic of early brain damage, we hope that the various approaches and multiple levels of analyses presented in the two volumes will contribute to a better understanding, for all readers regardless of their backgrounds or theoretical orientations, of the consequences of early brain damage. It is hoped that the topics covered in *Early Brain Damage* will clarify some of the perplexing and pertinent issues in this field, will increase appreciation of the difficulties and complexities involved in comparing brain-damaged groups of different ages, and will stimulate new research to answer at least some of the important unanswered questions about brain damage sustained early in life.

Contents of Volume 2

Neurobiology and Behavior

III. Variables Interacting with Early Brain Damage

Early Brain Damage

Volume 1

Research Orientations and Clinical Observations

I

Research Strategies and Theoretical Issues

1

Intermodal Compensation following Damage or Deprivation: A Review of Behavioral and Neural Evidence

Thomas H. Burnstine,
William T. Greenough,
and Richard C. Tees

Introduction

The idea that the function of one modality may be altered to compensate for the loss of another has a long history. Extensive use of terms such as *behavioral substitution, sensory substitution,* and *vicariate of the senses* attests to its acceptance as a partial explanation of recovery of function after sensory damage. At a more practical level, therapies and prosthetic devices have been developed to enhance or embellish the function of intact modalities. Behavioral research has provided some support for the existence of such compensatory phe-

EARLY BRAIN DAMAGE, Volume 1
Research Orientations and Clinical Observations

Copyright © 1984 by Academic Press, Inc.
All rights of reproduction in any form reserved.
ISBN 0-12-052901-7

nomena, and recent studies of the nervous system have provided some insight into their possible substrates.

For organizational purposes we define three terms. *Intermodal compensation* (IC) refers to the behavioral phenomenon in which capacities emerge in an intact modality that are superior in or unique to individuals who have been damaged or deprived in one or more other modalities. (*Intramodal compensation,* involving different abilities within a modality, is also occasionally described.) *Compensatory hypertrophy* (CH) refers to one type of proposed neural substrate of intermodal compensation, in which reorganization takes place within the neural tissue normally associated with an intact modality, adding new functional capacity. *Functional reallocation* (FR) refers to a second proposed neural substrate of behavioral compensation, in which tissue normally used for one purpose is used for a different purpose (e.g., visual cortex processing auditory information). In this chapter we first discuss behavioral evidence regarding IC; we then review findings indicating central nervous system (CNS) reorganization in intact modalities following damage or deprivation in others; and finally we consider mechanisms whereby the maturing and the mature CNS may remain amenable to reorganization.

Intermodal Compensation

Intermodal compensation (IC) is not a recent idea. In the eighteenth century, Diderot wrote of heightened tactile and auditory sensitivity in the blind:

> The blind man of Puisaux judges of his nearness to the fire by the degrees of heat; of the fullness of vessells by the sound made by liquids which he pours into them; of the proximity of bodies by the action of air on his face. He is so sensitive to the atmospheric change that he can distinguish between a street and a closed alley (Diderot, 1749/1916, p. 78).

These feats were attributed not to mysterious powers but to the attention to and different uses of the remaining senses. Of the same blind man he wrote, "He has a surprising memory for sounds, and can distinguish as many differences in voices as we can in faces. He finds in these an infinite number of delicate gradations which escape us because we have not the same interest in observing them" (Diderot, 1749/1916 p. 75). Experimental work in the ensuing two and one-third centuries has provided some support for Diderot's views.

LONG-TERM IC STUDIES IN HUMANS

Table 1 summarizes human studies involving long-term damage to one or more modalities. Most involve intact modalities of blind or deaf subjects. Taken as a whole the data in Table 1 are rather confusing. Even though the early reports are discounted due to methodological inadequacies and small sample sizes, about half of the remainder find evidence for IC, one fourth do not, and the remaining fourth report the opposite effect; such a distribution might be expected from chance alone, especially when one assumes that negative studies are less frequently published.

However, a different picture emerges for studies that have provided sufficient data if two hypotheses are considered:

1. Damage to a modality places additional demands on or allows greater attention to nondamaged modalities.
2. In some instances an ability (e.g., spatial) is broadly based and depends on information that is optimally acquired through a particular modality (and possibly at or by a particular age). Compensation will thus be greater (or may only occur) in those who have had the opportunity to gain such information.

Turkewitz and Kenny (1982) recently summarized support for these views in the context of a theory of neuroperceptual development. They argue that the emergence of modalities must be temporally distinct from each other during ontogenesis to allow more concentrated attention to each and to allow later-maturing modalities to more effectively utilize information from previously organized ones. They note that tactile development precedes vestibular development and that audition and vision are further delayed. For example, they suggest that the eyes stay closed postnatally in some species to allow other modalities to establish themselves. In passing, they observe that IC may be a reflection of decreased interference by another modality. They propose that competition for attention or competition of the type seen within developing modalities at the level of neural connections (e.g., LeVay, Wiesel, & Hubel, 1980) may underlie IC effects and may be reduced by maturational staggering of the organization of modalities.

This theory suggests two possible outcomes for a modality that is damaged or deprived. First, if relatively little information from the damaged modality is required for organization of some capacity in

TABLE 1

Long-Term Deprivation or Damage Effects on Other Modalities: Human Studies

Authors/date	Measures or procedures[a]	Results	Comments
Hall, 1879	Vibratory, tactile abilities of Laura Bridgeman (blind, deaf) (onset: 2 yr)	Heightened vibratory, tactile sensitivity	Compared to population averages
Jastrow, 1894	Tactile measures in Helen Keller (blind, deaf) (onset: 2 yr)	Higher verbal memory; heightened tactile stimulus reaction time	Compared to world's fair attendees
Griesbach, 1899; cited by Kunz, 1908	1. Sound localization 2. 2-Point limen (blind, deaf vs. sighted children)	1. No differences 2. Sighted slightly superior; braille finger *less* sensitive in blind	Matching of controls unclear
Kunz, 1908	Spatial abilities (blind vs. sighted children)	No difference between blind and sighted	Matching of controls unclear
Sylvester, 1913	Form board test (spatial) (congenitally, early, and late-blind adolescents)	Latency, errors decreased with increasing prior vision	Controls not matched for sex or intelligence
Seashore and Ling, 1918	Sound localization, intensity discrimination, weight and pressure discrimination (blind vs. sighted adolescents)	Blind slightly superior at sound localization; inferior at weight, pressure, surface-irregularity discrimination	Controls not age matched
Koch (unpublished) cited by Carr, 1921	Stylus maze learning (blind vs. sighted adults)	Congenital blind took more trials and made more errors	Sighted subjects reported visual image of maze
Brown and Stratton, 1925	Distance between posts on a board (blind and sighted children)	Blind superior; totally blind superior to partially blind	Axelrod, 1959 noted similarity of test to braille
Koch and Ufkess, 1926	Stylus maze learning (blind and sighted adolescents and adults)	Congenitally blind inferior; no differences between later blind and controls	Large sample; controls not matched for sex

Knotts and Miles, 1929	Finger and stylus maze learning (blind vs. sighted adolescents)	Blind as good or better overall; age of onset effect as in Koch and Ufkess, 1926	Large sample
Hayes, 1933, 1935	1. Auditory acuity 2. Auditory recognition of objects in shaken box (sighted and blind children)	1. No differences 2. Sighted faster	
Tilney, 1929	Olfactory, tactile, motion, temperature, vibratory abilities of Helen Keller	Concluded no evidence for "passive" compensation	Disputes control groups of Hall, 1897; Jastrow, 1894
Renshaw, Wherry, and Newlin, 1930	Cutaneous localization (congenitally blind vs. sighted, ages 8–14, early 20s)	Blind adults better than sighted adults; the opposite at age 8–14	
Duncan, 1934	Finger maze learning (blind vs. sighted adolescents and adults)	Little difference between blind and sighted overall (age of onset more important than present vision)	Large sample
Blumenfeld, 1937	Perception of curvature of rulers (blind vs. sighted)	Sighted superior to blind in some cases	$N = 4$
Crewdson and Zangwill, 1940	Similar to Blumenfeld, 1937	Similar to Blumenfeld, 1937	$N = 1$
Supa, Cotzin, and Dallenbach, 1944	Ability to locate walls in an open area; manipulated auditory and tactile cues (2-yr, 5-yr onset)	Blind superior at detecting and approaching walls more closely without touching; auditory cues primary; sighted improved with practice	$n = 2$ blind, 2 sighted
Teuber, Krieger, and Bender, 1949	Two-point limens on amputated stumps and unamputated counterparts (adults)	Greater acuity on amputated stumps; most pronounced distally	Intramodal
MacFarland, 1952	Maze learning (blind vs. sighted)	Sighted superior	

(continued)

TABLE 1 (*Continued*)

Authors/date	Measures or procedures[a]	Results	Comments
Hunter, 1954	Perception of curvature of rulers (blind vs. sighted adolescents) (see Blumenfeld, 1937)	Sighted less able to detect curvature when ends bent toward them and were more variable in performance	Large sample
Haber, 1955	Two- and 3-point limens, light touch threshold on stump and intact arm in upper-arm amputees, compared with intact controls	Greater stump sensitivity on all measures, compared to intact arm or to intact controls; no differences between intact arms of amputees and controls; distal stump most sensitive; greatest sensitivity when phantom limb retracted into stump	Systematic replication of Teuber *et al.*, 1949; intramodal
Drever, 1955	Tactile recognition of geometric figures, spatial position in rotated pegboard, recognition of unique arrangements of pegs (early, <4 yr, and late blind vs. sighted, 9–19 yr)	Sighted and late blind superior to early blind; late blind superior to sighted; blind primarily used shape whereas sighted counted pegs	
Rosenstein, 1957	Discrimination of rhythmic vibratory patterns on fingertips (11–13 yr-old blind, deaf, aphasic, and control children)	Blind superior to other groups, which did not differ; only blind and controls improved with practice	
Axelrod, 1959	1. Light touch and 2-point threshold (index and ring fingers of preferred hand) 2. Tactile abstraction	1. Early blind males more touch sensitive than sighted males on ring finger—opposite for females; early	Noted that braille experience could affect his (and others') index-finger results

	3. Ability to pick correct object from sound or verbalized principles Early (<2 yr) and late (>2 yr) blind vs. sighted (9–19-yr old)	blind better 2-point acuity than sighted on right index finger 2. Sighted superior to early blind on metal, but no length- or softness-tactile abstraction 3. Sighted superior to early blind; late blind superior to early blind on verbal–tactile test	
Ewart and Carp, 1963	Match-to-sample shape recognition of geometric blocks	High-intelligence blind superior to low-intelligence blind and to both high- and low-intelligence sighted	Authors suggest intelligent blind develop better rectangular concept
Stellwagen and Cuthbert, 1963	Tactile discrimination of embossed complex patterns (blind vs. sighted)	No significant differences; blind slightly superior	Large sample
Hunter, 1964	1. Estimating linear circumference of cylinders 2. Matching spatial pattern of objects 3. Estimating size of rooms (auditory cues masked) (congenitally blind vs. sighted)	1. and 2. Sighted superior 3. No difference	
Sterritt, Camp, and Lipman, 1966	Auditory and visual temporal-pattern reproduction (severe to profound hearing impaired)	Blind inferior in both modalities	Authors suggest audition primary source of temporal-pattern information

(*continued*)

TABLE 1 (*Continued*)

Authors/date	Measures or procedures[a]	Results	Comments
Blank and Bridger, 1966	Cutaneous form sensitivity (deaf vs. hearing children, 5–6 yr)	Deaf superior to hearing	
Hartlage, 1968	Spatial and nonspatial reasoning (congenitally blind vs. sighted children)	Sighted superior to blind in spatial reasoning	
Rice, 1969	Ability to detect and locate disks of various sizes at short distance, using oral sounds; immediate memory span for brief, multisite tactile stimulation	Early blind superior to late blind and sighted	$N = 1$ Early blind
Aftanas and Zubek, 1971	Visual flicker fusion frequency in unilateral arm amputees vs. intact controls	Slight (borderline significance) differences favoring amputees	
Spigelman, 1976	Sound (tones) localization 360° around head; (congenitally and late blind, and sighted)	Early blind equalled sighted; late blind inferior to both	Large sample
Zihl, 1980	Detection of position of flash in adults with geniculostriate-path damage	Ability improved with practice presumably through nongeniculostriate paths	Small N; intramodal
Landau, Gleitman, and Spelke 1981	Determining shortest path between two objects (blind and sighted children, and sighted adults)	No differences among children; adults more accurate	Small N; not gestationally age-matched; sex not given

[a]Subjects were adults except as noted. Where relevant, sighted controls were tested without visual cues.

an undamaged modality, then that capacity should either develop normally or be enhanced. Second, if the damaged modality normally provides information crucial to development of a capacity of another, then that capacity will be impaired. Moreover, in the second case the impairment should be greater with congenital or early damage to the contributing modality than with later or postmaturational damage.

The studies in Table 1 that provide information regarding onset age can generally be interpreted to support these predictions. For instance, development of cutaneous sensitivity might be expected to require little input from other modalities and to undergo increased functional demand (e.g., due to Braille usage; Axelrod, 1959) in the blind. The better controlled studies tend to support the view that cutaneous sensitivity is greater in blind than in sighted subjects (e.g., Axelrod, 1959; Brown & Stratton, 1925; Renshaw, Wherry, & Newlin, 1930; Rosenstein, 1957). Moreover, Axelrod (1959) reported touch threshold to be lower in the early but not in the later blind, as would be predicted from reduced intermodal competition. Although there is evidence that such changes in sensitivity may occur quite rapidly with practice (Renshaw, 1930; Renshaw *et al.*, 1930; Volkmann, 1858/1955), their stability in the absence of continued practice does not appear to have been described. An enhanced ability to localize above-threshold skin sensations in congenitally blind people (Renshaw *et al.*, 1930) and in blind people of unspecified onset (Rice, 1969) might also be predictable, if we assume that the body's surface would be known only tactually by the blind, whereas awareness of visual location would actually compete with the tactile sense in the sighted, as argued by Hayes (1941). Indeed, Rock and Victor (1964) found that visual images tend to predominate over conflicting tactual information in sighted adults. And sighted adults were inferior to sighted children in the Renshaw *et al.* (1930) study, whereas the opposite prevailed with blind subjects. Moreover, McKinney (1964) reported that (in children) rotating the hand away from the position in which it was held when a tactual stimulus was presented interfered with its subsequent localization in both blind and sighted, and returning to the original position restored performance in the sighted but further impaired performance in the blind. McKinney argued that the sighted children had a visual image of the hand, which was affected by movement away from the original position and restored when the original position returned. Also, while cutaneous localization seems to improve rapidly with practice (Renshaw, 1930), the sighted adults remain slightly poorer than untrained blind adults, who also improve with practice. For more visually dependent tactile abilities, such as shape discrimination, on the other hand, one might expect early visual experience to be of value. (Visual imagery continues to dominate thought after blindness onset in the later but not in the earlier blind; Schlaegel, 1953.) Thus, reports that the sighted are superior to early but not to late blind subjects on aspects of tactile abstraction and object recognition would be predicted from the preceding second hypothesis (Axelrod, 1959; Drever 1955). Ewart and Carp (1963) found no overall blind–sighted difference in shape matching (the high-IQ blind were superior to all sighted subjects), but age of onset was not considered in this report. It could be argued that the matching-to-sample procedure used by Ewart and Carp may be less sensitive than those of other investigators.

Spatial knowledge might be expected to be particularly lacking in the congenitally blind, because it is primarily through vision that one generates a coherent, analog concept of the surrounding space and especially a "feel" for the existence of distant objects, as several authors in Table 1 note (see also Critchley, 1953). Thus, authors of better controlled studies have typically expressed little surprise at the general superiority of the sighted to the blind on tasks with a spatial component, particularly in the case of the early or the congenitally blind (Carr, 1921; Drever, 1955; Duncan, 1934; Hartlage, 1968; Hunter, 1964; Koch & Ufkess, 1926; MacFarland, 1952). One exception to this pattern of findings (Knotts & Miles, 1929), in which the blind were as good as or better than the sighted, still found poorer performance in the congenitally blind. Overall, these findings generally fit well with the Turkewitz and Kenny (1982) view that information in one modality is used in organization of another, although in the case of spatial knowledge a later-developing modality provides information to an earlier one.

Necessity again seems the mother of extravisual intervention in the case of environmental orientation; however, data indicating both heightened cutaneous sensitivity (Blank & Bridger, 1966) and no difference in sensitivity (Rosenstein, 1957) in deaf relative to hearing subjects are harder to interpret in this way. Unfortunately, these studies cannot be interpreted in terms of the attention–competition developmental model, because they did not indicate onset age of deafness. However, possible visual enhancement in adult arm amputees (Aftanas & Zubek, 1971) hints that intermodal compensation may not be limited to development. Another study indicates that audition may provide general information used to develop extramodal information processing in the Sterritt, Camp, and Lipman (1966) report that congenital and early onset hearing-impaired subjects were inferior to the hearing in both auditory and visual–temporal pattern reproduction.

One type of spatially-related performance that does not seem to fit this pattern is object perception in the blind. The remarkable ability of many of the blind and even the blind–deaf to travel about in a familiar environment has often been noted (e.g., Supa, Cotzin, & Dallenbach, 1944; Worchel & Dallenbach, 1947). Supa *et al.* (1944) found that their blind subjects were generally superior to blindfolded, sighted subjects in locating walls and partitions accurately. This ability improved with practice in both blind and sighted subjects (Supa *et al.*, 1944; Worchel & Mauney, 1951). Indoors, self-generated auditory cues were primary, whereas outdoors tactile air-movement perception, olfaction, and perhaps other abilities could be used (Ammons, Worchel, & Dallenbach, 1953; Supa *et al.*, 1944). Similarly, the blind have been found to be superior to the sighted in detecting and locating small, nearby objects using self-generated sound cues (e.g., Rice, 1969), although auditory localization in general is not always superior. In contrast to earlier positive reports (Griesbach, 1899; Seashore & Ling, 1918), Spigelman (1976) found the late blind to be inferior to the early blind and to the sighted (who did not differ) in localizing an experimentally generated sound. Studies of the tactile ability to detect curvature (seemingly a spatial perceptual capacity) have provided conflicting results. Several investigators (Blumenfeld, 1937; Crewdson & Zangwill, 1940; W. F. Hunter, 1964) found the sighted to be superior to the blind in tactile detection of curvature in edges and surfaces, whereas I. M. L. Hunter (1954) found the blind to be superior. W. F. Hunter (1964) used subjects who were blind from birth, whereas I. M. L. Hunter (1954) included later-blind and partially sighted subjects, which may explain this discrepancy.

In general, these studies are compatible with the view that IC may occur under conditions in which intact modalities are not dependent upon damaged ones for organizational information or when the damaged modality is intact during early periods of organization of perceptual abilities. An issue not resolved is whether the positive IC results arise from functional demand, from relatively passive redistribution of attention, or through some other facet of altered competitiveness from other modalities.

Long-Term IC Studies in Animals

Animal research, shown in Table 2, has in general provided less clear-cut evidence of IC, but it has strongly supported the idea that information gained through one modality may be important to an-

TABLE 2

Long-Term Deprivation or Damage Effects on Other Modalities: Animal Studies

Source	Measures or procedures	Results	Comments
Wolf, 1943	Auditory or visual deprivation at ear (10d) or eye (12–15d) opening or at 26, 50, or 75d for $1\frac{1}{2}$ to 2 wk in rats. Tested in competition, running for food using visual or auditory cue	At all ages, rats more likely to win when cued in nondeprived (competitor's deprived) modality	
Hebb, 1949	Maze learning in early- vs. late-blinded rats	Late blinded superior	
Hymovitch, 1952	Maze learning in early- vs. late-blinded rats reared in complex or standard housing	Age of blinding not significant; complex environment enhanced performance	No test for interaction
Gauron and Becker, 1957	Substantially similar to Wolf, 1943	Substantially similar to Wolf, 1943	
Tees and Cartwright, 1972	Sensory preconditioning using auditory–auditory, auditory–visual, or visual–visual cues in dark-reared vs. light-reared rats	Deprived rats inferior in auditory–visual and visual–visual tasks	
Turkewitz, Gilbert, and Birch, 1974	Visual-cliff performance in kittens with or without neonatal vibrissae removal	Earlier discrimination of visual cliff in deprived kittens	
Spigelman, 1976	1. Sound localization in Y maze in early-blind, late-blind, and sighted rats 2. Tone discrimination in equivalent groups 3. As in 1, varying onset and duration of blindness	1. Late blind superior to early blind, sighted intermediate 2. Early blind superior to late blind; sighted intermediate 3. Age of onset, not duration, important	

other and to intermodal integration. Wolf (1943) reported that visually deprived rats were inferior to auditorially deprived rats at running to food upon presentation of a visual signal, and vice versa (auditorially deprived—auditory signal). Gauron and Becker (1959) essentially confirmed this, but whether this represents a deficit in the deprived modality or enhancement of the other is uncertain, although the late deprivation effects in the Wolf study, as well as the short-term effects discussed in the following section, suggest possible enhancement. Early blindness yielded deficits relative to late blindness in various spatial tasks (Hebb, 1949; Spigelman, 1976; Tees, Midgley, & Nesbit, 1981; nonsignificant tendency, Hymovitch, 1952), whereas the early blind were superior to the late blind in a nonspatial frequency discrimination (Spigelman, 1976). Whisker removal in kittens appeared to accelerate visual development (Turkewitz, Gilbert, & Birch, 1974). Several reports suggest that blind, whiskerless or auditorially deprived animals exhibit greater exploration of novel environments (Glickman, 1958; MacDougall & Rabinovich, 1972; Zucker & Bindra, 1961). However, the finding is neither universal (Spigelman, 1976) nor interpretable in strictly exploratory terms, given possible affects of sensory impairment or deprivation on measures of affective responses, thereby affecting exploratory behavior, given that the deprivation procedures may alter exploration by affecting "emotionality" (cf. Denenberg, 1967).

A problem with most of these studies is that a laboratory cage does not place demands on the subjects comparable to those placed on blind or deaf humans who must somehow deal with their complex surroundings. The neonates' laboratory environment may differ little from feral conditions, but the differences between the laboratory and nature become increasingly pronounced as the organism matures. In one attempt to examine this question, Rogowski and Greenough (personal communication, 1982) compared neonatally blinded mice with sighted mice. Each had been reared with various objects in the maternal cage prior to weaning and had been reared together after weaning in a large cage with a changing pattern of toys, elevated ramps, shelves, and so forth. Informal observation indicated that the blind mice negotiated the environment quite well, and that they used their whiskers extensively. After 36 days the mice were tested for whisker-triggered forepaw extension by suspending them by the tail in a device in which a clear Plexiglas shelf could be slowly raised toward their dangling head and forepaws. The sighted animals' eyes were dilated with atropine and the task was run in dim red light to prevent visually triggered extension. The dependent variable was the distance between the shelf position at the first forepaw extension and

TABLE 3

Whisker-Triggered Placing[a]

	n	Mean (mm)	*SEM*
Sighted	6	1.4	.39
Blind	6	3.2	.30

[a]Mean distance between first placing response and first touch (see text for details). Difference significant by t test ($p < .01$). There was no overlap between groups.

its position when the mice first were able to touch it. As Table 3 shows this distance was nearly 2 mm greater in the blinded mice, suggesting that they were more sensitive to whisker sensations; however, the possibility that their whisking pattern was altered so that the sweep extended further forward could not be ruled out. Although this result could merely indicate greater attention to somatosensory input, it certainly suggests that IC might be more evident in animal studies with more demanding conditions, both in the rearing environment and in the test situation.

Much human research also seems to have been oriented away from those IC phenomena that are routinely used in coping with handicaps. In the blind, simple techniques call upon other modalities in new ways and must require new functional organizational patterns in the brain for initial processing and integration of the information: step counting and auditory recognition of specific location-associated sounds (detailed descriptions appear in Hayes, 1941, and in Villey, 1930), use of simple prosthetics such as canes; changes in the manner of acquisition of detailed information as in the use of Braille or more modern electronic text-scanning devices (Tobin & James, 1974), or in the use of lip reading (Helen Keller could understand speakers by placing fingertips over the larynx, lips, and nostrils; Keller, 1903/1947; Villey, 1930). These changes need not be reflected in simple threshold shifts, but are evident in the everyday behavior of those with damaged modalities.

Short-Term Deprivation Studies

An important question is whether IC phenomena represent relatively short-term effects of a competition for current attention or longer-term adaptations to demand or use. Several reports (e.g., Renshaw *et al.,* 1930; Supa *et al.,* 1944) describe improvement with practice in intact subjects, but they generally fall short of the performance of the handicapped. Reduced sensory thresholds following short-term deprivation (see Harper and Bross, 1978, for review) suggest that increased sensitivity in other modalities may occur in the absence of functional demand. But because of the variety of measures that have been used (e.g., Gibby, Gibby, & Townsend, 1970; Nagatsuka, 1965; Vernon & McGill, 1961; Zubek, Bross, & Gelfant, 1973) it is difficult to determine whether the degree of threshold shift is equivalent to that reported in blind or deaf subjects. At best, this phenomenon seems likely to account only for threshold shifts and not for the other apparent forms of IC in Table 1. The heightening of sensitivity of nondeprived modalities, which may outlast the deprivation period for a considerable time, has most often been attributed to an attempt to maintain an optimal overall level of input (Harper & Bross, 1978), although attention-splitting notions similar to that of Turkewitz and Kenny (1982) have also been entertained. The preceding exploratory behavior findings have been similarly interpreted (See Tees, 1980).

Compensatory Hypertrophy in the CNS

The CNS evidence for extramodal change following long-term deprivation or damage has been more consistent than the behavioral research, possibly because the changes observed reflect altered information-processing capacities (e.g., facial vision and other IC not tapped by the laboratory studies) as well as simple threshold shifts. Gyllensten, Malmfors, and Norrlin (1966) examined mice reared in the dark (DR) either from birth to 4 months or from 4 to 7 months. Relative to diurnal light-housed mice (LR), after an initial decline in the younger group, both DR groups had increased internuclear material (presumably axons, dendrites, and neuronal and glial somata) in the primary auditory cortex. The initial decline in the younger animals may reflect nutritional factors. Total darkness upsets maternal circadian rhythms, reducing the milk supply (Eayrs & Ireland, 1950; Mos, 1976), and Gyllensten *et al.* and others have noted lower weight in DR pups. The initial decrease in internuclear material was also much greater in the visual than in the auditory cortex, suggesting that more of the nutrient supply was devoted to the active sense.

In a study without nutritional complications Ryugo, Ryugo, Globus, and Killackey (1975) removed either the eyes or the whiskers of 1-day-old rats. At 25 days of age, after either treatment, the frequency of spines (post-synaptic structures) on apical dendrites of Layer V auditory cortex pyramidal neurons in Layer IV was increased. Comparable measures in the somatosensory cortex were not affected by eye removal nor was visual cortex affected by whisker removal. Ryugo *et al.* proposed that hypertrophy might be initially limited to the auditory system due to its early development and use (Kasatkin, 1967; Sewell, 1968). However, studies of development of the whisker area of the neocortex suggest that sensitivity to whisker removal occurs within the first 5 postnatal days—well before the ears open (Woolsey & Wann, 1977). Thus the delayed development of the auditory system seems more likely to account for the difference.

In seeming contrast, Meyer, Feo Ramos, and Ferres-Torres (1976) did not find temporal cortex-spine differences between DR and LR rats at 36–45 days of age. This may reflect early undernutrition. Meyer *et al.* did, however, find increased spine density in the dentate gyrus and CA1 hippocampus in the DR rats, a result not suggestive of malnutrition (or very compatible with the spatial-maze findings of Tees *et al.*, 1981).

We have completed preliminary studies of the auditory cortex in DR and blinded rats and of the dentate gyrus in DR rats. Our DR situation gave the mother access to a cage placed in diurnal light through a tunnel; three tunnel curves ensured that light did not reach the pups (DeVoogd, 1979). The lighted cage was divided in half, and each half was connected to a separate maternal dark cage to discourage mothers from carrying their pups into this shared environment. None of 8 mothers, observed for over 50 hours, was ever seen carrying a pup to the light cage. At 16 days, about 2–3 days before pups could enter the tunnels themselves, they were sealed off. Results for auditory cortex dendritic branching are shown in Figure 1 (Burnstine, Beck, Pierre-Jerome, & Greenough, in progress). Our DR procedure nearly equalized body weight to LR controls, and auditory cortex dendritic branching showed at most a borderline increase at 25 days of age in blinded rats and a borderline decrease in DR rats. These results suggest that even when nutrition is controlled, hypertrophy may not occur immediately. We are currently studying older animals to determine whether additional hypertrophy occurs in this measure. A parallel study (Greenough & Schwark, personal communication) of 6 LR and 5 DR rats at 25 days of age indicated no significant or apparent difference in total dendritic length of dentate gyrus granule cells. It should be noted that these results involve a different

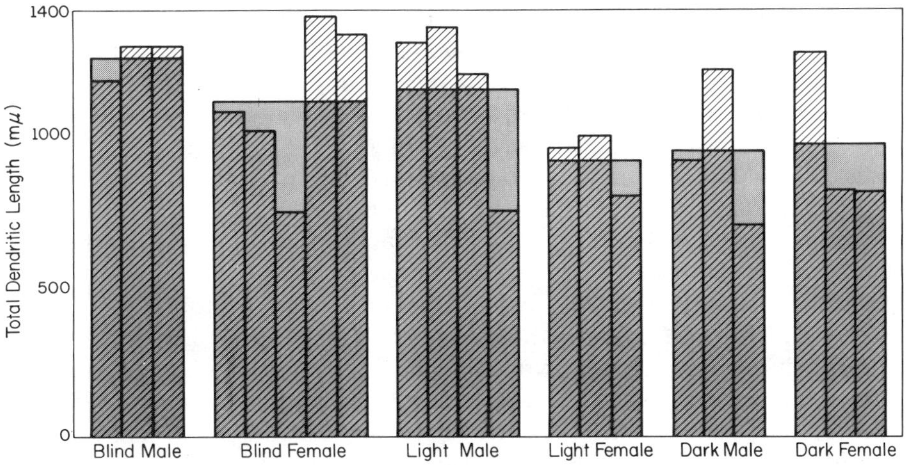

Figure 1. Effects of enucleation and dark rearing on auditory-cortex Layer III–IV pyramidal-cell dendritic fields. Cross hatched bars represent data for individual subjects; shaded bars represent mean for each group (Burnstine *et al.*, in progress.

measure than the spine frequency described by Ryugo *et al.* (1975) and Meyer *et al.* (1976), and there is some evidence that the sensitivity of spine frequency to experience may be greatest in the first 3–4 weeks of postnatal life in the rat (e.g., Schapiro & Vukovich, 1970). Taken with prior findings, our results suggest that hypertrophy in a measure that is sensitive to other environmental influences (reviewed, Greenough & Green, 1981) may be relatively slow to develop. The sort of change predicted by Gyllensten *et al.* (1966) may arise gradually as a result of behavioral demands placed on the auditory system by the absence of vision.

Evidence that behavioral demand may affect CH has been presented by Krech, Rosenzweig, and Bennett (1963). Rats blinded at 25 days of age were raised in complex or isolated environments. Blinding reduced the weight of the visual cortex in both rearing conditions. However, blinded rats reared in the complex environment had a heavier somesthetic cortex with greater activity of the neurotransmitter-related enzyme acetylcholinesterase (ACHE) than similarly reared, sighted rats. MacNeill and Zubek (1967) failed to find similar weight effects, but they speculated that this difference may have been due to the difference in complexity of the environment. Krech *et al.* (1963) also suggested that a prior result (Krech, Rosenzweig, & Bennett, 1960), in which damage to one cortical hemisphere increased ACHE activity in the other, may also reflect increased functional demand.

Further structural and metabolic evidence for CH has come from studies of the motor cortex after visual deprivation. Busniuk (1978) reported greater pyramidal neuron soma size and increased activity of glutamate dehydrogenase in Layers III and V of the motor cortex of DR rats relative to LR rats. Glutamate dehydrogenase activity could reflect increased general metabolism (Krebs-cycle activity) or increased neurotransmitter activity. (Glutamate and a compound into which it is converted, gamma-aminobutyric acid, are both neurotransmitters.) Gerstein (1976) similarly found increased amounts and concentrations of cytoplasmic protein and greater cytoplasmic area in Layer III and V of pyramidal cells in the motor cortex of DR rabbits. This contrasts with reports by Vrensen and DeGroot (1974, 1975) that motor cortex synapses had fewer vesicles in DR rabbits. Both Busniuk and Gerstein argue that visual deprivation complicates the task of moving about in the environment and thus increases the functional demand on the motor cortex.

An example interpreted to be CH with associated behavioral IC has been reported by Norton and Culver (1977), who studied rats exposed to carbon monoxide on postnatal Day 5. After an initial lag, spine frequency on caudate Golgi type II neurons increased to above-control levels at 8 weeks and further increased through 7 months of age. After carbon monoxide exposure (Culver & Norton, 1976) the rats became hyperactive, peaking at 6 weeks, and then returned to normal at 3 months. Norton and Culver propose that carbon monoxide damages an unspecified inhibitory center and that the hypertrophy in the caudate increases its inhibitory output. Caudate stimulation elicits inhibitory postsynaptic potentials in other basal ganglia regions (Levine, Hull, and Buchwald, 1974; Yoshida, Rabin, & Anderson, 1972).

Putative evidence for CH has also come from electrophysiological studies. Feinsod, Bach-y-Rita, and Madey (1973) found that in subjects trained to use Braille and the tactile vision substitution system (described here later) somatosensory evoked response peaks to index-finger stimuli occurred at shorter latency than they did in sighted controls. This suggests a change in the way in (or at least the rate at) which the brain processes information. Further evidence for brain-organization changes was presented by Neville, Schmidt, and Kutas (1983), who examined the visual evoked response (VER) in the congenitally deaf and in hearing adults. Amplitude of an early negative peak was greater over the frontal, anterior, temporal, and occipital cortices to peripheral, but not to foveal, retinal stimuli, and a later positive peak increased over the occipital and the parietal cortices to either peripheral or foveal stimuli in the deaf subjects. When deafness occurred after 4 years of age these enhanced VERs were not seen over auditory areas (Neville, in press). Neville *et al.* (1983) note the increased importance of peripheral vision to the deaf, who cannot use audition as an alerting modality, and they suggest that early deafness alters the intermodal organization of the brain. Decreased input in one modality may be more likely to affect others that are related to the orienting or localizing functions normally provided by the damaged modality. This work can also be interpreted in terms of the X, Y, and W components of the visual system. In animals such as cats the fovea contains almost exclusively X and W types with Y cells predominantly restricted to the periphery (Stone, Dreher, & Leventhal, 1979). The Y system appears to be more plastic than the X system and suffers more decrement after visual deprivation. Thus, in animals, the peripheral retinal aspect of the visual system is more experience sensitive, and such a difference in humans could account for the Neville *et al.* results. A physiological study in animals also provided evidence for CH. Postnikova (1978), investigating aversive conditioning in rabbits, found shorter latency and increased amplitude of auditory evoked potentials over cortical auditory regions and a similar smaller effect over somatosensory regions.

CNS Evidence for Functional Reallocation

Functional reallocation (FR) refers to tissue that is used for a nonnormal purpose. At least between modalities, this is probably the most controversial of the three basic concepts discussed here. Some evidence can be interpreted to indicate FR. Krech *et al.* (1963), who described somatosensory cortical CH in blinded animals, also reported increased visual cortex ACHE, which could indicate visual cortex reorganization for nonvisual function. Neville *et al.* (1983) found increased responsiveness to visual stimuli over nonvisual areas of the cortex in congenitally deaf humans.

If reallocation is involved there must be some way for information from alternate modalities to influence reallocated areas. In this regard, it is of interest that bimodal and trimodal cortical and subcortical neurons have been demonstrated in sensory systems (Fishman & Michael, 1973; Murata, Cramer, & Bach-y-Rita, 1965: Rhoades, Dellacroce, & Meadows, 1981; Wickelgren, 1971). Evidence also exists for thalamocortical (Benevento & Ebner, 1971) and corticocortical (Jones & Powell, 1970) polysensory pathways. Such nonprimary input appears to be specific rather than a reflection of a nonspecific general arousal system. Morrell (1972) noted spatial specificity in acoustic projections to visual association areas; Fishman and Michael (1973) found that acoustically responsive visual cortex cells were selective for direction and spatial location, and Wickelgren (1971) found that visual and auditory receptive fields of superior colliculus neurons were similarly spatially located. In intact organisms these multimodal cells may be involved in cross-modal integration (Skya & Straschill, 1968; Spinelli, Starr, & Barrett, 1968; Wickelgren, 1971). However, in the absence of input from the primary modality, dominance by extramodal inputs could increase, providing, in effect, substitute information and hence functionally reallocating the neurons, and those to which they project, to the secondary modalities. Rhoades *et al.* (1981) have demonstrated such a shift. Following unilateral eye removal in neonatal hamsters, there was an increase in the somatosensory dominance of units in the contralateral superior colliculus. Similarly, Cynader (1979) has reported increased auditory and tactile dominance of superior colliculus units in DR kittens.

Such takeover need not involve previously existing connections. A dramatic example of novel connections has been presented by Graziadei, Levine, and Monti Graziadei (1978), who found that, after unilateral olfactory bulbectomy in mice, olfactory epithelial axons invaded the forebrain, forming glomerular connections typical of those in the intact bulb. Moreover, Wright and Harding (1982) demonstrated that these connections are behaviorally functional. As they formed, an olfactory aversion, learned prior to bulbectomy, reappeared. Anomalous connections in other afferent systems after removal of the primary central target have been reported (e.g., Schneider, 1979), and it could be argued that in development, a peripherally functional modality deprived of normal central representation finds ways to reallocate central tissue to its purposes.

In some cases the distinction between FR and CH may not be absolutely clear. Schaefer and Meyer (1973, 1974) and Giretti (1971) studied recovery from head deviation and visual nystagmus after peripheral vestibular destruction. These two systems recede at different rates after unilateral labyrinthectomy in young and adult guinea pigs, and recovery is facilitated by contact with the floor. Cortical and cerebellar lesions as well as spinal transection slow recovery of head deviation but barely affect nystagmus, and spinal transection reinduces both symptoms after recovery is complete (Azzena, 1969). Thus other regions and somatosensory submodalities subserve vestibular reflexes, probably via the same brainstem nuclei and pathways. The role of vision in recovery provides a clearer case of compensatory change. Visual input is necessary for recovery from nystagmus, head tilt, and postural deficits following hemilabyrinthectomy (Courjon, Jeannerod, Ossuzio, & Schmid, 1977; Putkonen, Courjon, & Jeannerod, 1977). Following hemilabyrinthectomy, ipsilateral vestibular-nuclei activity is depressed and contralateral activity increases due to release from inhibition. Recovery from nystagmus parallels an increase in ipsilateral activity and a contralateral decrease. Courjoun *et al.* (1977) propose that vision restores balance in the vestibular system via cerebellar paths.

Does the lack of an absolute distinction between FR and CH suggest that the distinction may not be meaningful? Several studies suggest that the FR concept is useful in describing what appear to be true reallocation processes. Bonaventure and Karli (1968, 1969) found larger visual cortex evoked responses (ERs) to auditory stimuli in surgically blinded mice and in mice with congenital retinal degeneration. Although these responses occurred in older surgically blinded mice, they tended to decrease with increasing onset age of blinding, which suggests that the phenomenon does not merely reflect reduced volume–conducted visual EEG noise in the auditory average relative to the sighted controls. Similarly, Rebillard, Carlier, Rebillard, and Pujol (1977) found enhanced ERs to photic stimuli over the auditory but not the somatosensory cortex of adult cats that were either congenitally deaf or surgically deafened at 1 week of age. Deafening at 2 months did not produce this result. These studies are among the best evidence for considering FR as a separate explanatory–descriptive concept which suggest that capacity for this sort of change decreases with age. Studies of the effects of early lesions have also suggested a role for FR in development. Howarth, Meyer and Meyer (1979) found that extravisual cortex damage had much more severe effects in animal subjects that had received visual damage in infancy than in those that had received damage in adulthood. Likewise, Hata, Diaz, Gibson, Jacobs, Meyer, and Meyer (1980) found that visual cortex lesions produced greater deficits in rats that had suffered extravisual damage in infancy.

Other work, however, suggests that FR may also occur in adults. Scheff, Wright, Morgan, and Bowers (1977) found that following successive unilateral lesions to the occipital cortices, which promoted recovery of visual discrimination performance relative to simultaneous bilateral lesions, secondary extravisual lesions contiguous to the damaged visual cortex diminished performance more than distal lesions in the serial but not the simultaneous group. Scheff and

Wright (1977) found that VERs in the contiguous extravisual cortex were more frequent in the serial-lesion group, which appeared, from the secondary-lesion results, to be using the contiguous region more than the simultaneous group in performing the task. The implication of these results (see Chapter 6 Almli, Volume 2, for further support) is that when serial lesions facilitate recovery they may do so by allowing recruitment of adjacent tissue. It should be noted, however, that nonadjacent cortical tissue can also by recruited, at least in early development (Goldman-Rakic, 1981; Kalaska & Pomeranz, 1979), and that a possible basis for this is a more extensive developmental connectivity pattern in which some connections are eliminated, apparently through a competition process, by adulthood.

Reallocation has also been described within modalities. In 1- to 5-day-old mice, Woolsey and Wann (1977) found that when a row of mystacial vibrissae in the periphery was removed, the somatosensory cortex regions subserving adjacent rows expanded, taking over most of the available cortical tissue. This did not occur if vibrissae were removed after 7 days postpartum, suggesting that the central representation of this part of the somatosensory periphery becomes stable quite early. A similar but probably dysfunctional effect occurs in the auditory system with unilateral deprivation: a deprived ear relinquishes control of medial superior olivary nucleus neurons to an experienced ear (Feng & Rogowski, 1980). Such phenomena may arise through modulation of an early overproduction of connections in development with selective preservation or even expansion of a subset dependent upon functional activity (Feng & Rogowski, 1980; Ivy, Akers, & Killackey, 1979) as has been reported in developing visual systems (Land & Lund, 1979; LeVay *et al.*, 1980). A number of similar phenomena have been noted after damage in early development (e.g., Goldman-Rakic, 1981; Kalaska & Pomeranz, 1979; Rothblat & Hayes, 1982).

In some parts of the somatosensory system this sort of phenomenon is not limited to early development, and the results have suggested the presence of both silent overlapping connections in the adult and a capacity for the formation of new connections at some point along somatosensory input pathways. Continuing plasticity has been described in the central somatosensory representation of adults. Damage to pathways subserving hindlimb input in the brainstem results in expanded forelimb representation in the somatosensory thalamus and the cortex within days (Wall & Egger, 1971). Destruction of lumbar (hindlimb) spinal roots (Millar, Basbaum, & Wall, 1976) or peripheral hindlimb nerves (Kalaska & Pomeranz, 1982) causes similar shifts in the brainstem representation of the somatosensory periphery. Some reversible changes are seen immediately after damage or conduction block produced by cooling, but further changes occur more slowly with irreversible spinal-nerve damage, such that the system may take weeks or months to establish a stable central representation (Dostrovsky, Millar, & Wall, 1976). Similar reversible effects occur in the somatosensory cortex (Metzler & Marks, 1979). Wall (1977) suggests that such phenomena reflect both the "unmasking" of existing overlapping connections and either the growth of new connections or a more gradual loss of lateral inhibition. Merzenich and Kaas (1982) described similar alterations in the central representation of the forelimb in monkeys and found that in some cases the expanded central representation of a reduced periphery is associated with smaller receptive fields and greater acuity. Rasmusson (1982) has reported similar central representation shifts in raccoons after digit removal. Some clinical reports suggest similar phenomena after peripheral nerve damage in humans. For example, Denny-Brown (1965) noted that subjects experience novel sensations in intermediate zones of skin between areas of total anesthesia, and Rudel, Teuber, and Twitchell (1966) reported localized hyperesthesia in some congenitally encephalopathic children. The reports of higher acuity on the stumps of amputated limbs (Haber, 1955; Teuber, Krieger, & Bender, 1949; see Table 1, present volume) may reflect a similar process.

Prosthetic Facilitation of Compensatory Processes

Behavioral and neural indications of IC suggest that such processes may be facilitated by devices which assist undamaged modalities in receiving information normally available through others. Of course techniques such as braille reading and newer electronic tactile text-translating systems such as the Optacon (Schoof, 1975; Tobin & James, 1974) are widely used. It should be noted that both Braille and Optacon skills are greatest in those trained at younger ages, and that Braille ability predicts Optacon learning rate (Tobin & James, 1974). A particularly ambitious prosthetic device is the tactile vision substitution system (Bach-y-Rita, 1971, 1975), in which images from a television camera are transformed into a vibrotactile pattern on the abdomen or back. Subjects can perceive such patterns as images in front of them and can recognize objects and faces and even use visual spatial cues such as motion parallax for depth. Bach-y-Rita suggests that blind subjects can interpret tactile information in truly visual terms with this system and proposes that tactile input that is normally filtered out or ignored becomes attended to because of its new importance or meaning. Whether this system calls upon multimodal channels that actually involve central portions of the deprived visual system, is unclear.

Possible Neural Bases for Active Reorganization

In preceding sections we have referred both to latent capacities for FR and CH (e.g., nondominant modality takeover of multimodal neurons) and active (e.g., experience-dependent or learned) reorganization processes. Mechanisms for active reorganization have been previously suggested. In the developing brain, in addition to the projections that are present in the developing system but are absent or reduced in adulthood noted above, there appears to be a greater capacity for axonal sprouting into denervated regions (e.g., Nadler, Cotman, & Lynch, 1977) and perhaps for axonal regeneration or redirection (e.g., Grafe, 1983; Graziadei *et al.*, 1978; Hicks & D'Amato, 1970; Reh & Kalil, 1982). Furthermore, studies of the intact adult nervous system response to experience and training suggest that the brain retains the capacity to form new connections throughout most of the lifespan (reviewed, Greenough & Green, 1981). The functional demand in these cases is potentially comparable to the demand placed on an intact modality by sensory damage. The new connections could result from modulation of continuing synapse turnover in the adult brain, as suggested elsewhere (e.g., Greenough & Green, 1981), or they could involve activity-dependent generation of new synapses, as suggested by electrical-stimulation studies (Chang & Greenough, in press; Lee, Oliver, Schottler, & Lynch, 1980).

Summary and Conclusions

Behavioral evidence for IC appears less controversial when the data are viewed from the perspectives of intermodal competition and when we recognize the possibility that in specific cases information derived from experience in one modality may be expected to play a role in the later development of others. The limits of IC have yet to be explored in laboratory studies of either humans or animals. Recent research indicates both evidence for and possible neural mechanisms of CH and FR. The effects of functional demand upon structural and functional plasticity in the CNS in intact adults, sensorially deprived or damaged adults, and developing young indicate potential compensatory capacity well beyond that previously predicted. The potential for prosthetic devices that take advantage of these forms of plasticity is enormous, and it seems likely that they will receive increased attention.

Acknowledgment

We thank Scott Krause for assistance with translation, C. Bartle for excellent typing, and B. A. Rogowski, R. Uslander and I. Shasha for library assistance. The work in progress cited was supported by the Retirement Research Foundation and NSF BNS 82-16916.

References

Aftanas, M., & Zubek, J. P. (1971). The CFF in unilateral arm amputees. *Perceptual and Motor Skills, 32,* 881–882.

Ammons, C. H., Worchel, P., & Dallenbach, K. M. (1953). Facial vision: The perception of obstacles out of doors by blindfolded and blindfolded-deafened subjects. *American Journal of Psychology, 66,* 519–553.

Axelrod, S. (1959). Effects of early blindness: Performance of blind and sighted children on tactile and auditory tasks. *American Foundation for the Blind Research Series,* Whole No. 7.

Azzena, G. B. (1969). Role of the spinal cord in compensating the effects of hemilabyrinthectomy. *Archives Italienes de Biologie, 107,* 43–53.

Bach-y-Rita, P. (1971). Neural substrates of sensory substitution. In R. Klinke & O. J. Grusser (Eds.), *Pattern recognition in the biological and technical systems* pp. 130–142. New York: Springer-Verlag.

Bach-y-Rita, P. (1975). Plastic brain mechanisms in sensory substitution. In O. Creutzfeldt & G. C. Galbraith (Eds.), *Cerebral localization* (pp. 204–216). New York: Springer-Verlag.

Benevento, L. A., & Ebner, F. F. (1971). The contribution of the dorsal lateral geniculate nucleus to the total pattern of thalamic terminations in striate cortex of the Virginia opossum. *Journal of Comparative Neurology, 143,* 243–260.

Blank, M., & Bridger, W. H. (1966). Conceptual cross modal transfer in deaf and hearing children. *Child Development, 37,* 29–38.

Blumenfeld, W. (1937). The relationship between the optical and haptic construction of space. *Acta Psychologica Amsterdam, 2* 125–174.
Bonaventure, N., & Karli, P. (1968). Apparition au niveau du cortex visuel, de potentiels évoqués d'origine auditive chez la Souris privée de photorécepteurs. *Journal de Physiologie Paris, 60,* 407.
Bonaventure, N., & Karli, P. (1969). Nouvelles données sur les potentiels d'origine auditive évoqués au niveau du cortex visuel chez la Souris. *Comptes Rendus des Seances de la Societe de Biologie Paris, 163,* 1705–1708.
Brown, M. S., & Stratton, G. M. (1925). The spatial threshold of touch in blind and in seeing children. *Journal of Experimental Psychology,* , 434–442.
Burnstine, T. H., Beck, D., Pierre-Jerome, F., & Greenough, W. T. (in progress). Effects of neonatal visual deprivation on dendritic branching in rat auditory cortex.
Busniuk, M. M. (1978). The change in activity of glutamate hydrogenase in the neurons of the motor cortex of the brain in the presence of visual deprivation. *Zhurnal Vysshei Nervnoi Deyatel'nosti Imeni I. P. Pavlova, 28,* 402–407. (In Russian)
Carr, H. A. (1921). The influences of visual guidance on maze-learning. *Journal of Experimental Psychology, 4,* 399–417.
Chang, F.-L. F., & Greenough, W. T. (in press). Transient and enduring morphological correlates of synaptic activity and efficacy change in the rat hippocampal slice. *Brain Research.*
Courjon, J. H., Jeannerod, M., Ossuzio, I., & Schmid, R. (1977). The role of vision in compensation of vestibulo- ocular reflex after hemilabyrinthectomy in the cat. *Experimental Brain Research, 28,* 235–248.
Crewdson, J., & Zangwill, O. L. (1940). A note on tactual perception in a blind subject. *British Journal of Psychology, 30,* 224–229.
Critchley, M. (1953). Tactile thought with special reference to the blind. *Brain, 76,* 19–35.
Culver, B., & Norton, S. (1976). Juvenile hyperactivity in rats after acute exposure to carbon monoxide. *Experimental Neurology, 50,* 80–98.
Cynader, M. (1979). Competitive interactions in the development of the kitten's visual system. In R. D. Freeman (Ed.), *Developmental neurobiology of vision.* New York: Plenum.
Denenberg, V. (1967). Stimulation in infancy, emotional reactivity and exploratory behavior. In D. C. Glass (Ed.), *Neurophysiology and emotion.* New York: Rockefeller University Press.
Denny-Brown, D. (1965). The release of deep pain by nerve injury. *Brain, 88,* 725–738.
DeVoogd, T. J. (1979). *Effects of dark-rearing and enucleation on the development of visual cortex in rats.* Unpublished Ph.D. dissertation, University of Illinois, Urbana-Champaign.
Diderot, D. (1749/1916). Letter on the blind for the use of those who see. In M. Jourdain (Ed. & Trans.), *Diderot's early philosophical works* (pp. 68–141). New York: Burt Franklin. (Original work published 1749)
Dostrovsky, V. O., Millar, J., & Wall P. D. (1976). The immediate shift of afferent drive of dorsal column nucleus cells following deafferentation: A comparison of acute and chronic deafferentation in gracile nucleus and spinal cord. *Experimental Neurology, 52,* 480–495.
Drever, J. (1955). Early learning and the perception of space. *American Journal of Psychology, 68,* 605–614.
Duncan, B. K. (1934). A comparative study of finger-maze learning by blind and sighted subjects. *The Pedagogical Seminary and Journal of Genetic Psychology, 44,* 69–95.

Eayrs, J. T., & Ireland, K. F. (1950). The effects of total darkness on the growth of the newborn albino rat. *Journal of Endocrinology, 6,* 311–337.

Ewart, A. G., & Carp, F. M. (1963). Recognition of tactual form by sighted and blind subjects. *American Jouranl of Psychology, 76,* 488–491.

Feinsod, M. P., Bach-y-Rita, P., & Madey, J. M. J. (1973). Somatosensory evoked responses: Latency differences in blind and sighted persons. *Brain Research, 60,* 219–233.

Feng, A. S., & Rogowski, B. A. (1980). Effects of monaural and binaural occlusion on the morphology of neurons in the medial superior olivary nucleus of the rat. *Brain Research, 189,* 530–534.

Fishman, M. C., & Michael, C. R. (1973). Integration of auditory information in the cat's visual cortex. *Vision Research, 13,* 1415–1419.

Gauron, E. F., & Becker, W. C. (1959). The effects of early sensory deprivation on adult rat behavior under competition stress: An attempt at replication of a study by Alexander Wolf. *Journal of Comparative and Physiological Psychology, 52,* 689–693.

Gerstein, L. M. (1976). An interferometric investigation in the reaction of the neurons in the motor regions of the brain cortex to early visual deprivation. *Tsitologiya, 18,* 48–52. (In Russian)

Gibby, R. G., Jr., Gibby, R. G., Sr., & Townsend, J. L. (1970). Short term visual restriction in visual and auditory discrimination. *Perceptual and Motor Skills, 30,* 15–21.

Giretti, M. C. (1971). Spinal compensation of cerebral release phenomena. *Experimental Neurology, 30,* 459–466.

Glickman, S. E. (1958). Effects of peripheral blindness on exploratory behavior in the hooded rat. *Canadian Journal of Psychology, 12,* 45–51.

Goldman-Rakic, P. S. (1981). Development and plasticity of primate frontal association cortex. In F. O. Schmitt, F. G. Worden, G. Adelman, & S. G. Dennis (Eds.), *The organization of the cerebral cortex.* Cambridge, MA: MIT Press.

Grafe, M. R. (1983). Developmental factors affecting regeneration in the central nervous system: Early but not late formed mitral cells reinnervate olfactory cortex after neonatal tract section. *Journal of Neuroscience, 3,* 617–630.

Graziadei, P. P. C., Levine, R. E., & Monti Graziadei, G. A. (1978). Regeneration of olfactory axons and synapse formation in the forebrain after bulbectomy in neonatal mice. *Proceedings of the National Academy of Sciences, U.S.A., 75,* 5230–5234.

Greenough, W. T., & Green, E. J. (1981). Experience and the changing brain. In J. L. McGaugh, J. G. March, & S. B. Kiesler (Eds.), *Aging: Biology and behavior* (pp. 159–200). New York: Academic Press.

Griesbach, H. Vergleichende untersuchungen über die sinnesschärfe blinder und sehender. *Pflüger's Archiv,* 1899, *74,* 577–638; 1900, *75,* 365–429, 523–573.

Gyllensten, L., Malmfors, T., & Norrlin, M. L. (1966). Growth alteration in the auditory cortex of visually deprived mice. *Journal of Comparative Neurology, 126,* 463–470.

Haber, W. B. (1955). Effects of loss of limb on sensory functions. *Journal of Psychology, 40,* 115–123.

Hall, G. S. Laura Bridgeman. *Mind,* 1879, *4,* 149–172.

Harper, D. W., & Bross, M. (1978). The effect of unimodal sensory deprivation on sensory processes: A decade of research from the University of Manitoba. *Canadian Psychological Review, 19,* 128–144.

Hartlage, L. C. (1968). Deficits in space concepts associated with visual deprivation. *Journal of Learning Disabilities, 1,* 21–23.

Hata, M. G., Diaz, C. L., Gibson, C. F., Jacobs, C. -E., Meyer, P. M., & Meyer, D. G.

(1980). Perinatal injuries to extravisual cortex enhances the significance of visual cortex for performance of a visual habit. *Physiological Psychology, 8,* 9–14.

Hayes, S. P. (1933). New experimental data and the old problem of sensory compensation. *The Teachers Forum, 6,* 22–24.

Hayes, S. P. (1935). Where did that sound come from? *Teachers Forum, 7,* 47–51.

Hayes, S. P. (1941). *Contributions to a psychology of blindness.* New York: American Foundation for the Blind.

Hebb, D. O. (1949). *The organization of behavior.* New York: Wiley.

Hicks, S. P., & D'Amato, C. J. (1970). Motor-sensory and visual behavior after hemispherectomy in newborn and mature rats. *Experimental Neurology, 29,* 416–438.

Howarth, H., Meyer, D. R., & Meyer, P. M. (1979). Perinatal injuries to the visual cortex enhance the significance of extravisual cortex for performance of a visual habit. *Physiological Psychology, 7,* 163–166.

Hunter, I. M. L. (1954). Tactile–kinaesthetic perception of straightness in blind and sighted humans. *Quarterly Journal of Experimental Psychology, 6,* 149–154.

Hunter, W. F. (1964). An analysis of space perception in congenitally blind and in sighted individuals. *Journal of General Psychology, 70,* 325–329.

Hymovitch, B. (1952). The effects of experimental variations on problem solving in the rat. *Journal of Comparative and Physiological Psychology, 45,*313–321.

Ivy, G. O., Akers, R. M., & Killackey, H. P. (1979). Differential distribution of callosal projection neurons in the neonatal and adult rat. *Brain Research, 173,* 532–537.

Jastrow, J. (1894). Psychological notes on Helen Keller. *Psychological Review, 1,* 356–362.

Jones, E. G., & Powell, T. P. S. (1970). An anatomical study of converging sensory pathways within the cereberal cortex of the monkey. *Brain, 93,* 793–820.

Kalaska, J., & Pomeranz, B. (1979). Chronic paw denervation causes an age-dependent appearance of novel responses from forearm in "paw cortex" of kittens and adult cats. *Journal of Neuroscience, 42,* 618–633.

Kalaska, J., & Pomeranz, B. (1982). Chronic peripheral nerve injuries alter somatotopic organization of the cuneate nucleus in kittens. *Brain Research, 236,* 35–47.

Kasatkin, N. I. (1967). Personal communication cited in Y. Brackbill and M. M. Koltsova. Conditioning and learning. In Y. Brackbill (Ed.), *A handbook and guide to human development* (pp. 207–288). New York: Free Press.

Keller, H. (1903/1947). *The story of my life.* London: Hodder & Stoughton. (Original work published 1903)

Knotts, J. R., & Miles, W. R. (1929). The maze-learning ability of blind compared with sighted children. *Pedagogkal Seminary and Journal of Genetic Psychology, 36,* 21–50.

Koch, H. L., & Ufkess, J. (1926). A comparative study of stylus maze learning by blind and seeing subjects. *Journal of Experimental Psychology, 9,* 118–131.

Krech, D., Rosenzweig, M. R., & Bennett, E. L. (1960). Interhemispheric effects of cortical lesions on brain biochemistry. *Science, 32,* 352–353.

Krech, D., Rosenzweig, M. R., & Bennett, E. L. (1963). Effects of complex environment and blindness on rat brain. *Archives of Neurology, 8,* 403–412.

Kunz, M. (1908). Physiology of the blind. *Volta Review, 10,* 465–493.

Land, P. W., & Lund, P. D. (1979). Development of the rat's uncrossed retinotectal pathway and its relation to plasticity studies. *Science, 205,* 698–700.

Landau, B., Gleitman, H., & Spelke, E. (1981). Spatial knowledge and geometric representation in a child blind from birth. *Science, 213,* 1275–1278.

Lee, K. S., Oliver, M., Schottler, F., & Lynch, G. (1980). Brief bursts of high-frequency stimulation produce two types of structural change in rat hippocampus. *Journal of Neurophysiology, 44,* 247–258.

LeVay, S., Wiesel, T. N., & Hubel, D. H. (1980). The development of ocular dominance columns in normal and visually deprived monkeys. *Journal of Comparative Neurology, 191,* 1–51.

Levine, M. S., Hull, C. D., & Buchwald, N. A. (1974). Pallidal and entopeduncular intracellular responses to strial, cortical, thalamic, and sensory inputs. *Experimental Neurology, 44,* 448–460.

MacDougall, J. C., & Rabinovich, M. S. (1972). Early auditory deprivation and exploratory activity. *Developmental Psychology, 7,* 17–20.

MacFarland, D. C. (1952). An exploratory study comparing the maze learning ability of blind and sighted subjects. *New Outlook for the Blind, 46,* 259–263.

McKinney, J. P. (1964). Hand schema in children. *Psychonomic Science, 1,* 99–100.

MacNeill, M., & Zubek, J. P. (1967). Effects of progonged visual deprivation (dark-rearing) on the weight of the sensory cortex of the rat. *Canadian Journal of Psychology, 21,* 177–183.

Metzler, J., & Marks, P. S. (1979). Functional changes in cat somatic sensory-motor cortex during short-term reversible epidural blocks. *Brain Research, 177,* 379–383.

Merzenich, M. M., & Kaas, J. H. (1982). Reorganization of mammalian somatosensory cortex following peripheral nerve injury. *Trends in Neuroscience, 5,* 434–436.

Meyer, G., Feo Ramos, J. J., & Ferres-Torres, R. (1976). Respuesta morfofuncional del hipocampo y corteza temporal al estímulo deprivación visual. *Anales de Anatomía (Madrid), 25,* 539–544.

Millar, J., Basbaum, A. I., & Wall, P. D. (1976). Restructuring of the somatotopic map and appearance of abnormal neuronal activity in the gracile nucleus after partial deafferentation. *Experimental Neurology, 50,* 658–672.

Morrell, F. (1972). Visual systems view of acoustic space. *Nature, 238,* 44–46.

Mos, L. P. (1976). Light rearing effects on factors of mouse emotionality and endocrine organ weight. *Physiological Psychology, 4,* 503–510.

Murata, K., Cramer, H., & Bach-y-Rita, P. (1965). Neuronal convergence of noxious, acoustic, and visual stimuli in the visual cortex of the cat. *Journal of Neurophysiology, 28,* 1223–1240.

Nadler, J. V., Cotman, C. W., & Lynch, G. (1977). Histochemical evidence of altered development of cholinergic fibers in the rat dentate gyrus following lesions. I. Time course after complete unilateral entorhinal lesions at various ages. *Journal of Comparative Neurology, 171,* 561–568.

Nagatsuka, Y. (1965). Studies of sensory deprivation: III Part 2. Effects of sensory deprivation upon perceptual functions (3). *Tohoku Psychologica Folia, 23,* 56–59.

Neville, H. J. (in press). Effects of early sensory and language experience on the development of the human brain. In J. Mehler & R. Fox (Eds.), *Neonate cognition: Beyond the blooming, buzzing confusion.* Hillsdale, NJ: Erlbaum.

Neville, H. J., Schmidt, A., & Kutas, M. (1983). Altered visual evoked potentials in congenitally deaf adults. *Brain Research, 266,* 127–132.

Norton, S., & Culver, B. (1977). A Golgi analysis of caudate neurons in rats exposed to carbon monoxide. *Brain Research, 132,* 455–465.

Postnikova, N. N. (1978). The formation of a defensive conditioned reflex to acoustic stimuli in rabbits after early visual deprivation. *Zhurnal Vysshei Nervnoi Deyatel'nosti Imeni I. P. Pavolva, 28,* 293–297. (In Russian)

Putkonen, P. T. S., Courjon, J. H., & Jeannerod, M. (1977). Compensation of postural effects of hemilabyrinthectomy in the cat. A sensory substitution process? *Experimental Brain Research, 28,* 249–257.

Rasmusson, D. D. (1982). Reorganization of raccoon somatosensory cortex following removal of the fifth digit. *Journal of Comparative Neurology, 205,* 313–326.

Rebillard, G., Carlier, E., Rebillard, M., & Pujol, R. (1977). Enhancement of visual responses in the auditory cortex of the cat after early destruction of cochlear receptors. *Brain Research, 129,* 162–164.

Reh, T., & Kalil, K. (1982). Functional role of regrowing pyramidal tract fibers. *Journal of Comparative Neurology, 211,* 276–283.

Renshaw, S. (1930). The errors of cutaneous localization and the effect of practice on the localizing movement in children and adults. *Pedagogical Seminary and Journal of Genetic Psychology, 38,* 223–238.

Renshaw, S., Wherry, R., J., & Newlin, J. C. (1930). Cutaneous localization in congenitally blind versus seeing children and adults. *Pedagogical Seminary and Journal of Genetic Psychology, 38,* 239–248.

Rhoades, R. W., Dellacroce, D. D., & Meadows, I. (1981). Reorganization of somatosensory input to superior colliculus in neonatally enucleated hamsters: Anatomical and electrophysiological experiments. *Journal of Neurophysiology, 46,* 855–877.

Rice, C. E. (1969). Perceptual enhancement in the early blind? *Psychological Record, 19,* 1–14.

Rock, I., & Victor, J. (1964). Vision and touch: An experimentally created conflict between the two senses. *Science, 143,* 594–596.

Rosenstein, J. (1957). Tactile perception of rhythmic patterns by normal, blind, deaf, and aphasic children. *American Annals of the Deaf, 102,* 399–403.

Rothblat, L. A., & Hayes, L. L. (1982). Age-related changes in the distribution of visual callosal neurons following monocular enucleation in the rat. *Brain Research, 246,* 146–149.

Rudel, R. G., Teuber, H. L., & Twitchell, T. E. (1966). A note on hyperesthesia in children with early brain damage. *Neuropsychologia, 4,* 351–356.

Ryugo, D. K., Ryugo, R., Globus, A., & Killackey, H. P. (1975). Increased spine density in auditory cortex following visual or somatic deafferentation. *Brain Research, 90,* 143–146.

Schaefer, K. P., & Meyer, D. L. (1973). Compensatory mechanisms following labyrinthine lesions in the guinea-pig. A simple model of learning. In H. P. Zippel (Ed)., *Memory and transfer of information* (pp. 203–232). Plenum.

Schaefer, K. P., & Meyer, D. L. (1974). Compensation of vestibular lesions. In H. H. Kornhuber (Ed.), *Handbook of sensory physiology* (Vol. 6 *Vestibular system* (Part 2): *Psychophysics, applied aspects and general interpretation* (pp. 463–490). New York: Springer-Verlag.

Schapiro, S., & Vukovich, K. R. (1970). Early experience effects upon cortical dendrites: A proposed model for development. *Science, 167,* 292–294.

Scheff, S. W., & Wright, D. C. (1977). Behavioral and electrophysiological evidence for cortical reorganization of function in rats with serial lesions of the visual cortex. *Physiological Psychology, 5,* 103–107.

Scheff, S. W., Wright, D. C., Morgan, W. K., & Bowers, R. P. (1977). The differential effects of additional cortical lesions in rats with single or multiple-stage lesions of the visual cortex. *Physiological Psychology, 5,* 97–102.

Schlaegal, T. F., Jr. (1953). The dominant imagery in blind as compared to sighted adolescents. *Journal of Genetic Psychology, 83,* 265–277.

Schneider, G. E. (1979). Is it really better to have your brain lesion early? A revision of the Kennard principle. *Neuropsychologia*, 557–583.

Schoof, L. T., II (1975, June). An analysis of Optacon usage. *American Foundation for the Blind Research Bulletin, 29,* 33–50.

Seashore, C. E., & Ling, T. L. (1918). The comparative sensitiveness of blind and seeing persons. *Psychological Review Monographs, 25,* 148–158.

Sewell, G. D. (1968). Ultrasonic communication in rodents. *Nature, 217,* 682–688.

Skya, J., & Straschill, M. (1968). Activation of superior colliculus neurons and motor responses after electrical stimulation of the inferior colliculus. *Experimental Neurology, 22,* 75–84.

Spigelman, M. N. (1976). A comparative study of the effects of early blindness on the development of auditory–spatial learning. In Z. S. Jastrzembska (Ed.), *The effects of blindness and other impairments on early development* (pp. 29–45). New York: American Foundation for the Blind.

Spinelli, D. N., Starr, A., & Barrett, T. W. (1968). Auditory specificity in unit recordings from cat's visual cortex. *Experimental Neurology, 22,* 75–84.

Stellwagen, W. T. & Culbert, S. S. (1963). Comparison of blind and sighted subjects in the discrimination of texture. *Perceptual and Motor Skills, 17,* 61–62.

Sterritt, G. M., Camp, B. W., & Lipman, B. S. (1966). Effects of early auditory deprivation upon auditory and visual information processing. *Perceptual and Motor Skills, 23,* 123–130.

Stone, J., Dreher, B., Leventhal, A. (1979). Heirarchical and parallel mechanisms in the organization of visual cortex. *Brain Research Reviews, 1,* 345–394.

Supa, M., Cotzin, M., & Dallenbach, K. M. (1974). Facial vision: The perception of obstacles by the blind. *American Journal of Psychology, 57,* 133–183.

Sylvester, R. H. (1913). The mental imagery of the blind. *Psychological Bulletin, 10,* 210–211.

Tees, R. C. (1980). The effect of sensory deprivation on the behavior of infrahuman organisms. In P. Suedfeld (Ed.) *Restricted environmental stimulation* (pp. 160–190). New York: Wiley.

Tees, R. C., & Cartwright, J. (1972). Sensory preconditioning in rats following early visual deprivation. *Journal of Comparative and Physiological Psychology, 81,* 12–20.

Tees, R. C., Midgley, G., & Nesbit, J. C. (1981). The effect of early visual experience on spatial maze learning in rats. *Developmental Psychobiology, 14,* 425–438.

Teuber, H. L., Krieger, H. P., & Bender, M. B. (1949). Reorganization of sensory function in amputation stumps: Two-point discrimination. *Federation Proceedings,* 1949, *8,* 156.

Tilney, F. A. (1929). A comparative sensory analysis of Helen Keller and Laura Bridgeman. II. Its bearing on the further development of the human brain. *Archives of Neurology and Psychiatry, 21,* 1237–1269.

Tobin, M. J., & James, W. R. K. (1974, October). Evaluating the Optacon: General reflections on reading machines for the blind. *American Foundation for the Blind Research Bulletin, 28,* 145–157.

Turkewitz, G., Gilbert, M., & Birch, H. C. (1974). Early restriction of tactile stimulation on visual functioning in the kitten. *Developmental Psychobiology, 7,* 243–248.

Turkewitz, G., & Kenny, P. A. (1982). Limitations on input as a basis for neural organization and perceptual development: A preliminary theoretical statement. *Developmental Psychobiology, 15,* 357–368.

Vernon, J., & McGill, T. E. (1961). Sensory deprivation and pain thresholds. *Science, 133,* 330–331.

Villey, P. (1930). *The world of the blind.* New York: Macmillan.

Volkmann, A. (1858/1955). Ueber den enfluss der uebing auf das erkennen raumlicher distanzen. *Ber. d. sachs. ges. d. wiss. Math. Phys. Abth., 10,* 38–69. [As quoted by Gibson, J. J., & Gibson, E. J. (1955). Perceptual learning: Differentiation or enrichment. *Psychological Review, 62,* 132–141.]

Vrensen, G., & DeGroot, D. (1974). The effect of dark rearing and its recovery on synaptic terminals in the visual cortex of rabbits. A quantitative electron microscopic study. *Brain Research, 78,* 263–278.

Vrensen, G., & DeGroot, D. (1975). The effect of monocular deprivation on synaptic terminals in the visual cortex of rabbits. A quantitative electron microscopic study. *Brain Research, 93,* 15–24.

Wall, P. D. (1977). The presence of ineffective synapses and the circumstances that unmask them. *Philosophical Transactions of the Royal Society London Series B, 278,* 361–372.

Wall, P. D., & Egger, M. D. (1971). Formation of the new connexions in adult rat brains after partial deafferentation. *Nature, 232,* 542–545.

Wickelgren, B. G. (1971). Superior colliculus: Some receptive field properties of bimodally responsive cells. *Science, 173,* 69–71.

Wolf, A. (1943). The dynamics of the selective inhibition of specific functions in neurosis: A preliminary report. *Psychosomatic Medicine, 5,* 27–38.

Woolsey, T. A., & Wann, J. R. (1977). Areal change in mouse cortical barrels following vibrissal damage at different postnatal ages. *Journal of Comparative Neurology, 170,* 53–66.

Worchel, P., & Dallenbach, K. M. (1947). "Facial vision:" Perception of obstacles by the deaf-blind. *American Journal of Psychology, 60,* 502–553.

Worchel, P., & Mauney, J. (1951). The effect of practice on the perception of obstacles by the blind. *Journal of Experimental Psychology, 41,* 170–176.

Wright, J. W., & Harding, J. W. (1982). Recovery of olfactory function after bilateral bulbectomy. *Science, 216,* 322–324.

Yoshida, M., Rabin, A., & Anderson, M. (1972). Monosynaptic inhibition of pallidal neurons by axon collaterals of caudato-nigral fibers. *Experimental Brain Research, 15,* 333–347.

Zihl, J. (1980). "Blindspot": Improvement of visually guided eye movements by systematic practice in patients with cerebral blindness. *Neuropsychologia, 18,* 71–77.

Zubek, J. P., Bross, M., & Gelfant, W. (1973). Cutaneous sensitivity during prolonged visual deprivation: The role of interpolated testing. *Perceptual and Motor Skills, 36,* 823–826.

Zucker, I., & Bindra, D. (1961). Peripheral sensory loss and exploratory behavior. *Canadian Journal of Psychology, 15,* 237–243.

2

Evolutionary Advantages and Limitations of Early Plasticity*

Robert B. Glassman
and William C. Wimsatt

Prologue

The greatest gap in brain research today is an inadequately developed physiological psychology. Chemistry and physics are advanced sciences not only because of highly developed empirical methods but also because of a richly developed body of theory—including both entities and laws—that is based on variously long routes of inference from the data. In contrast, in much of neuroscience there is an obsession with parsimony that sanctions only a short theoretical tether.

One cause of this circumstance is the reasonable fear of orbits of philosophizing uncoupled from wordly reality. Another cause is that many of the entities that underlie mental functioning are actually

*The second author gratefully acknowledges the support of his research by the Systems Development Foundation and by the National Science Foundation (grant # SES 82-07519.)

Copyright © 1984 by Academic Press, Inc.
All rights of reproduction in any form reserved.
ISBN 0-12-052901-7

visible in their tangible reality, on gross dissection or with the minimal mediation of a microscope. This benefit of neuroscience research is also a distraction. Physics and chemistry have done well without this luxury. Evidence of molecules, atoms, subatomic particles, and the laws of interaction of all these things are highly indirect. Importantly, the data base for such inference is always in more macroscopic phenomena.

Neuroscientists have too often skipped a level going both ways: in trying to understand the behavior of organisms on the basis of neurons and their projections, and conversely in trying on occasion to understand neurons on the basis of behavioral observations. More effort must go into the search for the larger subsystems within which neurons function. Discerning the form of these subsystems requires knowledge from direct measurements of anatomy and physiology—the presently prevailing bottom-up method—but it also requires, to a much greater extent than is now practiced, inferences from more macroscopic sources at the level of psychology and even inferences from imperfectly perceived global patterns and constraints of biological evolution (Bonner, 1982). Without information arising from such sources, we do not know where to begin to look for phenomena of neural organization.

Introduction: Evolution of Restricted Areas of Ontogenetic Flexibility in Higher Organisms

It is not surprising that early brain damage often leads to outcomes different from those of later brain damage, because young organisms are sensitive and flexible in a great variety of ways. These special characteristics of early ontogeny provide the substance of personality theories (Rychlak, 1981) and theories of cognitive development (Phillips, 1975). Early sensitive periods are largely determined by genetic factors; development is not merely a progressive elaboration of material written on blank mental slates, but a complex interaction of what Mayr (1974) called closed and open developmental programs. The clearest empirical proofs of this proposition are based on deprivation experiments, in which animals are prevented from having experiences that could conceivably be relevant (such as objects allowing trial-and-error learning, or adult models) until an age when they would normally show the behavior in question. In a large number of such experiments reasonable facsimiles of the normal behavior emerge at the usual age; genetic information is their only possible source (Eibl-Eibesfeldt, 1975).

Phylogenetically higher species take over the earth as natural selection stumbles toward solutions of the neural arrangement problems associated with learning. Individual higher organisms can cope with a wider variety of circumstances because in them the grainy creative process of natural selection (Wimsatt, 1980a) is partially replaced by moments of pleasure and pain, the educational surrogates for life and death called vicarious selectors by Campbell (1974a). The richly varied and detailed studies of the ethologists suggest that the capacity to learn might better be thought of not as a diffuse enhancement but as a collection of specific successively elaborated dispositions. That is, where lower animals have certain rigidly innate stimulus–response patterns, higher animals have particular categories of flexibility; these flexibilities rigidify as learned commitments are made, in a succession of critical developmental stages.

A most interesting evolutionary change that pertains to neuropsychological flexibility is *neoteny,* the extension of some of the features of the youth of ancestors into older ages of the modified descendant species (de Beer, 1958; Gould, 1977). Such extension might not only allow early flexibilities to last longer but might also detain critical periods for learning until later in life (Eibl-Eibesfeldt, 1975).

Evolution, in its random searches, might also do the opposite of neotenic extension by closing down certain flexibilities or by condensing later ontogenetic developments into earlier parts of the life cycle. Flexibilities in cultural transmission and trial-and-error learning allow modes of acquisition of adaptive information that cannot be provided by genetic programming, but when the environment is sufficiently stable and other conditions are met (Mayr, 1974), learned information can over the course of many generations become incorporated into the genome by a non-Lamarckian process of genetic assimilation of acquired characteristics, the Baldwin Effect. This effect depends on the fact that learning can induce animals in one generation to change their ecological niche; this change then tends to select for new variants of the species (e.g., Hardin, 1972).

Because natural selection operates most strongly on early development through the reproductive age, and because idiosyncrasies of prior learnings cumulate, later ontogenetic critical periods must show more variability in age of appearance and other aspects. The success of longevity well beyond reproductive years (unequivocally evident in women) suggests that older individuals play significant roles in the adaptation of social species. Insofar as such roles require processing of information in a very different way from earlier roles, a case of early blindness to certain distracting sources of information followed by an opening of sensitivity and responsiveness to these sources, might be adaptive. Nature would be expected to select for late critical periods if their repercussions worked to the advantage of offspring (kin selection) or of others in a closed group (reciprocal altruism and group selection; see Wade, 1978; Wilson, 1975; Wimsatt, 1981).

Conservativeness in the Origins and Maintenance of Information

Energy, Information, and Organization

Concepts of information (see Weaver, 1949) are central to genetic and evolutionary theory. Furthermore, there are processes in evolution which tend to conserve the amount of adaptive information in the genome, or at least to constrain its rate of change to relatively low levels over relatively short evolutionary time periods. Thus, reliable transmission in asexual reproduction amounts to replication of the genome and conservation of its information. While different sexual genotypes contain different information, which is combined in sexual reproduction, the mechanism of meiosis generally results in a preservation of the number and character of the chromosomes, aided in part by intense selection against almost all major changes in information content. Natural tendencies for the degradation of information (derived from an extended application of the second law of thermodynamics) are opposed by selection forces because most of these degradations are unfit (Williams, 1966). Most major changes or additions of information are similarly unfit (Wimsatt, 1981), so there is a net tendency toward the conservation of information that parallels the conservation of energy of the first law of thermodynamics. In evolution, however, this is not an absolute constraint—if it were, evolution would be impossible—but a conservative tendency that affects the character of all evolutionary products.

The concept of information required to consider genetic information is not the channel capacity of Shannon–Weaver information theory, but functional information—the content of a message that tells the phenotype to do something—and this is related to biological organization. An adequate quantitative explication of information is not available, but there are numerous suggestive attempts to deal with this matter (e.g., Buckley, 1968; Lorenz, 1977; Schrödinger, 1956; Wimsatt, 1974).

Derivations from the Principle that Information Is Conserved

The conservativeness of evolution suggests these inferences about the brain:

1. Living systems—and brains in particular—will evolve approximately hierarchial structures comprising levels of control and boundaries within boundaries of modules that are partially decomposable conceptually and empirically.
2. Although new biological structures do evolve, in general newness comprises modifications of similar structures across species. These modifications are based largely on phylogenetic changes in the ontogenetic timing (delay or acceleration) of development of one subsystem with respect to the others (Gould, 1977), on changes in relative size of systems, or on reduplication of already existing subsystems (Glassman, 1978).
3. Such innovations in the nervous system must be made possible by the existence of diffuse excitations or inhibitions imposed on older subsystems by newer ones. That is, it is worthwhile to distinguish between evolutionary changes in *organization,* which take place slowly, and changes in *bias,* which have to accompany each step along the way to organizational change.
4. Any given category of information will be processed by a system that, compared to the universe of conceivable systems, is made of relatively few nerve cells and a relatively small variety of nerve cells. A corollary of this "conservation of neurons" principle is that, whenever possible, behavioral functions will share neural systems. A number of factors provide a constant selection pressure towards smallness of the burden of brain size. These are the need for concealment from enemies, agility in attack or defense, energy demands, and other aspects of self-maintenance in the environment and internal maintenance of orderliness (Glassman & Malamut, 1977). In humans, selective pressures in regard to locomotion by organisms having a larger pelvic passageway must yield a secondary restrictive pressure on head size.
5. Whenever possible, adaptive information will be left in the en-

vironment until it is absorbed during a critical period of development. Mayr (1974) considers in detail the conditions under which this is evolutionarily advantageous.

The following sections expand upon these inferences.

Subsystems and Hierarchical Structure

Loose Coupling in Nature

Although organisms appear to be marvelously integrated wholes, evolution by random variation and selective retention could not take place if all of the component parts or subsystems of organisms were tightly joined (Ashby, 1960) instead of being partly decomposable or loosely coupled (Glassman, 1973a; Lewontin, 1978; Simon, 1962/1969, 1973; Wimsatt, 1981). In some ways living systems have to be much more decomposable than are most machines, whose parts are so highly interdependent that a random change at a randomly selected point, like the proverbial monkey wrench, is likely to make the whole thing fail totally. Philosophers of biology have discussed this and other hierarchial aspects of nature (e.g., Buckley, 1968; Burhoe, 1981; Miller, 1978; Wimsatt, 1974, 1976).

Strict Causality Continues to Operate in Hierarchical Structures

Hierarchial structures allow subsystems to express their inherent ranges of variation until such times as they happen to organize into a stable aggregate or reform into a new semistable aggregate. It is important always to bear in mind that because wholes cannot escape the causality inherent in their parts such aggregation or reformation generally involves modifications of the parts that have come together. One might think of the sources of these modifications as cases of "downward causation" from the evolutionary contexts that are provided by larger entities to their component parts (Campbell, 1974b), or as cases of emergence of dramatic and visible alterations at the higher level, which thereby serve as a sort of amplifier of much more subtle alterations of the parts. The authors just cited manage to maintain their general-systems views without implying any deus ex machina or other mysticism in emergence (Glassman, 1983a). To some degree this is accomplished by recognizing that although the fundamental indeterminacy of elementary particles probably plays no significant role in entities as large as neurons one can meaningfully speak of lower-level subsystems behaving in part at random *with respect to* other subsystems to which they are loosely coupled.

The nervous system is often considered to be hierarchial in structure—not only in the simple senses of enclosure of cells and functional aggregates of cells but also in the more abstract sense that later phylogenetic innovations appear to control the fragments of behavior that are based on the workings of earlier phylogenetic structures.

Naturally Selected Systems Never Reach Perfection

The random aspect of evolutionary change suggests that the nervous system's hierarchial structure cannot be neat. Two analogies will help.

First, Hughlings Jackson (1884/1958) offered an analogy between the nervous system and a hierarchy of command in the navy. In a variation of this analogy, if upper level function is lost, the lower levels carry on—but in a fragmented way that is likely to lead them to cross-purposes. This idea that neural systems are more analogous to social systems than to machines is intriguing. In social systems more information resides in individual, relatively loosely coupled parts. But the evolved brain must be ordered more haphazardly than a human-planned naval hierarchy. Our guess is that the brain is not as haphazardly organized as is a democracy, but rather that it is more like a Byzantine bureaucracy: a prominent monarchial, egotistical subsystem with many ad hoc lines of communication that cut across levels and even with some subsystems that can surprisingly take command under particular circumstances (Arbib, 1972; Glassman & Glassman, 1980; Levins, 1979; Wimsatt, 1974).

Second, in structured programming one builds hierarchially, using distinct modules and explicitly defined subroutines within subroutines. But naturally selected organic hardware has arisen by a less planned process than has computer software or hardware. The brain must be organized more like the program of a beginner who inserts things as they occur to him, in a confusing array of ad hoc additions, loops, and overlapping subroutines that make the program difficult to understand and that make any further sensible modification difficult. Both of these analogies suggest a reason why new hierarchial levels such as the cortex arise in evolution: to conquer the older brain's Byzantine bureaucracy by subsuming it under a diffuse inhibitory influence, only to disinhibit what is needed, when it is needed, from the relics.

Two Mathematical Analogies

The selective pressures that tend to maintain hierarchial structure are powerful ones. Simon (1962/1969, 1973) offers two analogies of his own:

1. Parable of the watchmakers: Two watchmakers, Hora and Tempus, each manufacture fine watches of 1000 parts. Tempus puts his watches together in one long operation that cannot be interrupted without the partially assembled watch falling apart into its smallest pieces. Hora first makes up 100 stable subassemblies of 10 parts each, assembles each of these into 10 higher order stable subassemblies, and then assembles these 10 to make the finished watch. Each watchmaker has random interruptions caused by the calls of customers to order watches. If the mean time between interruptions is significantly less than the time it takes to assemble a watch, Hora will do far better than Tempus because of the design of his watches. While Tempus loses all of the progress he has made since he began to assemble a watch, Hora loses at most 9 assembly operations because his partially assembled parts just fall apart into the next-lowest level stable subassemblies. The difference can be enormous. Simon (1962/1969) calculates that if they are interrupted an average of once every 50 assembly operations Hora will complete 4000 watches for each one that Tempus makes.

Simon devised this parable to illustrate the immense significance of stable subassemblies and hierarchial structure for the rate of evolution, in response to Tempus-like calculations by H. Jacobson that purported to show that because of the thermodynamic improbability of large macromolecules there could not have been sufficient time for evolution. Simon's calculation applies not only to the rate of production of a given complex structure, but also to the expected time until one of that type is first produced. Thus, he argues, the first replicating entities almost certainly had a hierarchial structure. Jacobson's mistake is gleefully recreated by modern creationists in their arguments against evolution, and even occasionally by physicists and mathematicians who should know better.

2. The combination-lock analogy: Consider two cylindrical combination locks, each with a row of 10 wheels on which there are 10 positions. There are thus 10^{10} possible combinations, only one of

which is correct. In the first or complex lock, there are no clues for partial solutions, and so the expected number of trials needed to get the correct combination is half of 10^{10}, or 5×10^9. In the second or simple lock, one can hear a faint click when each wheel reaches its right position, so the expected number of trials is 5 per wheel, or 50. The advantage of decomposability in this problem is the ratio of the number of trials for each lock, or $10^8 : 1$.

Simon (1962/1969) introduced this analogy to illustrate the advantages of decomposing a complex problem into a set of simpler subproblems, each of which can be solved independently, and then combining these partial solutions to solve the complex problem. It is often the case, unlike the second lock, that the partial solutions do not fit together perfectly: But they can still constitute good first approximations to the behavior of the components in the context of the whole. In this case the complex problem can be treated as nearly decomposable, and the solution can be nearly as simple as that of the simpler lock (Simon, 1962/1969). Indeed, this is the reason for the effectiveness of reductionistic problem-solving, in which the strategy is to study the parts of a system in isolation and then to attempt to explain the behavior of the whole system in terms of the interactions of these parts (see Wimsatt, 1980b). This is a good strategy if two conditions are met: (1) if the decomposition of the system into parts is the right decomposition for the problem or the behavior in question, and (2) if the behavior of the parts in the context of the system is not significantly different than their behavior when studied in isolation. Errors in research on functional localization in the brain, in chromosomes, and in other systems frequently occur because of failure to meet these conditions.

This is directly analogous with an evolutionary constraint first discussed by Lewontin (1978). Lewontin argues that for evolution as we know it to be possible the phenotype must show quasi-independence for many of its characters, at least for small variations. His argument is that if changes in one character were always accompanied by changes in other characters almost all changes would be deleterious and it would be impossible to select for minor improvements in individual characters. But such minor improvements are required for adaptation to local environmental changes, and they are ultimately the stuff of evolution. Wimsatt (1981) argues that this constraint is formally equivalent to the requirement that there must exist (locally) additive variance in fitness. (The absence of such quasi-independence is equivalent to *genetic epistasis,* or nonadditive variance in fitness.) This requirement is theoretically central to the mathematical theory of evolution: Fisher's (1930/1958) fundamental theorem of natural selection states that the rate of evolution is proportional to the additive variance in fitness and implies that selection cannot act upon nonadditive variance in fitness because such variance is not heritable.

The argument of the combination lock and the parable of the watchmakers are complementary. The combination-lock example shows that top-down constraints (applying at the level of whole organisms) require at least quasi-independent parts and will select for that kind of organization even if organisms do not initially possess it (Wimsatt, 1981). The parable of the watchmakers suggests that there is a bottom-up constraint on assembly of the same sort. Both suggest a hierarchial organization for the adaptive design of organisms. The only complication is that in development, and in most cases of evolution, organisms are constructed not by aggregation but by differentiation and growth. There is thus no guarantee that the top-down and the bottom-up constraints will pick out the same modules, and in general they will not. But this is a matter for another occasion.

These points about hierarchial structure underlie the following arguments. Importantly, these arguments pertain not only to evolutionary change but also to the random changes and the ensuing adjustments wrought by instances of brain damage in an individual organism.

Least Underlying Change: Resemblances between Ontogeny and Phylogeny

Recapitulation and Differentiation in Evolution

Biologists of the nineteenth century were interested in ontogeny largely for what embryology might teach about the origins and taxonomy of organisms. Darwin's evolutionary theory cast the facts of comparative embryology in a new light and restructured the debate about whether organisms in their early ontogeny recapitulated the morphology of their ancestors. Von Baer's position in the nineteenth-century debate about ontogeny and phylogeny (de Beer, 1958; Gould, 1977) helps to provide a perspective both for the special sparing of function that sometimes follows early brain damage and for the unusually severe losses that can also follow interferences with early development.

Von Baer marshalled vast quantities of comparative embryological evidence in arguing that it often looks as if ontogeny recapitulates phylogeny because development proceeds from the general to the specific. In the classic example something resembling gill slits appears in both fish embryos and mammal embryos not because developmentally we are adult fish before we become infant mammals, but rather because all species appear more and more similar at earlier stages in their development; both ontogeny and phylogeny comprise progressive differentiation. Indeed, at the early extreme all multicellular creatures start as single fertilized ova; and one such single cell looks much like another.

Devastating Early Anomalies

An explanation for the qualitative character of von Baer's law can be derived from a model that combines Simon's two locks discussed earlier (see Wimsatt, in press). The "developmental lock" is a combination of these two locks—a simple lock if worked from left to right, but a complex lock if worked from right to left. Suppose that each wheel has its correct position (indicated by a click), but that this (correct) position depends upon the positions (whether correct or not) of any wheels to the left of it. If worked from left to right the first wheel is a simple problem with a probable number of 5 trials before success, because there are no wheels to the left of it. Given that this position has now been set, the solution of the next wheel is also a simple problem and so forth, and the probable number of trials for the lock is 50. If the lock is worked from the other end the last wheel is solved in a probable number of 5 trials, but when one moves to the next to the last wheel there is a probability of only 1 in 10 that the correct solution to that wheel will also be a correct solution to the last wheel and a probability of 9 in 10 that the correct solution will scramble the solution to the last wheel. Similar arguments show that the probability that the correct solution for a wheel m positions from the right will also be a correct solution for all subsequent wheels is 1 in 10^m. Thus, working from right to left, the probability that one is not scrambling the partial solution already arrived at for the first m wheels decreases exponentially as one moves to deeper and deeper levels.

This developmental lock is unrealistic in an organic context in many respects—especially in that it assumes only one correct solution, whereas the number of successful types of organism is enormous. This feature is readily modeled by supposing that there are 100 positions on each wheel, 10 of which are right. There are now 10^{20}

possible combinations, 10^{10} of which are correct. All other consequences of the model remain the same, except that we now speak of the probability of getting *a* correct solution rather than *the* correct solution. The different possible correct combinations correspond to the variety of actual and possible adaptive organisms.

Now consider this lock as a model of development, with the wheels being developmental stages: The leftmost wheel corresponds to the earliest stage, and sequentially later stages are mapped onto wheels further to the right. Suppose that expression of a mutation at a given stage of development corresponds to a random resetting of that wheel. The idea that earlier wheels set correct combinations for later wheels corresponds to the idea that the proper development of features at later stages presupposes or depends on the occurrence of given features at earlier stages. Suppose that the probability of getting a correct solution for that stage is k (rather than $\frac{1}{10}$) and that the correctness of a solution at one stage is independent of its correctness at other stages. Suppose finally that a given random mutation in the genes has an equal probability of being first expressed at any stage of development. The probability that a mutation will be advantageous at that stage and at all m subsequent stages is then k^m. But this means that a greater conservatism for evolutionary changes at earlier stages of development is likely.

This sequential dependence of developmental features also provides an explanation for frozen accidents in evolution. (Other extensions of this model are discussed in Wimsatt, in press.) Using this model we can now understand why an anomaly in early embryonic development often leads to spontaneous abortion or to devastating abnormalities as growth proceeds, and why early brain damage or abnormal early experiences often lead to profound changes. Moreover, the largely caudo-rostral development of the brain implies that at any age a given amount of damage to caudal and deeper structures will usually cause more debilitating behavioral disorders than the same amount of damage to phylogenetically newer and ontogenetically later, "higher" structures. In this regard, it is worth drawing a correspondence between two meanings of the word *general.* Older, lower brain functions have more generality both in the sense of being shared by more creatures and in the sense of having broader significance for the individual; that is, the necessity for their proper functioning is a shared feature of much of the individual's higher behavior (Wimsatt, 1981). For examples that fit both meanings of the word *general,* consider that there is not much any lower or higher organism can learn or do without arousal, breathing, and the basic movements involved in ingestion and locomotion. All these functions depend strongly on the brainstem.

The Sparing Effect

How is this abstract approach relevant to that other frequent outcome of early brain damage—the sparing phenomenon (Finger & Stein, 1982)? The lock has so far been a metaphor for serial development. But in living systems many subsystems (either different designs or iterations of the same design) often act in parallel. Such parallel processes may be largely independent of each other, or they may interact in a variety of orderly, adaptive ways that involve feedback controls. Interacting, compensating parallel systems might be compared not to one but to a set of developmental locks. Why should earlier damage sometimes be less harmful than later damage? Suppose that a perturbation of any one developmental stage may be fully compensated by a complementary change in the corresponding stage in some of the parallel systems. Let us label h the probability that an adequate compensation will occur in one or more of the parallel systems within that level, and let us make the further simplifying assumption that the same probability obtains at all the other levels. We then have an outcome quite the reverse of that which occurs with the serial system. With parallel systems the earlier an anomaly occurs the more chances there are for compensations, because there are still many following stages. If the anomaly occurs m levels down (assuming independence and equality and disregarding a possible devastating effect, as in the previous section) then the probability of compensation is the sum of probabilities at each level mh.

Other Empirical Relevancies

If effects of early brain damage are equal in adulthood to those of later damage, this must be because the damage was too small to significantly impair any stage in a serial developmental system or because it extracted one or more of a larger number of parallel subsystems that were already at the latest stage of development. Thus, in cats, early damage to the cortical nexus of the lemniscal and pyramidal systems in the sigmoid gyrus leads to the same degree of partial recovery and of long-term deficit in hopping and contact-placing reflexes as is seen with adult damage (Glassman, 1973b).

The idea that development proceeds from the general to the specific may apply to the finding of Almli, Hill, McMullen, and Fisher (1979), who noted that lateral hypothalamic damage causes sensorimotor deficits in young rats when it occurs at a later age than damage that causes consummatory deficits. Consummatory function might be seen as more general or similar across species and individuals. Postural, locomotor, and orientational behaviors are not needed until later in the rat's life, when it must begin to negotiate on its own and must face more particular contingencies.

In a similar vein Hughlings Jackson (1898/1958) commented:

> A man deeply comatose from sucking raw spirits out of a cask . . . recovers because the "vital" centres of his lowest level are very strongly organised and go on working . . . . If the "vital" centres of the lowest level were not strongly organised at birth, life would not be possible; if the centres of the highest level . . . were not little organised and therefore very modifiable we could only with difficulty and imperfectly adjust outselves to new circumstances.

Also possibly fitting von Baer's rule is the finding of Wolgin, Hein, and Teitelbaum (1980) that in both development and recovery from hypothalamic damage in cats, four categories of stimulation come to elicit forelimb placing, in the following order: vestibular, "proprioceptive" (including crude pressure), tactile, and visual. This order puts responsiveness under the control of progressively more distal stimuli. The cruder, earlier responses would probably serve almost any terrestrial creature, whereas later, finer responses to more distal stimuli require functioning that is more attuned to the bodily shape and behavior of a particular species and individual.

Although we have discussed why things should go from the general to the specific in development, it is not obvious why this direction should appear in certain cases of recovery, unless it is just a question of reconstructing the crudest, easiest things first. Another important possibility is that the hypothalamus, too small to do much detailed information processing by itself, serves primarily as a source of diffuse bias on the structures that process sensorimotor information. Perhaps a higher inhibitory bias on the most complexly differentiated functions somehow serves to ensure accurate responsiveness. According to Marshall (1975), ventromedial hypothalamic damage causes a sensorimotor hypersensitivity; thus it seems to be in dynamic balance with the lateral hypothalamus in biasing sensorimotor neural functions. The system as a whole may have a greater tendency to shut down than to function hyperactively. This safety feature would be adaptive in the same manner as that of a machine designed to shut off whenever the human operator releases his deliberate grip (Ashby, 1960).

Biasing Subsystems Costs Less Than Organizing Them

The nervous system is a highly organized structure. Undoubtedly, many cases of behavioral loss following damage are due to loss of the necessary information-processing apparatus. However, it is an old idea that recovery of some behaviors may follow brain damage because the relevant neural structures were not destroyed but only secondarily inhibited (see, e.g., Finger & Stein, 1982, on diaschisis; Glassman & Malamut, 1977). Such an inhibition might be dissipated more easily than an intricately structured organization could be rebuilt.

It is helpful to recognize a more general form of the idea of diaschisis; this is the notion of bias. In electronics the base of a transistor or the grid of a vacuum tube must be held at a particular dc voltage in order for the unit to remain within an optimal range of responsiveness. With too little bias the output subsystem is unresponsive to the voltage changes of the input that are superimposed on the bias, and with too much bias the system fails to respond because it is already saturated. In many physical systems there is a middle range of approximately linear responsiveness, and a declining sensitivity at the low and high ends, at which the response curve is asymptotic.

The most obvious neural instance of something like electronic bias is the resting potential of a neuron; however, there are as many analogies to bias as there are means of neural coding. For example, there may be optimal norms of resting rates of firing of single neurons or there may be norms of spatial position of maximal excitation in a topographically ordered neural array. In different cases such norms might be maintained locally or be imposed by some remote physiological monitor. Thus there must be a variety of ways in which different neural systems can be shifted out of their optimal range and as many ways in which recovery can be facilitated through simple bias readjustments.

Perhaps these factors underlie the efficacy (sometimes questioned) of cerebellar stimulation in relieving spasticity or emotional disorders (Ivan & Ventureyra, 1982) and the reemergence of organized responsiveness in some brain-damaged animals following administration of amphetamine (Meyer & Meyer, 1977). Considerations of set-point changes in food regulation and in irritability with damage to the lateral or ventromedial hypothalamus are also relevant (Keesey & Powley, 1975). In some such cases the bias shift is small enough that the animal remains alive, albeit less healthy and less prepared to deal with the environment. Similarly, neuroleptics and antidepressant drugs might be thought to work basically by rebiasing the relevant neurotransmitter systems, because it is inconceivable that a simple drug administration could contain any spatially or temporally organized recoding of adaptive information.

A shift in bias of certain neural structures might easily lead to a loss of one or more of the behavioral abilities which share dependence upon the same structure. Exceptions may occur in cases where the dynamic range of neural firing or other coding in the structure is greater than that needed for one of the behavioral functions. In some such cases accidental rebiasing may shift the neural system from the behavioral function that it would ordinarily serve under the test conditions to a different behavioral function that shares the neural system (see following section).

Because systems cannot function outside of the proper range of bias, establishment of bias in neural systems must be a prerequisite for the finer aspects of the ontogenetic growth of behavioral competencies. Because the information burden on the genes is minimized if as much information as possible is left in the environment until needed (see Introduction), the finer aspects of biasing must be left to feedback relations with the environment in learning and imprinting. If we knew where and how to look in the brain we would probably see much early ontogenetic variability as a hunt for the proper bias. For example, this may be the best interpretation of the fact that EEG rhythms are bigger and slower during early life, during some phases of sleep, and during recovery from brain damage (Glassman and Malamut, 1977).

This particular source of early flexibility must underlie some cases of sparing that follow early brain damage. Because proper later development depends on the fine tuning of earlier stages (recall the developmental-lock analogy), the generators of many system biases must lose flexibility later in development. Thus irreversible, deranged bias settings in one or several systems following adult brain damage might give the appearance—and indeed the fact—of irreversible disorganization. This analysis has obvious implications for research into methods of remediating early brain damage.

Conservation of Neurons and the Crowding Hypothesis

What Is the Evolutionary Path of Least Resistance?

Throughout this chapter we are concerned with the problem of how the stumbling, inefficient process of natural selection yields instances of organized complexity within plausible evolutionary times. Such examples of complexity are provided by hierarchially structured living systems—in their relations among levels. In this section we argue that in the brain this form of organization is efficient because it allows for a lesser degree of intricacy *within* levels. Indeed, it is possible to conceptualize levels of neural systems which can accomplish much on the basis of small numbers of subsystems, within each of which the rule of interaction is simply excitatory spatial summation. As suggested earlier, it is also efficient for information to be left in the environment until it can be absorbed during a critical period. In this section, we argue that such absorption may simply comprise early setting of biases and parameters of excitation in the just-mentioned subsystems. This section thus provides a more detailed general framework for considering sequelae of early brain damage.

A Prototypical Hierarchical System: Orientation–Localization

We leave consideration of inhibitory connections and other complications for another time, but to see the potential power of the basic method of analysis, consider a hypothetical neural system serving the ability of cats to orient the mouth toward tactile stimulation of any part of the body.

In cutaneous orientation–localization there is a well-defined, unique response to each of a large variety of stimuli. The responses are bound to the stimuli in an interesting way that goes beyond exclusive reflexive linkage between specific muscles and particular receptors to which they are dedicated; rather, many members of the same set of muscles participate in a large variety of well-defined movements. This is closely related to the scheme of functional multiplexing developed by Winograd and Cowan (1963) in an extension of von Neumann's work for the design of optimally reliable systems using a minimum of unreliable components. For these reasons this example can be used as a prototype that suggests a neural model having applicability to a much broader realm of behaviors.

Blindfolded cats are readily induced by food reward to orient and move the mouth into contact with any stimulated point on the body surface. The possible responses in this behavioral system may be analyzed—in a modification of the manner of those who engineer industrial robot-arm devices—into three subsystems, concerned with (1) moving the head up or down (pitch), (2) turning the head left or right (yaw), and (3) locating the point of maximal bend in the spine that will bring the head to the required position along the anterior–posterior axis.

A hypothetical primitive organism might accomplish orientation–localization by means of a highly differentiated single level of input–output connections. If the organism had some total number s of discriminable areas on the skin and some total number r of independently controllable muscle groups, then orientation–localization could be accomplished with a total number sr of all possible connections between the discriminable areas and the muscles. Each muscle would simply be excited in proportion to its utility in bringing the head into contact with the stimulated area.

Many of these connections could be eliminated in a system that had a single additional, hierarchial associative level. If each discriminable skin area and each muscle group were connected to each of three associative subsystems, as suggested by the pitch, yaw, and spinal-bend functions, then a total of only $3s + 3r$ connections would be needed. Since both s and r are much greater than 3, there is a tremendous saving of neural connections. In either the system of direct stimulus–response connections or the hierarchial system, excitatory synaptic spatial summation is a sufficient rule of association to accomplish the basic task. Some empirical evidence that suggests this mechanism is given in Glassman (1983b), where it is also argued that an associative subsystem need not be an isolated set of neurons that serves only one function.

Generalization of the Argument

Consider that wherever muscle groups were referred to in the preceding discussion, one might imagine any set of output units, and wherever discriminable areas on the skin were referred to, one might imagine any set of input units. Thus, in a multilevel hierarchial system any three consecutive levels may be described in the same manner of input level–associative level–output level. Also, this analysis so far involves an approximation in discrete units of continuously variable input–output relations. Accordingly, it remains viable for input and output categories that do not lend themselves to description on continua or even to ordinal scaling, but for which it is possible to assign unique joint values of neural excitations in a small set of subsystems at an interposed level. It is not even necessary that a given subsystem be dedicated to a single category. This point is a possible explanation of why easily describable deficits are not necessarily evident even after extirpation of what seems to be a unitary anatomical or physiological system (like a precisely bounded cytoarchitectural region, a system with well-defined neuronal response characteristics, or a system using a single neurotransmitter substance). When ablation of such a system has not revealed a simple behavioral localization, physiological psychologists have sometimes attributed the failure to fibers of passage or to other technical problems preventing a neat extirpation. The same methodological issues arise with other local manipulations such as electrical stimulation. But the problem of shared behavioral function probably runs deeper than this. Evolution may well have yielded some ad hoc mergers.

REPRESENTATION OF OTHER SORTS OF BEHAVIOR

Emotional behavior is not as neatly analyzable into terms of a few dimensions as is spatial orientation. A partial précis of perceptual categories and effector categories involved in emotional behavior might read as follows:

Effector categories: locomote toward, locomote away, cringe, jump up, vocalize, bite, solicit friendly contact, strike with forelimbs, copulate. Note that each of these behavioral categories is continuously variable in one or more aspects, as is each of the three dimensions of orientation–localization. Some of these categories can be further analyzed into qualitatively distinct components, each of which is continuously variable, but in some cases there are threshold discontinuities along what would otherwise be an intensity continuum (e.g., change in gait as speed increases). Each of these categories or subcategories might be represented in the brain by a diffusely excitable subsystem. The sum total of such subsystems would define a level.

Input categories: visual size of stimulus object, its speed of motion, its direction, its degree of proximity, intensity of particular components of its odor. The various possible states of motivation might also be considered input categories with respect to effector systems or with respect to some intermediate level. Note that more than one effector category and more than one input category are generally active at once. Thus, for example, a large object may elicit locomotion toward or away at various speeds, depending on its odor or its speed. These interactions are analogous to the simultaneous excitation of three dimensions of input and three parameters of output in orientation–localization.

Determinants of the Number of Subsystems at a Given Level

The multiplicity of muscles and joints involved in orientation–localization provides a model of multiplicity in associative levels. Many such levels may require more than the theoretical minimum number of subsystems required for a single function. Thus for orienting and localizing cats might have eventually evolved an efficient information-processing apparatus and body structure like robot arms, which from fixed bases can reach any point in a volume if they have one joint with two articulations (e.g., pitch and yaw, in the manner of a simplified primate shoulder) and a second joint with one articulation (e.g., an elbow, or a cylinder extending and retracting in a housing). Because the cat must locomote and manipulate using the same machinery as it uses in orientation–localization it has more muscles and joints than the minimum for any one of these functions. Analogous contingencies must contribute to the multiplication of the number of associative subsystems within levels of the brain.

In addition, natural selection can only make use of what already exists. An adaptive advantage that leads to new speciation may be the result of an inefficient, barely adequate mutational change. We might expect subsequent evolution to lead to greater efficiencies but for two factors, the evolutionary route to greater efficiency might require an improbable leap, and evolutionary progress in other subsystems might freeze accidents that become more refractory to change with the passage of evolutionary time.

The Structure of Crowded Information

The immature nervous system comprises a roughed-in structure whose levels and subsystems are poised for coding of certain categories. The subsystems are neither wholly flexible nor wholly predestined players in a ballistic ontogenesis. We have given reasons why evolution is likely to crowd subsystems with functions. But a fuller framework must be provided to explain how neural lines may repack aspects of information at one level into subsystems at other levels. Moreover, the notion that evolution, ontogeny, and recovery are sometimes analogous processes suggests that early brain damage may sometimes lead this redistribution to yield more than the usual functional crowding in subsystems.

As an abstract illustration of the possibility of crowding, consider a simple square shape having x and y axes and divided into 100 cells labeled systematically x_1y_1, x_2y_1, x_3y_1, . . ., $x_{10}y_1$; x_1y_2, ... These cells could easily be remapped into a line of cells by any of a variety of rules, for example the rule just used in listing the cells on a line of type.

This argument readily generalizes to cover convergence of any number of categories or dimensions into any smaller number of dimensions. The cells in the abstract example may be considered representative of any neural code—the spatial position of topographically organized neurons or groups of neurons such as columns or barrels, the firing rate of single neurons or of mass-acting groups of neurons, the difference or ratio of activity levels of two neurons or sets of neurons in dynamic balance, the concentration of a neurotransmitter, the voltage of a steady potential, and possibly others. Two or more interactions of each of these examples acting jointly can define higher dimensional subsystems.

The division of dimensions into discrete units, as suggested by the abstract example, is representative of limits of resolution. Remappings into lower dimensional subsystems can take place only if the structure embodying the condensed dimension has a broader range of values than do the structures converging onto it or if the system can tolerate reduced resolution. Resolution is not much of a problem for categories with very few different meaningful values. For instance, recalling the example of emotional behavior, discriminations of stimulus size must often be little more than a binary matter of "too big" or "small enough" as the animal judges whether to attack, defend, flee, or prey. For this reason many emotional behavioral functions may fit in the same neural structures.

It seems unlikely that the abstract mapping closely represents something that can have evolved naturally. Rather, the lower dimensional target system must first appear with values near its center that represent the most frequently encountered combinations of x and y inputs. Later its dynamic range may stretch to increase resolution or to admit a greater number of possible values.

This mechanism of crowding is a logically possible partial explanation of what has sometimes been said to occur ontogenetically with regard to linguistic and cognitive functioning of patients who have sustained left hemispherectomy early in life. Although there is some dramatic empirical evidence to the contrary (Smith & Sugar, 1975), the previous arguments on conservation suggest that on the average we need all the brain that we have and therefore that crowding and consequent reduced functioning of some sort must be present even in apparently exceptional cases. If individuals do have vast amounts of spare neural capacity, we must revise our notions of the implications of natural selection.

References

Almli, C. R., Hill, D. L., McMullen, N. T., & Fisher, R. S. (1979). Newborn rats: Lateral hypothalamic damage and consummatory-sensorimotor ontogeny. *Physiology & Behavior, 22,* 767–773.

Arbib, M. A. (1972). *The metaphorical brain: An introduction to cybernetics as artificial intelligence and brain theory.* New York: Wiley (Interscience).

Ashby, W. R. (1960). *Design for a brain.* New York: Wiley.

Bonner, J. T. (Ed.) (1982). *Evolution and development.* New York: Springer-Verlag.

Buckley, W. (Ed.) (1968). *Modern systems research for the behavioral scientist.* Chicago: Aldine.

Burhoe, R. W. (1981). *Toward a scientific theology.* Ottawa, Ontario: Christian Journals.

Campbell, D. T. (1974a). Unjustified variation and selective retention in scientific discovery. In F. J. Ayala & T. Dobzhansky (Eds.), *Studies in the philosophy of biology* (pp. 139–161). Berkeley: University of California Press.

Campbell, D. T. (1974b). 'Downward causation' in hierarchically organised biological systems. In F. J. Ayala & T. Dobzhansky (Eds.), *Studies in the philosophy of biology* (pp. 179–186). Berkeley: University of California Press.

deBeer, G. (1958). *Embryos and ancestors* (3rd ed.). New York: Oxford University Press.

Eibl-Eibesfeldt, I. (1975). *Ethology: The biology of behavior* (2nd ed.). New York: Holt, Rinehart & Winston.

Finger, S., & Stein, D. G. (1982). *Brain damage and recovery: Research and clinical perspectives.* New York: Academic Press.

Fisher, R. A. (1930/1958). *The genetical theory of natural selection* (2nd ed.) New York: Dover (Original work published 1930).

Glassman, R. B. (1973a). Persistence and loose coupling in living systems. *Behavioral Science, 18,* 83–98.

Glassman, R. B. (1973b). Similar effects of infant and adult sensorimotor cortical lesions on cats' posture. *Brain Research, 63,* 103–110.

Glassman, R. B. (1978). The logic of the lesion experiment and its role in the neural sciences. In S. Finger (Ed.), *Recovery from brain damage: Research and theory* (pp. 3–31). New York: Plenum.

Glassman, R. B. (1983a). Free will has a neural substrate: Critique of Joseph F. Rychlak's Discovering free will and personal responsibility. *Zygon Journal of Religion and Science, 15,* 133–154.

Glassman, R. B. (1983b). Dissociation of vertical and horizontal components of somesthetic orientation - localization during recovery from cortical damage: Implication regarding central associative functions. *Physiological Psychology, 11,* 47–53.

Glassman, R. B., & Glassman, H. N. (1980). Oral dyskinesia in brain-damaged rats withdrawn from a neuroleptic: Implication for models of tardive dyskinesia. *Psychopharmacology, 69,* 19–25.

Glassman, R. B., & Malamut, B. L. (1977). Does the brain actively maintain itself? *BioSystems, 9,* 257–268.

Gould, S. J. (1977). *Ontogeny and phylogeny.* Cambridge: Harvard University Press.

Hardin, G. (1972). Genetic consequences of cultural decisions in the realm of population. *Social Biology, 19,* 350–361.

Hughlings Jackson, J. (1884/1958). Evolution and dissolution of the nervous system, Lecture II. In J. Taylor (Ed.), *Selected writings of John Hughlings Jackson* (Vol 2, pp. 53–63). London: Staples Press. (Original work published 1884)

Hughlings Jackson, J. (1898/1958). Relations of different divisions of the central nervous system to one another and to parts of the body. In J. Taylor (Ed.), *Selected writings of John Hughlings Jackson* (Vol. 2, pp. 422–443). London: Staples Press. (Original work published 1898)

Ivan, L. P., & Ventureyra, E. C. G. (1982). Chronic cerebellar stimulation in cerebral palsy. *Applied Neurophysiology, 45,* 51–54.

Keesey, R. E., & Powley, T. L. (1975). Hypothalamic regulation of body weight. *American Scientist, 63,* 558–565.

Levins, R. (1979). Coexistence in a variable environment. *American Naturalist, 114,* 765–783.

Lewontin, R. C. (1978). Adaptation. *Scientific American, 239,*(3), 212–230.

Lorenz, K. (1977). *Behind the mirror: A search for a natural history of human knowledge* (R. Taylor, Trans.). New York: Harcourt.

Marshall, J. F. (1975). Increased orientation to sensory stimuli following medial hypothalamic damage in rats. *Brain Research, 86,* 373–387.

Mayr, E. (1974). Behavior programs and evolutionary strategies. *American Scientist, 62,* 650–659.

Meyer, D. R., & Meyer, P. M. (1977). Dynamics and bases of recoveries of functions after injuries to the cerebral cortex. *Physiological Psychology, 5,* 133–165.

Miller, J. G. (1978). *Living systems.* New York: McGraw-Hill.

Phillips, J. L., Jr. (1975). *The origins of intellect: Piaget's theory* (2nd ed.). San Francisco: Freeman.

Rychlak, J. F. (1981). *Introduction to personality and psychotherapy* (2nd ed.). Boston: Houghton.

Schrodinger, E. (1956). *What is life: And other scientific essays.* Garden City, NY: Doubleday.

Simon, H. A. (1962/1969). The architecture of complexity. *Proceedings of the American Philosophical Society, 106,* 467–482. Reprinted in H. A. Simon (1969). *The sciences of the artificial* (pp. 84–118). Cambridge: MIT Press.

Simon, H. A. (1973). The organization of complex systems. In H. H. Pattee (Ed.), *Hierarchy theory* (pp. 1–27). New York: Braziller.

Smith, A. & Sugar, O. (1975). Development of above normal language and intelligence 21 years after left hemispherectomy. *Neurology, 25,* 813–818.

Wade, M. J. (1978). A critical review of the models of group selection. *Quarterly Review of Biology, 53,* 101–114.

Weaver, W. (1949). Companion essay. In C. E. Shannon & W. Weaver (Eds.), *Mathematical theory of communication.* Urbana: University of Illinois Press.

Williams, G. C. (1966). *Adaptation and natural selection: A critique of some current evolutionary thought.* Princeton: Princeton University Press.

Wilson, E. O. (1975). *Sociobiology: The new synthesis.* Cambridge: Harvard Univeristy Press.

Wimsatt, W. C. (1974). Complexity and organization. In K. F. Schaffner & R. S. Cohen (Eds.), *Boston studies in the philosophy of science* (Vol. 20, pp. 67–86). Dordrecht, Netherlands: Reidel.

Wimsatt, W. C. (1976). Reductionism, levels of organization, and the mind-body problem. In G. G. Globus, G, Maxwell, & I. Savodnik (Eds.), *Consciousness and the brain: A scientific and philosophical inquiry* pp. 199–267). New York: Plenum.

Wimsatt, W. C. (1980a). Randomness and perceived-randomness in evolutionary biology. *Synthese, 43,* 287–329.

Wimsatt, W. C. (1980b). Reductionistic research strategies and their biases in the units of selection controversy. In T. Nickles (Ed.), *Scientific discovery* (Vol. 2): *Historical and scientific case studies* pp. 213–259). Dordrecht, Netherlands: Reidel.

Wimsatt, W. C. (1981). Units of selection and the structure of the multi-level genome. *Proceedings of the Philosophy of Science Association, 2,* 122–183.

Wimsatt, W. C. (in press). Von Baer's law of development, generative entrenchment, and scientific change. *Philosophy of Science,* in press.

Winograd, T., & Cowan, J. D. (1963). *Reliable computation in the presence of noise.* Cambridge: MIT Press.

Wolgin, D. L., Hein, A., & Teitelbaum, P. (1980). Recovery of forelimb placing after lateral hypothalamic lesions in the cat: Parallels and contrasts with development. *Journal of Comparative and Physiological Psychology, 94,* 795–807.

3

Lesion-Induced Neuroplasticity and the Sparing or Recovery of Function following Early Brain Damage*

Oswald Steward

Introduction

Interest in the mechanisms of recovery following central nervous system (CNS) injury is long standing, evolving from a clinical concern with the functional sequellae of brain injury and from an experimental interest in the relation between brain and behavior. Certainly one of the central tenets of research in functional recovery following brain injury is that the functional consequences of injury depend on the age of the organism at the time of the injury. In most cases better

*The author's research is supported by NSF grant #BNS80-21865, NIH grant NS 12333, and Research Career Development Award NS 00325. I thank Barry Fass for his helpful discussions of the problems of behavioral sparing and recovery of function, and for his helpful comments on this manuscript.

Copyright © 1984 by Academic Press, Inc.
All rights of reproduction in any form reserved.
ISBN 0-12-052901-7

recovery or better sparing of function is observed if lesions are incurred early in development (for a discussion of the terms *recovery* and *sparing of function,* see Laurence & Stein, 1978). This represents the so-called Kennard Principle, after the initial study that demonstrated greater functional return after lesions in developing monkeys than after similar lesions in mature monkeys (Kennard, 1938). Why it may be better to have one's brain lesion early, as H. L. Teuber has put it (for a discussion, see Schneider, 1979), is still not clear despite almost a half-century of research.

Several types of cellular mechanisms for developmental effects have been proposed. I do not review all of these here, however. Rather, I concentrate on one of the currently popular hypotheses: namely, that rearrangements of neuronal connections that occur following brain injury might be functionally significant, contributing to sparing or behavioral recovery, and differences in the extent or nature of this lesion-induced neuroplasticity might account for the differences in the functional consequences of injury in young and old animals. The present chapter reveals some experimental strategies that have previously been used for evaluating relationships between remodeling of CNS connections and behavioral sequellae following brain injury (Steward, 1982); here the focus is on the extent to which these strategies can be applied to analysis of the sequellae of brain injury in young animals.

Evolution of the Hypothesis

The hypothesis that the behavioral consequences of brain injury might be related to a reorganization of surviving circuitry does not have a long history. Until about 1970 most researchers considered the reorganization of circuits following injury to be at best a rare curiosity and perhaps impossible in most situations. At most, any reorganization that did occur was generally considered to be abortive, failing in the establishment of functionally meaningful connections. Since 1970 this view has changed radically. Indeed, anatomical reorganization of circuitry has been observed in virtually all brain regions, and following lesions at all ages. Furthermore, numerous studies within the past decade have explicity or implicitly considered the possibility that a reorganization of surviving circuitry contributes to the behavioral changes observed after brain injury.

Why is this suddenly an attractive possibility? The answer may lie in the ubiquity of the reorganizational events, in the fact that a cellular mechanism can be suggested that seems reasonable, or in the fact that some of the rules of reorganization resemble the rules of behavioral change following injury. Specifically, studies of anatomical reorganization following lesions have suggested principles that are in many ways reminiscent of the principles that have been derived from studies of recovery or sparing of function. There are anatomical parallels of the central tenet that animals with brain damage early in development often exhibit more recovery or sparing than animals with apparently identical lesions at maturity; the capacity of the brain to reorganize itself anatomically following a given kind of injury also seems greater in developing animals. Indeed, lesions in developing animals often result in the construction of aberrant pathways that would not be constructed following lesions at maturity. This is particularly true in the case of pathways that do not exist at all in intact animals, but are induced by lesions—*ectopic pathways*. Completely ectopic interconnections rarely form except after lesions in developing animals. Postlesion anatomical reorganization in mature animals is for the most part limited to enlargement or remodeling of connections that are normally present. When a given type of reorganization occurs in both developing and mature animals, the extent of the reorganization is typically greater in developing animals. Numerous examples of these generalizations may be found in the literature. Thus, perhaps the keystone of the hypothesis that recovery is related to anatomical reorganization following early brain injury is the observation that damage in developing organisms typically results in greater amounts of both.

Functional Significance of Lesion-Induced Reorganization of Circuitry

It is important to recall that by definition anatomical rearrangements following lesions result in the establishment of abnormal circuits. These may either be entirely ectopic or may be exaggerated versions of pathways which normally exist. Why would the production of an abnormal circuit contribute to a sparing or recovery of function? In a broad sense the operational significance of any pathway depends on the information that it carries and the ability of its interconnected neurons to make use of this information. If abnormal pathways were very unlike those which normally existed, it would not be immediately apparent how these abnormal circuits could contribute to appropriate function. As we will see, however, it is possible to conceive of situations in which abnormal circuits might be functionally beneficial.

For example, if a neuron loses its normal synaptic input as a consequence of a lesion, and is later reinnervated by fibers that arise from a structure that is anatomically homologous and physiologically analogous with the structure that normally innervates the denervated neuron, then it is at least conceivable that the reinnervation could be useful. The construction of aberrant but homologous circuits is probably not as unusual as might be supposed. An example of a frequent situation in which aberrant but homologous circuits are formed is illustrated in Figure 1. The left side of the figure is a schematized bilaterally symmetrical neuron chain, the components of which are for the most part unilaterally distributed. Numerous examples of this type of bilaterally symmetrical but unilaterally projecting system can be cited, including components of most sensory and motor systems and many other pathways as well. A very frequent pattern of reorganization following lesion is illustrated on the right side of the figure. A lesion at Station C induces an abnormal crossing of pathways that are normally unilateral. At Station D, cells that have lost their normal synaptic inputs are reinnervated by fibers originating from the contralateral (wrong) side of the brain. These connections are homologous with the normal ones, although inappropriate with regard to laterality. Similarly, axons from cells in Station A that are deprived of their normal targets in C cross the midline and reinnervate the contralateral Station C. Many examples of just these sorts of rearrangements may be found in the literature, and in fact, all of these examples may be found in the case of the reorganization of projections following unilateral destruction of the superior colliculus of the developing hamster (see Schneider, 1973; and Schneider & Jhaveri, 1974). Interestingly, the two types of abnormal circuits could lead to a reestablishment of throughput on the right side. As illustrated in Figure 2, the double crossing of the projections from A to C and then from C to D result in a potential reconnection between A and D on the right side, which normally connects by projections which are exclusively ipsilateral.

The preceding illustrations suggest that a postlesion reorganization could contribute to a restoration of normal throughput, which might further result in a restoration of information processing along interrupted pathways. In many cases, however, reorganization can contribute to improved function independent of the specific informa-

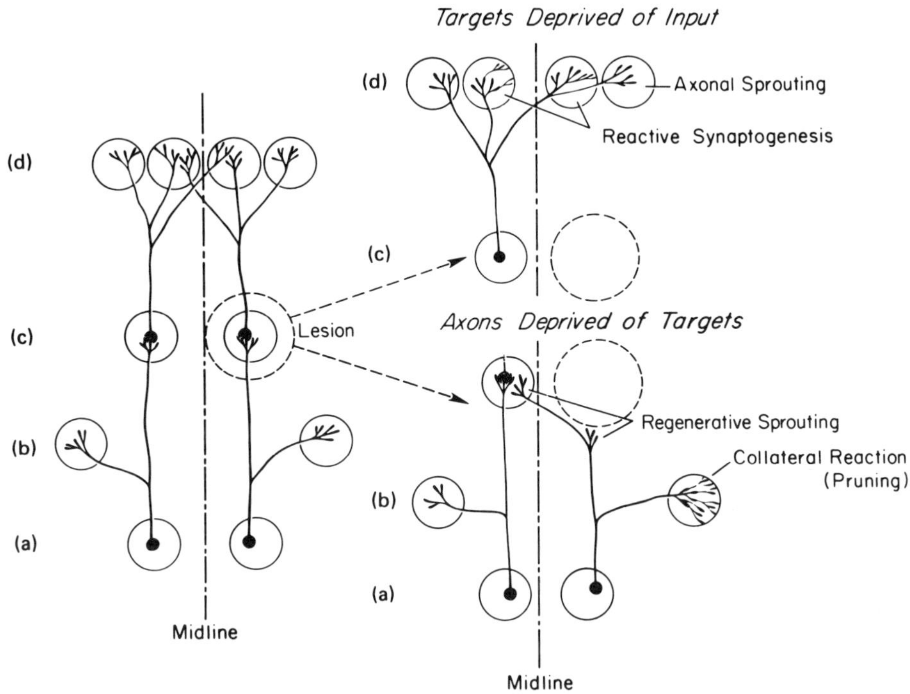

Figure 1. Changes in CNS connectivity following lesions. The left side of the figure is a schematized neuronal circuit with several stations (A–D). The hallmark of this idealized circuit is that it is bilaterally symmetrical with most of the connections being unilateral. Some typical types of remodeling of connections that might occur following damage at one station are illustrated on the right. The lesion at station (c) deprives cells at station (a) of normal targets and cells at station (d) of normal synaptic inputs. The various types of reactive changes that are illustrated restore input to denervated cells or provide alternate targets for cells deprived of their normal sites of termination. Note that many of the reorganizational events result in a loss of the normal laterality of projection. (Reproduced from Steward, 1982.)

tion conveyed. For example, cells that have been deprived of their normal targets may not be capable of normal physiological operation even at portions of their circuitry that are spared by the lesion. This is particularly true if the lesion amputates a major axon collateral of the neuron. Similarly, it is likely that cells that have been extensively denervated will be incapable of normal physiological operation even if they retain input from some other source. If the lost connections are excitatory a decrease in the level of tonic excitation may make it impossible for these cells to respond to other inputs. If the lost connections were inhibitory the neurons may fire in an uncontrolled

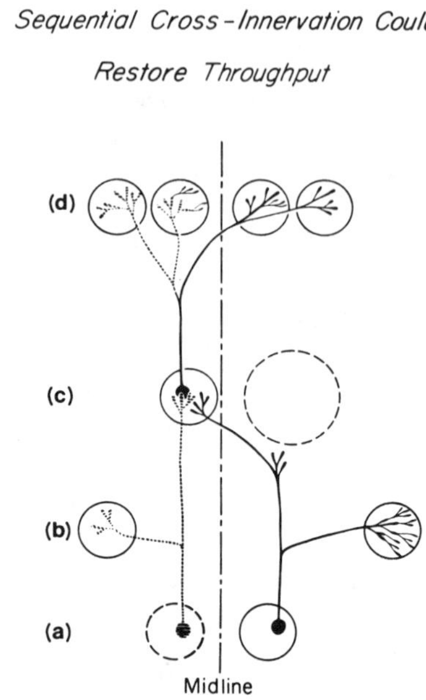

Figure 2. Normal throughput through two abnormal circuits. The reorganization illustrated in Figure 1 results in an abnormal crossing of axons from station (a) to station (c) and an abnormal innervation of the right side of station (d) by axons originating from cells in station (c). This recrossing might result in the restoration of throughput from station (a) to station (d) on the left side (emphasized by the solid lines). The normal projections that would survive the lesion are indicated by the broken lines. This type of remodeling is consistent with known examples of reorganization of circuitry in the visual system. (For a discussion, see Steward, 1982. Figure reproduced from Steward, 1982.)

fashion. To the extent that postlesion remodeling restores inputs of a similar physiological sign to the denervated cells (excitatory or inhibitory) and provides alternate targets for cells that have lost their normal ones, the functional capacity of the surviving neurons may be improved. This may occur even if the information that is carried by the connections is functionally meaningless.

Consider for example the denervated neuron at Station D of Figure 1. If this neuron is involved in circuitry other than that illustrated, then this other circuitry may be totally unaffected by the lesion, but transmission along the other pathway may be compromised. As a simple consequence of the loss of an excitatory input, the cells at Station D may be no longer capable of discharging in response to other excitatory inputs because of a loss of excitatory tone. In this case, reinnervation by any other excitatory afferent, regardless of the specific information that this alternate input conveys, may contribute to a return of tonic excitation and thus a processing via intact pathways. This hypothetical example is only slightly modified from the hypothesis of diaschisis originally proposed by von Monakow (1910, and see von Monakow, 1969). A similar disruption may occur in the case of neurons in Station A that lose their normal targets. In this case transmission to Station B may be disrupted as a consequence of the damage to a remote collateral. The reestablishment of connections by the collateral which normally projected to C might simply heal the wound of the neuron, enabling it to return to processing via circuitry which it retained, for example, the connection from A to B. In either of these cases the simplest contribution that the postlesion remodeling would make is the reversal of the deleterious effects of denervation and target loss independent of the specific information that these abnormal connections carry.

Strategies for Evaluating the Functional Consequences of Lesion-Induced Growth

As the preceding discussion indicates, it is reasonable to think that some types of lesion-induced rearrangements of circuitry could be functionally beneficial. Exploring the relationships between anatomical reorganization and function depends on the evolution of experimental strategies, however. In the remainder of this chapter I consider the extent to which two strategies that have been used for evaluating the relation between anatomical reorganization and function following injury in mature animals are applicable to young animals.

The basic issues that need to be addressed in any such analysis have been discussed in more detail in a previous review (Steward, 1982). At the outset it is important to define one's experimental perspective; that is, whether one is interested in defining the mechanisms of functional recovery or the functional significance of a given cellular event. If these two were perfectly correlated—if behavioral recovery depended exclusively on a certain type of anatomical reorganization—then these general perspectives would approach the same relation from opposite directions. If, however, recovery is a multifaceted process, and if anatomical reorganization has multiple functional consequences, then each approach generates a quite different data base. Studies of the mechanisms of functional recovery would almost certainly reveal factors other than anatomical reorganization that contribute to recovery. Similarly, defining the functional consequences of growth would almost certainly reveal examples in which anatomical reorganization was functionally neutral or resulted in a derangement of normal function. Indeed, given types of growth could be both adaptive and maladaptive. In the now classic example in which damage to the spinal cord results in sprouting of dorsal root projections, sprouting may contribute to the development of spasticity and thus may be considered maladaptive (McCouch, Austin, Liu, & Liu, 1958). Yet, as noted by Goldberger (1974), the same spastic hyperreflexia can actually contribute to the return of useful function in the affected limb. My favorite example, however, is the case of reorganization of retinotectal projections. If one removes one tectum along with the eye that normally projects to the surviving contralateral tectum, the surviving eye reroutes its projections and innervates the surviving tectum (Schneider, 1973; Schneider and Jhaveri, 1974). This is an example of an aberrant but homologous connection; the eye projects to its normal target area (the tectum) but is inappropriate with respect to laterality. The consequence of this miswiring is that the animal orients incorrectly when presented with a visual stimulus to the affected eye. Is this misorientation adaptive or maladaptive? If one considers accurate orientation the miswiring is maladaptive. In a case of escape from a potential predator, however, these connections may be adaptive. They would at least make the animal aware of something in its environment and permit an escape response. In many cases any information along a pathway may be better than no information at all. In either case the connections are functional.

In the following sections I adopt the second of the two preceding general approaches, asking whether there are functional consequences of specific types of anatomical reorganization. Two principle experimental strategies have been previously outlined for investigating this question in the case of injury in mature animals (Steward, 1982). These have been termed the *neurological sequellae strategy* and the *sensor–motor system strategy.*

The Neurological Sequellae Strategy

The neurological sequellae strategy is one that we have used most extensively in our studies of the functional significance of postlesion rearrangement of circuitry in the hippocampal formation. It offers several advantages. The key to the strategy is the comparison of the time courses of neural and behavioral events. The principle criterion that must be met is that one must know the time course of any anatomical reorganization that occurs. One then asks whether there are behavioral changes that occur with a similar time course. The type of evidence that this strategy provides is illustrated in Figure 3. The time course of reinnervation of the dentate gyrus of the mature rat following destruction of its principle input from the ipsilateral entorhinal cortex can be defined in a variety of ways. Synapse replacement on the dentate granule cells can be evaluated ultrastructurally (Figure 3a). The sprouting of individual afferent systems may be traced with quantitative anatomical methods such as autoradiography (Figure 3b). In applying the neurological sequellae strategy one asks whether there are behavioral changes that evolve with a time course that is comparable to the anatomical events. As illustrated in Figure 3c, there is a behavior that meets this criterion; the performance of rats in a maze task that requires the short-term recollection of spatial cues is substantially disrupted by unilateral damage to the entorhinal cortex and recovers with a time course wich is comparable to the time course of the anatomical reorganization. Control studies have demonstrated that this recovery is a time-dependent and not a training-dependent process (Loesche & Steward, 1977; and see Steward, 1982 for a review).

In evaluating the temporal relation between the rearrangement of connections and particular behavioral capacities, it is important to consider the inherent limitations of each of the measures. For example, in evaluating the time course of synapse replacement at the electron-microscopic level, one would expect little functional benefit until synapses had formed. As illustrated in Figure 3a, there is an apparent proliferation of presynaptic processes several days prior to the formation of synapses. One might expect the proliferation of the presynaptic processes to be functionally insignificant. Yet there may be a problem with identification of immature synapses. The early stages of synapse formation may well involve functionally competent contacts which are not recognizable as synapses. For example, the contacts may have poorly developed postsynaptic specializations. As a consequence, some presynaptic processes that do not meet the criteria for synapses may nevertheless be functional. Physiological evidence (discussed below) suggests that this is the case; the time course of the increases in physiological efficacy correspond more closely to the terminal proliferation measured electron microscopically.

Tract-tracing methods also have serious limitations for time-

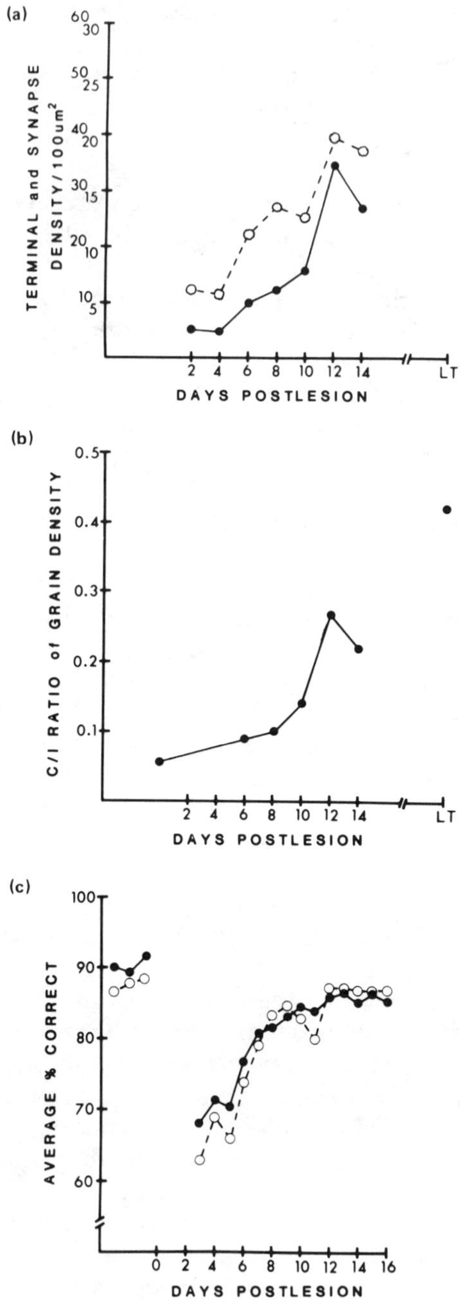
(a)
TERMINAL and SYNAPSE DENSITY/100um²
DAYS POSTLESION
LT
(b)
C/I RATIO of GRAIN DENSITY
DAYS POSTLESION
LT
(c)
AVERAGE % CORRECT
DAYS POSTLESION

course studies. Tracing reorganized pathways at early postlesion intervals by secondary degeneration methods is quite impossible. The degeneration products from the initial lesion confuse any analysis. Autoradiographic methods require the placement of injections some time prior to sacrifice. In the example of Figure 3b the injections of [^{3}H] proline that were used to trace the projections from the surviving entorhinal cortex were actually made 6 days prior to sacrifice. The projections revealed by the methods could be those that are present at the time of the injection or at the time of sacrifice, or they could be some integrated average over the postlesion survival interval. Probably the best methods for anatomical tracing are those that use some intrinsic property of the afferent, for example the content of transmitter or transmitter-related enzyme.

One way to circumvent some of the problems posed by anatomical methods is to measure the time course of the formation of new connections physiologically. This approach is particularly attractive, because one can ask when operational synapses form. In an elegant study, Reeves (1983) used chronic neurophysiological methods to measure the synaptic efficacy of the crossed projection from the entorhinal cortex to the dentate gyrus after unilateral entorhinal cortical lesions. By testing animals daily after the lesions, he was able to demonstrate dramatic increases in the efficacy of the crossed pathway during the same interval as the increases in terminal density as revealed by previous electron microscopic studies [see Figure 4(a)]. The same animals were also tested in a T maze alternation task; there was a striking correspondence between the increases in synaptic

---

Figure 3. Comparison of the time course of terminal proliferation and reactive synaptogenesis with the time course of recovery of maze performance. The time course of terminal growth (open circles) and synapse replacement (filled circles) in the dentate gyrus denervated by ipsilateral entorhinal-cortex lesions is illustrated in (a) (redrawn from Steward & Vinsant, 1983). LT refers to long-term postlesion (in this case, approximately 200 days). (b) illustrates the time course of proliferation of the projections from the contralateral entorhinal cortex following ipsilateral entorhinal lesions. The extent of the projection at various postlesion intervals is measured autoradiographically following injections of protein precursor ([^{3}H] proline) into the surviving entorhinal cortex contralateral to the lesion (redrawn from Steward & Loesche, 1977) (LT again indicates long term post-lesion). (c) illustrates the time course of recovery of rewarded alternation performance in a T maze. The animals are required to alternate between goal arms for reinforcement, and thus the task is a test of a form of spatial short-term memory (see Loesche & Steward, 1977; Steward, 1982; Steward, Loesche, & Horton, 1977). The data represented by the open circles is from the original study of Steward and Loesche (1977). The data represented by the solid circles is the average of all animals that have been tested in the rewarded alternation task after unilateral entorhinal lesions in our laboratory.

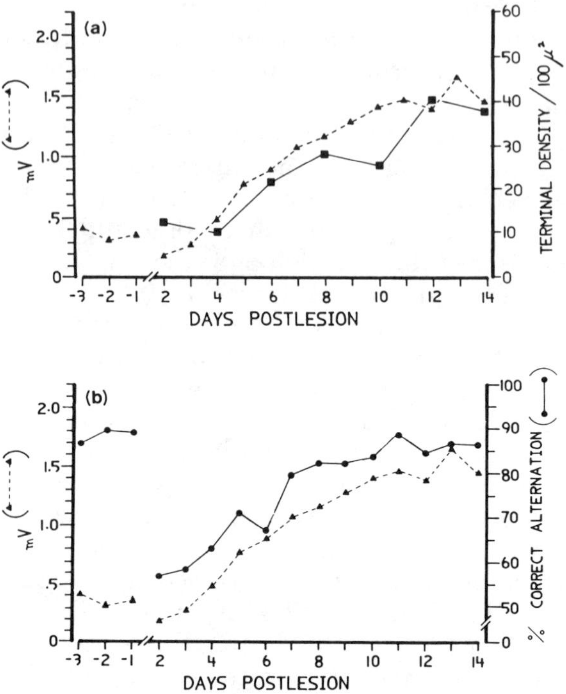

Figure 4. Comparisons between anatomical and physiological measures of sprouting and their relationship to post-lesion behavioral recovery. (a) The time course of lesion-induced terminal proliferation in the dentate gyrus following unilateral entorhinal cortical lesions is compared with the time course of increases in the physiological potency of one of the pathways that participates in the sprouting response. Filled squares represent the density of terminals (per 100μm²) in the denervated zone (referenced to the right-hand ordinate). These data are redrawn from Fig. 2, which is based on the data from Steward and Vinsant (1983). The synaptic efficacy of the crossed temporo-dentate pathway from the surviving entorhinal cortex contralateral to the lesion was evaluated with chronic neurophysiological techniques. Stimulating electrodes were placed in the surviving entorhinal area, and recording electrodes were situated in the denervated dentate gyrus. The amplitude of the monosynaptic "population EPSP" generated by the crossed pathway was plotted over time. Filled circles indicate the amplitude of the population EPSP in mV (referenced to the left-hand ordinate). (b) The time course of the increases in the synaptic efficacy of the crossed temporo-dentate pathway, from (a), is compared with the time course of recovery of alternation performance in a T maze. Filled circles indicate the percentage of alternation (referenced to the right-hand ordinate). (From Reeves, 1983).

efficacy of the sprouting pathway and the behavioral recovery [Figure 4(b)]. There is the potential reservation that some part of the increased synaptic efficacy could be related to a change other than the growth (i.e.denervation supersensitivity). The parallels between the anatomical and physiological measures argue against this interpretation, however.

Finally, one must be very concerned with the behavioral measurements. If a task used to assess the animal's functional ability is very easy, animals may be capable of performing flawlessly while they are still functionally incapacitated. Because most behavioral tests have ceilings (e.g., animals cannot perform above 100% correct) the time course of recovery may be artificially attenuated by task ceiling. As a consequence, the time course of recovery might appear to be much more rapid than it actually is. All of these issues underscore the fact that temporal correlations need not be perfect to suggest a relationship between two processes. Indeed, despite some apparent differences in the time course of the behavioral changes after unilateral entorhinal-cortex lesions and the time course of the anatomical events, we are confident that these two processes are related.

After establishing the initial hypothesis by correlating the time courses of anatomical reorganization and behavior, the contribution of specific pathways can be assessed by placing secondary lesions. Such secondary lesion studies provided strong support for the role of the contralateral entorhinal cortex in recovery following ipsilateral entorhinal lesions. In fact, several pathways participate in the reinnervation of the dentate gyrus after entorhinal-cortex lesions, and all of these appear to proliferate with approximately the same time course. The recovery of maze performance which occurs following unilateral entorhinal-cortex lesions (Figure 3c) is eliminated if the crossing projections from the entorhinal cortex are destroyed by midline transections (Loesche & Steward, 1977). Interestingly, similar midline transections in otherwise intact animals do not result in behavioral debilitation in the maze task. Thus we believe that it is the reinnervating fibers from the surviving contralateral entorhinal cortex that contribute to the recovery of certain performance abilities. The issue of whether the anatomical reorganization mediates the recovery is quite another matter and is considered further.

The neurological sequellae strategy is quite useful. Unlike the sensory–motor system strategy, the neurological sequellae strategy can be applied to any neural system. The secondary manipulations needed to assess the role of given systems may vary in difficulty, but the basic strategy is quite flexible for initial evaluation of brain–behavior relations following injury in mature animals. Unfortunately, this is not true in the case of injury in young animals. First, the strategy depends on a stable behavioral baseline. If behavior would normally change during the period in which anatomical reorganization is occurring, it is exceedingly difficult to assess the relative contribution of the anatomical reorganization; a lesion could induce a change in behavior superimposed upon changes due to development. Dissociating the two types of change may be problematic because the changes due to development and those due to recovery processes are almost certain to be nonadditive. In the case of developing animals, very few behaviors are stable. Other difficulties also arise. For example, anatomical reorganization in young animals, in addition to being more extensive than in mature animals, typically occurs much more rapidly. Indeed, in the hippocampal formation, aberrant fiber growth may occur within hours rather than days following deafferenting lesions (Gall & Lynch, 1978). Assessing behavioral capacities during this relatively short reorganization interval might be quite difficult. On the other hand, the rapidity of the reorganization alleviates to some extent the problem of a changing behavioral baseline. Even in rapidly developing animals it may be possible to obtain a stable behavioral baseline over a period of a few days which would permit an evaluation of behavioral change related to rapid anatomical reorganization. Unfortunately, an even more serious problem is that the rate of behavioral and neural development can be affected by brain injury; a behavioral baseline which is established in intact animals may not be appropriate for comparison with brain-injured animals. All of these facts make the application of the neurological sequellae strategy difficult in the study of the relationship between anatomical reorganization and function after injury in young animals. Application is not impossible; careful attention, however, must be paid to the nonstable baselines of both behavioral processes and anatomical distributions of the pathways in question. But as was noted earlier, the parallel between neural and behavioral changes need not be perfect to suggest a relationship. The advantages of the strategy are sufficient to make the effort worthwhile, particularly because this strategy can be used for evaluating almost any anatomical system or behavior.

The Sensory–Motor System Strategy

The sensory–motor system strategy requires that three criteria be met: (1) one must be able to define the nature of the postlesion growth, (2) the behavioral role of the neural systems involved in the growth must be well characterized, and (3) the function of the system must be closely related to its structural organization so that structural rearrangement will have predictable functional consequences. Because of the latter two requirements the strategy is almost exclusively limited to sensory and motor systems. The strategy can best be understood through an example.

Unilateral destruction of the superior colliculus in the developing hamster results in a redirection of the optic axons that would normally innervate the damaged side into the opposite colliculus (Schneider, 1973; Schneider & Jhaveri, 1974). If one simultaneously removes the contralateral eye, which is the normal source of retinal innervation of the surviving colliculus, the recrossing pathway is enhanced. The result of this double lesion is that virtually all retinotectal projections that survive are abnormal with regard to laterality (Schneider & Jhaveri, 1974). The nature of the postlesion reorganization is well characterized anatomically, fulfilling Criterion 1. The retinotectal system is known to play an important role in visual orientation, and accurate orientation depends on the orderly representation of visual space in the projection system, fulfilling Criterion 2. Finally, normal orientation depends on the topographic organization of the retinotectal projections. The connections between the eye and the wrong side of the brain would be expected to result not only in misdirection of visually guided behavior but also in responses toward the side opposite the actual site of stimulus presentation. This is exactly what is observed (Schneider & Jhaveri, 1974; So, Schneider, & Ayers, 1981). The key to applying the sensory–motor system strategy is an anticipated isomorphism between the reorganized circuitry and the resulting behavior. Connections to the wrong side result in responses to the wrong side.

Using this isomorphism criterion for the sensory–motor system strategy requires considerable prior knowledge about how the spatio-topic organization of a given system is expressed behaviorally and about how the remodeled circuit differs from the normal in terms of its spatio-topic organization. The approach has limited applicability because of the limited number of situations in which the assumption of isomorphism between the neural system and the behavior is reasonable. Examples that may be approached with the strategy include the dorsal root projection to the spinal cord that increases following deafferenting lesions and the cross-innervation that occurs in the corticospinal tract following unilateral motor-cortex lesions early in development. In the case of the increased dorsal root projections following hemisection or chronic unilateral dorsal rhizotomy, the assumption of isomorphism would predict an increased effect of sensory input on local cord reflexes. This is exactly what is observed

(Goldberger & Murray, 1974; Murray & Goldberger, 1974). In the motor system, unilateral lesions in developing animals induce the formation of an ipsilateral corticospinal tract. The surviving cortex thus form bilateral projections to the cord, whereas its normal projection is predominantly unilateral (Castro, 1975). With an assumption of isomorphism, any behavioral consequences of this bilateral projection would be expected to result in bilaterally symmetrical movements of the affected musculature. This expectation would be adjusted if the topographic specificity of the aberrant ipsilateral corticospinal tract did not match the normal, or if there was a cortical reorganization such that cells which project abnormally were activated independently of cells which project normally. In this regard, there are interesting examples from the clinical literature of mirror movements in patients who have suffered unilateral damage to the motor cortex in childhood (Woods & Teuber, 1978).

In all of these examples the behaviors predicted are abnormal variants of normal behaviors mediated by the structure in question. The key to identifying these behaviors as being related to specific types of anatomical change is the isomorphism between the remodeling and the behavior. It is worth emphasizing that the identification of the behavior is based on abnormality. As a consequence, this approach is not appropriate for detecting normal behavior that might be mediated by aberrant circuits. For example, if the sort of sequential cross-innervation in Figure 2 did contribute to normal throughput, and if these two afferent projections could together mediate some normal behavior, the isomorphism criterion would fail to identify those behaviors as being due to the remodeled circuitry. Furthermore, the isomorphism criterion will be entirely inappropriate for evaluating situations that involve *functional reorganization* (Kennard, 1938), in which animals make use of systems that are not normally used for a particular behavior. For example, if some circuit other than the surviving collicular circuitry were used for visual orientation after unilateral collicular damage, then a strategy that depended on the assumption that remodeling in the colliculus would affect visual orientation in a predictable fashion would fail.

Despite the preceding limitations, the sensory–motor system strategy with its requirement for isomorphism between brain and behavior is applicable to several kinds of reorganization that are particularly prominent after injury in developing animals. We have noted the frequent construction of aberrant crossing pathways following lesions in developing animals. These are particularly well suited to analysis by the sensory–motor system strategy as here defined, because responses are expected that are appropriate for the system but inappropriate with regard to laterality. While abnormal, some of these behavioral capacities could be adaptive (as noted previously in the case of misconnected retinotectal pathways.) However, unless the behaviors are abnormal variants of normal behaviors, that is, unless there is some element of abnormality in them, they will not be detected. Rather one will simply detect greater functional improvement in animals with lesions early in development. Establishing a role for this sort of neuronal reorganizational event would be impossible in the absence of some supplemental criteria (for a discussion of some ways to avoid this limitation, see Steward, 1982).

Conclusions

The neurological sequellae- and sensory–motor system strategies allow one to propose relations between neural and behavioral events. Great care must be taken, however, in the interpretation of these relations. If, for example, the evidence suggests that anatomical reorganization contributes to behavioral recovery, does this mean that the anatomical reorganization *mediates* the recovery? Another way to phrase the question is What amount of the behavioral variability can be accounted for by the anatomical change? Our present knowledge about brain–behavior relationships prohibits an answer to this type of question, particularly for complex behaviors. For example, in the case of the recovery of maze performance following unilateral entorhinal-cortex lesions in adult rats, behavioral recovery proceeds in parallel with the reinnervation—if considered on a population basis. On an individual-animal basis, however, this is certainly not the case. Some animals can perform flawlessly in the behavioral tasks that are used after unilateral damage to the entorhinal cortex; other animals exhibit persistent deficits. It is only on a population basis that the temporally well-defined recovery is observed. Although there may be some difference in the extent of the crossed projection from one entorhinal cortex to the contralateral side, this is certainly not sufficient to account for the variability.

There are at least two ways of interpreting this kind of variability. First, the behavior and the anatomical change may in fact not be related; the correlation may be spurious and due to some other event that occurs following the lesions. The other possibility is that the neural events (i.e., reorganization of pathways) only *contribute* to the recovery and indeed may contribute a relatively small amount to the total behavioral variance. Unless it is possible to eliminate the role of all other factors in performance, variability is inevitable. This does not mean that the variability is experimental. Indeed, after several years of attempting to revise our behavioral testing situation to improve the variability, we now believe that the variability is meaningful and indicates that numerous factors can contribute to the animals' performance in any task. In the day-to-day performance in a given behavorial task, the contribution of anatomical reorganization following lesions may be considerable or insignificant, depending on the relative contribution of other factors.

As brain scientists, these types of uncertainty should not disturb or even surprise us. If centuries of research have told us anything, it is that very rarely if at all is there a tight relationship between the brain and any given behavior. If one-to-one relationships between brain and behavior cannot be expected in intact animals, it is certainly not reasonable to expect similar relationships in animals responding to brain injury.

References

Castro, A. J. (1975). Ipsilateral corticospinal projections after large lesions of the cerebral hemisphere in neonatal rats. *Experimental Neurology, 46,* 1–8.

Gall, C., & Lynch, G. (1978). Rapid axon sprouting in the neonatal rat hippocampus. *Brain Research, 153,* 357–362.

Goldberger, M. E. (1974). Recovery of movement after CNS lesions in monkeys. In D. G. Stein, J. J. Rosen, & N. Butters (Eds.), *Plasticity and recovery of function in the central nervous system* (pp. 265–338). New York: Academic Press.

Goldberger, M. E., & Murray, M. (1974) Restitution of function and collateral sprouting in the cat spinal cord: the deafferented animal. *Journal of Comparative Neurology, 158,* 37–54.

Kennard, M. A. (1938). Reorganization of motor function in the cerebral cortex of monkeys deprived of motor and premotor areas in infancy. *Journal of Neurophysiology, 1,* 477–496.

Laurence, S., & Stein, D. G. (1978). Recovery after brain damage and the concept of localization of function. In: S. Finger (Ed.) *Recovery from Brain Damage.* 369–407. Plenum Press, New York.

Loesche, J., & Steward, O. (1977). Behavioral correlates of denervation and reinnervation of the hippocampal formation of the rat: Recovery of alternation performance following unilateral entorhinal cortex lesions. *Brain Research Bulletin, 2,* 31–39.

McCouch, G. P., Austin, G. M., Liu, C. N., & Liu, C. Y. (1958). Sprouting as a cause of spasticity. *Journal of Neurophysiology, 21,* 205–216.

Murray, M., & Goldberger, M. E. (1974). Restitution of function in the cat spinal cord: The partially hemisected animal. *Journal of Comparative Neurology, 158,* 19–36.

Reeves, T. M. (1983). Electrophysiological correlates of recovery from entorhinal lesions. Ph.D. thesis, Department of Psychology, Southern Illinois University (D. C. Smith advisor).

Schneider, G. E. (1973). Early lesions of superior colliculus: Factors affecting the formation of abnormal retinal projections. *Brain, Behavior and Evolution, 8,* 73–109.

Schneider, G. E. (1979). Is it really better to have your brain lesion early? A revision of the "Kennard Principle." *Neuropsychologia, 17,* 557–583.

Schneider, G. E., & Jhaveri, J. R. (1974). Neuroanatomical correlates of spared or altered function after brain lesions in the newborn hamster. In D. G. Stein, J. J. Rosen, & N. Butters (Eds.), *Plasticity and recovery of function in the central nervous system* (pp. 65–109). New York: Academic Press.

So, K. -F., Schneider, G. E., & Ayres, S. (1981). Lesions of the brachium of the superior colliculus in neonate hamsters: Correlation of anatomy with behavior. *Experimental Neurology, 72,* 379–400.

Steward, O. (1982). Assessing the functional significance of lesion-induced neuronal plasticity. *International Review of Neurobiology, 23,* 197–254.

Steward, O., Loesche, J., & Horton, W. C. (1977). Behavioral correlates of denervation and reinnervation of the hippocampal formation of the rat: open field activity and cue utilization following bilateral entorhinal cortex lesions. *Brain Research Bulletin, 2,* 41–48.

Steward, O., & Vinsant, S. L. (1983). The process of reinnervation in the dentate gyrus of the adult rat: a quantitative electron microscopic analysis of terminal proliferation and reactive synaptogenesis. *Journal of Comparative Neurology, 214,* 370–386.

von Monakow, C. (1910). *Neue Gesichtspunkte in der Frage nach der Lokalisation im Grosshirm* (pp. 1–21). Wiesbaden: Bergman.

von Monakow, C. (1969). Diaschisis. In K. Pribram (Ed.), *Mood, states, and mind.* Baltimore, MD: Penguine Books.

Woods, B. T., & Teuber, H. -L. (1978). Mirror movements after childhood hemiparesis. *Neurology, 28,* 1152–1158.

II

Animal Models of Pathological States

4

Early Brain Damage due to Hypoxia

Marcus W. van Hof and E. M. W. Wildervanck de Blécourt

Survival during Hypoxia

The notion that immature brains are more resistant to hypoxia than mature ones presumably emerged from the vacuum-pump experiments that Robert Boyle carried out in the middle of the seventeenth century. Among many other things, he discovered that newborn cats survive much longer under low air pressure than do adults (Frank, 1980). However, this experiment does not prove that the brain of the newborn animal has a relatively high resistance to hypoxia: a greater resistance of the heart could have the same effect (Dawes, Mott, & Shelley, 1959; Dawes, Mott, Shelley, & Stafford, 1963).

The oldest quantitative experiments showing that the brain of immature animals are genuinely more resistant to hypoxia were done by Legallois (1812) during the French Revolution. In *Experiences sur le principe de la vie* [Experiences regarding the principle of life] he

Copyright © 1984 by Academic Press, Inc.
All rights of reproduction in any form reserved.

ISBN 0-12-052901-7

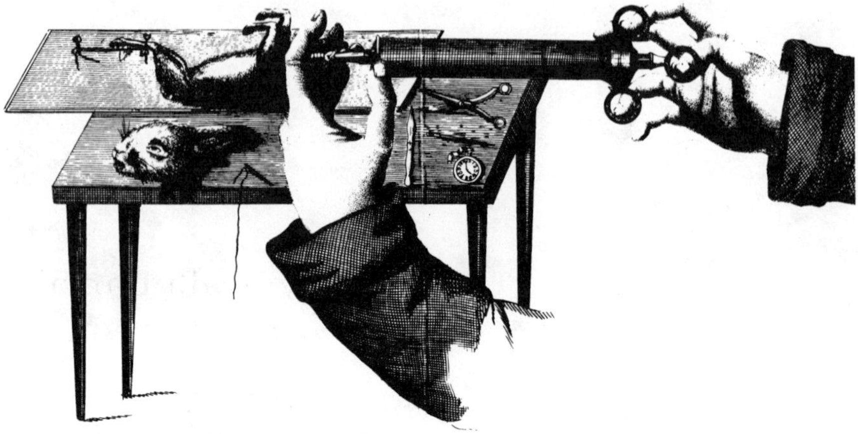

Figure 1. Illustration from LeGallois *Experience sur le principe de la vie* (1812).

described part of his work on the localization of the respiratory center. He discovered that after decapitation the heart continues to beat for a long time, provided that the lungs are artificially ventilated (Figure 1). In addition, he found that the head continues to make gasping movements for some time. By cutting the brainstem systematically Legallois managed to localize the respiratory center. The data from his table of the duration of gasping as a function of age are plotted in Figure 2.

Cerebral hypoxia was elicited in three different ways: submersion, opening of the thorax, and removal of the heart. In Figure 2 the duration of gasping is plotted as a function of the age of the rabbits. As the graph shows, the results were almost the same with all three methods. These data show that the neurons of the respiratory center are genuinely more resistant to hypoxia in immature rabbits than in adults. The postnatal development of the rabbit has been studied in various ways. The greatest increase of brainweight takes place 10 days before birth and continues until 5 days after birth (Harel, Watanabe, Linke, & Schain, 1972). Myelination begins at Day 10 and continues until the end of the third month. The postnatal development of the visual system has been studied in the developing rabbit by Chow and his collaborators. Spear, Chow, Masland, and Murphy (1972) recorded from units in the superior colliculus in the developing rabbit. Responses to light were not seen prior to 6 days of age. From 6 days on, there was a progressive increase in cells driven by light. All of the receptive-field types described in the adult animal

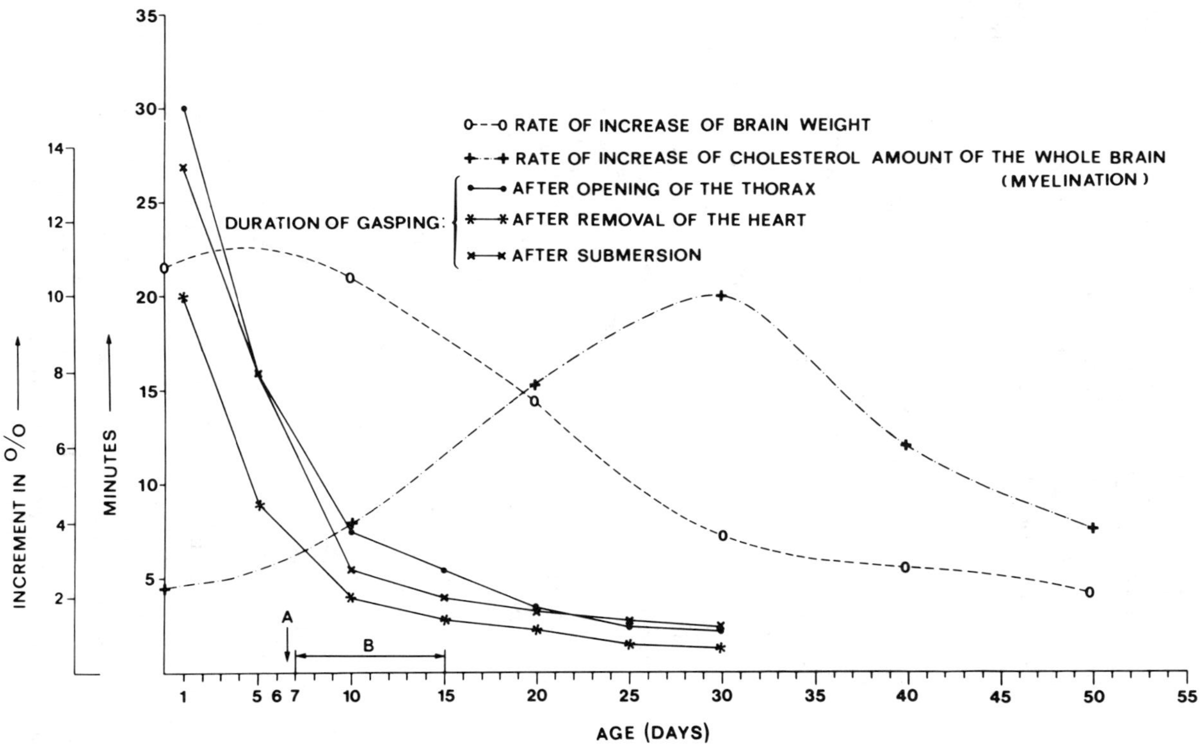

Figure 2. Mean duration of gasping in minutes after opening of the thorax, after removal of the heart, and after submersion plotted as a function of age in rabbits. (A) beginning of maturation of single units in the rabbit's visual system. (B) development of elementary motor behavior in the rabbit. For comparison with brain maturation, the rate of increase of brain weight and of amount of cholesterol of the whole brain (both measured as percentages of the adult value) are plotted. The cholesterol amount is a measure for the myelination of the brain.

could be identified by 9 days of age. In the visual cortex very few responses were found at Days 5–8, but a sharp increase during Days 9–10 followed. The development of the visual cortex was found to be markedly slower than that of the superior colliculus. In the visual cortex it was not until 18 days after birth that all adult receptive-field types could be found. Because the rabbit's retina is not well developed at birth, the question arises whether one is actually recording from an immature retina via a mature central system. This has been shown to be very unlikely (Chow, Masland, & Stewart, 1971; Grobstein, Chow, Spear, & Mathers, 1973; Mathers, Chow, Spear, & Grobstein, 1974; Rapisardi, Chow, & Mathers, 1975). Electrical stimulation of the optic nerve was found to elicit single-unit responses in the geniculate body as early as Day 2, but the responses were immature. None of the units recorded from this early age responded to receptive-field stimuli presented at rates higher than one every 10 seconds.

The rabbit motor system is also very immature during the first week after birth. Swimming behavior develops during the second week after birth (Stuurman & Van Hof, 1979). Because rabbits can swim after removal of the cortex it seems obvious that the development is an expression of subcortical maturation. This coincides with the development of the air-righting reflex (Schönfelder, 1978; Schönfelder, Asmussen, & Schaaf, 1977; Schönfelder & Schwartze, 1970).

All these findings can be summarized as follows: The relatively long duration of gasping after circulatory arrest can be found in that stage of postnatal development in which the growth rate of the brain is maximal, in which myelination has not yet started, and in which the motor system and the visual system are not yet functioning.

The great resistance to hypoxia is probably the reason that von Gudden (1886) was able to do large cerebral ablation experiments under undoubtedly very primitive circumstances. Stuurman, van Hof, and Hobbelen (1981) noted that newborn rabbits can stand anesthesia remarkably well and rarely die after ablation of the occipital lobe. However, lack of care by the doe causes the death of many animals a few days later.

As is the case with many scientific discoveries, the work of Legallois was either forgotten or did not cross language barriers. In 1929, Reiss and Haurowitz, working in Vienna, rediscovered the great resistance of newborn animals to hypoxia. In a study on mice they found that it took a relatively long time to kill newborn mice with CO or CO_2 or with neckclamping. In their brief article, the authors were convinced that they had made a fundamental discovery, one that had never been described before. Kabat (1940) noted that the brain of the young dog is also much more resistant to arrest of its circulation than that of the adult animal. Of particular interest is a comparative study by Fazekas, Alexander, and Himwich (1941) in rats, rabbits, cats, dogs and guinea pigs. The relatively great tolerance of the newborn was confirmed. However, the resistance was found to depend on the degree of physiological maturity at the time of birth. Newborn rats, which are without hair and teeth, survived for approximately 1 hour in pure nitrogen. On the other hand, the relatively mature newborn guinea pig survived for only 7 minutes under the same condition.

Many authors have described mechanisms by which the newborn animal would be able to survive hypoxia much longer than the adult. These proposed mechanisms have some important factors in common. First, they all point to the fact that the cerebral metabolism is much lower in the newborn than in the adult. The second important thing is that the newborn has more readily available glycogen sources: By breaking down this glycogen to glucose and then metabolizing the glucose anaerobically by forming lactic acid, the newborn would have a greater anaerobic energy supply on which to live during hypoxia than would the adult (Himwich, Bernstein, Herrlich, Chester, & Fazekas, 1942; Vannucci & Vannucci, 1980).

Although the preceding experiments show that neurons in the respiratory center of partially developed nervous systems have a relatively large tolerance to hypoxia, this does not mean that other nerve cells that become involved later in the development of other functions are not damaged by hypoxia. Theoretically, such immature cells could even be more susceptible to brain hypoxia.

Chronic Effects of Hypoxia

In 1861 the founder of the Royal Orthopaedic Hospital in London, W. J. Little (1861), gave a lecture for the Obstetrical Society of London entitled "On the influence of abnormal parturition, difficult labour, premature birth, and asphyxia neonatorum on the mental and physical condition of the child, especially in relation to deformities." In the minutes of the meeting we read that the "author introduced his subject by stating that pathology had gradually taught that the foetus in utero was subject to diseases similar to those which affect the economy at later periods of existence, and that this was particularly true as regards deformities." He said the object of his communication was "to show that the act of birth did occasionally imprint upon the nervous and muscular systems of the nascent organism very serious and peculiar evils. . . . Nearly twenty years ago the author had shown that premature birth, difficult labours, mechanical injuries during parturition to head and neck where life had been saved, and convulsions following the act of birth, were apt to be succeeded by a determinate affection of the limbs of the child," which he then designated "spastic rigidity from asphyxia neonatorum. . . . Medical writers," he continued, "seemed unaware that abnormal parturition, besides ending in death or recovery of the child, had another termination, namely, in other diseases." The discussion after the presentation is interesting in several ways. First of all, it becomes clear that the obstetricians of those days were unaware of the possibility of long-term effects of early asphyxiation. A certain Dr. Barnes said "that although not able from his own observations, to produce any facts in confirmation or negation of Dr. Little's theory, this might be due to his not having studied the subsequent history of children in connection with the phenomena attending their birth." "The difficulty there appeared to be in discussing this excellent paper, arose no doubt from the entire novelty and originality of the subject. Dr. Little had brought before the obstetric world new matter for inquiry of the highest interest." A Dr. Smith remarked that "he thought dentition the great source of paraplegia and hemiplegia in young children."

Interestingly, contrary to the obstetricians of the nineteenth century, laymen of the early seventeenth century were probably aware of possible long-term effects of difficult labor.

At the end of the discussion of the meeting of the Obstetrical Society, Little mentioned that "not having found any reference to the affections consequent on abnormal and premature parturition in the works of English medical writers, he had referred with some confidence, to Shakespeare, to ascertain whether any notions on the subject were contained in his works." "He said the description of the physical character of Richard III was exactly that of an individual affected with one kind of deformity originating at birth." He was convinced Shakespeare had drawn the picture from such an individual. Assuming that Little's interpretation is correct, it is surprising that the notion of long-term effects of early brain hypoxia disappeared after Shakespeare's time.

Experiments on chronic effects of early hypoxia have been carried out in a number of species. Of the common laboratory animals, the guinea pig has longest been used (Windle & Becker, 1943).

Fetuses were delivered through a midline incision, and the umbilical cord was compressed until the fetal heart had slowed or could no longer be palpated. The animals were resuscitated if necessary. All animals showed neurological symptoms such as motor weakness, decerebrate states, convulsions, tremor, and ataxia. The symptoms lasted for a few hours to more than a month. The animals that had been made anoxic were less irritable, less active, more docile, and showed little reaction to changes in the environment. They were quiet when picked up and did not try to escape when released. In a simple maze in which an alternation problem had to be learned in order to escape from electrical shock and reach a food reward, the asphyxiated animals made more errors. Considerable morphological abnormalities were found in histological studies of the brain (Windle, Becker, & Weil, 1944).

Windle was also the first to do similar experiments on the rhesus monkey. A review of his studies was published in 1968. The fetuses in near-term rhesus monkeys were delivered by caesarean section under local anesthesia. Asphyxia was elicited by clamping the umbilical cord and covering the head with a rubber bag. Later in life these animals developed severe motor disturbances. In learning experiments Sechzer (1969) found that asphyxiated monkeys at ages of 8–10 years were extremely handicapped in delayed-response learning.

Compared with the ubiquity of the laboratory rat, the number of papers on the chronic effects of early hypoxia in this species is relatively small. Several procedures have been followed and three examples are given here. Meier and Bunch (1950) studied learning and memory in rats that had been exposed to a condition of less than 3% oxygen for a period of 30 minutes within 3 hours after birth. When the animals were between 75 and 100 days of age, they were trained on a left turn or right turn position habit in a water T-maze. The only significant difference found between anoxic and normal animals was in reversal learning. The anoxic animals were inferior in immediate reversal, but they reversed the habit more quickly than the controls after an interval of 14 days. McCullough and Blackman (1976) exposed pregnant rats to an oxygen-depleted atmosphere in 2-hour daily sessions over the last 14 days of pregnancy. The progeny of these rats were later compared to normal control animals. In the Hebb–Williams maze, impairment of performance in the difficult problems was seen. In a paper on hyperactivity in rats following postnatal hypoxia (Speiser, Korczyn, Tepletzky, & Gitter, 1983), it was found that rats exposed to severe hypoxia within 24 hours following birth showed augmented motor activity in ambulation, sniffing, and rearing activities in an open field. Activity was significantly increased at 10 days of age, was maximal from 20 to 25 days, and returned to normal values at around 6 weeks of age.

To the best of our knowledge chronic effects of early hypoxia have never been studied in the rabbit.

The results obtained in rats give the impression that the chronic effects found in this species are less robust than those found in the guinea pig and the rhesus monkey. Either the oxygen-deprivation procedures followed in rat experiments were less drastic or the newborn guinea pig and monkey are more sensitive to hypoxia. There are no quantitative data, such as blood-oxygen measurements, that could indicate between these possibilities.

Relevance to Human Pathology

What do these experiments teach us about human pathology? This question is especially important for studies in pharmacological brain protection.

Pharmacological experiments are usually done in adult animals (Wauquier, Clincke, Ashton, & Van Reempts, 1981), but it is likely that the developing brain will receive attention in this respect. Therefore, the search for suitable animal models is of great importance. Survival during low oxygen pressure is a common method in pharmacological study (Wauquier *et al.* 1.c.). If a compound were found that shifted the duration of gasping curve plotted in Figure 2 to the right, it could only be concluded that the neurons of the respiratory center were protected. However, the experiment would not allow any conclusions to be drawn with respect to the immature neurons. Theoretically, it could well be that though such a drug enabled an animal to withstand an otherwise lethal period of low oxygen pressure, the long-term effects due to damage to immature neurons were even more severe. Therefore, experiments on the chronic effects, rather than on acute survival, seem more relevant.

As described before, chronic effects have been studied in various species. At first sight monkeys seem the most suitable animals. But with their decreasing availability, it is important to see whether there is a firm basis for this assumption.

First, there is no evidence that the neuronal elements in, for instance, a rat differ essentially from those in a human. The real difference is in the neuronal network and the number of neuronal ele-

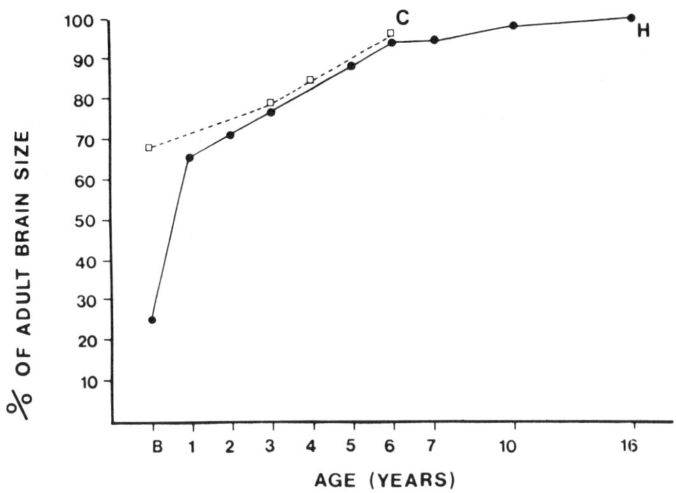

Figure 3. Percentage of adult brain weight plotted against age in the chimpanzee (C) and human (H).

ments. Rats and rabbits, for instance, do not show a hemiparesis after a unilateral cortical lesion, whereas animals with more complex nervous systems do. The rhesus monkey may be more suitable for copying human phenomenology. This by no means precludes the possibility that behavioral studies in lower mammals, provided that tests are used that fit into the animal's behavioral repertoire, can give us valuable information on the effects of early hypoxia on the structures involved in, for instance, learning and memory.

The assumption that the development of the brain of a monkey resembles that of a human is less well founded than one would intuitively assume. Even the brain of a newborn ape differs considerably from that in a human baby. This is shown in Figure 3. The data given in this graph were collected by I. S. Russell, University College London. The brain weight of the adult human is about three times that of an adult chimpanzee. However, the chimpanzee's brain at birth has already reached 65–70% of its adult weight, whereas this percentage is in on the order of 25% at human birth. In humans, rapid growth takes place during the first year.

This and the lack of evidence for essential differences between the neuronal elements of various mammalian species diminish support for the popular view that studies on long-term effects in simple laboratory animals are inferior to those obtained in monkeys.

In this review no attempt has been made to give a complete overview of the literature on this subject. Only typical examples of classes of experiments were given for support of the view that behavioral studies on chronic effects of early hypoxia in common laboratory animals deserve more attention than they have received.

Acknowledgment

The authors are greatly indebted to I. S. Russell, London for his data on the development of the brain in chimpanzees and humans.

References

Chow, K. L., Masland, R. H., & Stewart, D. L. (1971). Receptive field characteristics of striate cortical neurons in the rabbit. *Brain Research, 33,* 337–352.

Dawes, G. S., Mott, J. C., & Shelley, H. J. (1959). The importance of cardiac glycogen for the maintenance of life in foetal lambs and new-born animals during anoxia. *Journal of Physiology, 146,* 516–538.

Dawes, G. S., Mott, J. C., Shelley, H. J., & Stafford, A. (1963). The prolongation of survival time in asphyxiated immature foetal lambs. *Journal of Physiology, 168,* 43–64.

Fazekas, J. F., Alexander, F. A. D., & Himwich, H. E. (1941). Tolerance of the newborn to anoxia. *American Journal of Physiology, 134,* 281–287.

Frank, R. G., Jr. (1980). Boyle and vacuumpump experiments on respiration—Oxford, 1659. *Harvey and the Oxford Physiologists,* University of California Press.

Grobstein, P., Chow, K. L., Spear, P. D., & Mathers, L. H. (1973). Development of rabbit visual cortex: late appearance of a class of receptive fields. *Science, 180,* 1185–1187.

Harel, S., Watanabe, K., Linke, J., & Schain, R. J. (1972). Growth and development of the rabbit brain. *Biology of the Neonate, 21,* 381–399.

Himwich, H. E., Bernstein, A. O., Herrlich, H., Chester, A., & Fazekas, J. F. (1942). Mechanisms for the maintenance of life in the newborn during anoxia. *American Journal of Physiology, 135,* 387–391.

Kabat, H. (1940). The greater resistance of very young animals to arrest of the brain-circulation. *American Journal of Physiology, 130,* 588–599.

Legallois, M. (1812). *Expérience sur le principe de la vie,* Paris: Hautel.

Little, W. J. (1861). On the influence of abnormal parturition, difficult labour, premature birth, and asphyxia neonatorum on the mental and physical condition of the child, especially in relation to deformities. *The Lancet, 2,* 378–380.

McCullough, M. L., & Blackman, D. E. (1976). The behavioural effects of prenatal hypoxia in rats. *Developmental Psychobiology, 9(4),* 335–342.

Mathers, L. H., Chow, K. L., Spear, P. D., & Grobstein, P. (1974). Ontogenesis of receptive fields in the rabbit striate cortex. *Experimental Brain Research, 19,* 20–35.

Meier, G. W., & Bunch, M. E. (1950). The effects of natal anoxia upon learning and memory at maturity. *Journal of Comparative and Physiological Psychology, 43,* 436–441.

Rapisardi, S. C., Chow, K. L., & Mathers, L. H. (1975). Ontogenesis of receptive field characteristics in the dorsal lateral geniculate nucleus of the rabbit. *Experimental Brain Research, 22,* 295–305.

Reiss, M., & Haurowitz, F. (1929). Ueber das verhalten junger und alter tiere bei erstickung. *Klinische Wochenschrift, 1,* 743–744.

Schönfelder, J. (1978). The postnatal development of rabbit's air-righting reflex. *Agressologie, 19,* A, 5–6.

Schönfelder, J., Asmussen, G., & Schaaf, P. (1977). Zur postnatalen ontogenese der äusseren augenmuskeln des kaninchens. *Verhandlungen der Anatomischen Gesellschaft, 71,* 1187–1191.

Schönfelder, J., & Schwartze, P. (1970). Die entwicklung des fallumkehr reflexes in der ontogenese des kaninchens. *Acta Biologica Med. Ger., 25,* 109–114.

Sechzer, J. A. (1969). Memory deficit in monkeys brain damaged by asphyxia neonatorum. *Experimental Neurology, 24,* 497–507.

Spear, P. D., Chow, K. L., Masland, R. H., & Murphy, E. H. (1972). Ontogenesis of receptive field characteristics of superior colliculus neurons in the rabbit. *Brain Research, 45,* 67–86.

Speiser, Z., Korczyn, A. D., Teplitzky, D., & Gitter, S. (1983). Hyperactivity in rats following postnatal anoxia. *Behavioural Brain Research, 7,* 379–382.

Stuurman, P. M., & van Hof, M. W. (1979). The postnatal development of swimming behaviour in the rabbit. *Physiology and Behaviour, 23,* 185–186.

Stuurman, P. M., van Hof, M. W., & Hobbelen, J. F. (1981). Behavioural effects of early and late unilateral ablation of the occipital lobe in the rabbit. In M. W. van Hof & G. Mohn (Eds.) *Functional recovery from brain damage,* North-Holland: Elsevier, pp. 121–129.

Vannucci, S. J., & Vannucci, R. C. (1980). Glycogen metabolism in neonatal rat brain during anoxia and recovery. *Journal of Neurochemistry, 34*(5), 1100–1105.

Von Gudden, B. (1886). Ueber die Frage der Lokalisation der Funktionen der Grosshirnrinde. *Allgemeine Zeitschrift für Psychiatrie und Grensgebiete, 42,* 478–499.

Wauquier, A., Clincke, B., Ashton, D., & van Reempts, J. (1981). Considerations on models and treatment of brain hypoxia. In M. W. van Hof & G. Mohn (Eds.), *Functional recovery from brain damage,* North-Holland: Elsevier, pp. 95–114.

Windle, W. F. (1968). Brain damage at birth. *Journal of the American Medical Association, 206*(9), 1967–1972.

Windle, W. F., & Becker, R. F. (1943). Asphyxia neonatorum. *American Journal of Obstetrics and Gynaecology, 45*(2), 183–199.

Windle, W. F., Becker, R. F., & Weil, A. (1944). Alterations in brain structure after asphyxiation at birth. *Journal of Neuropathology and Experimental Neurology, 3,* 224–238.

5

The Ontogeny of Locomotor Behavior following Lesions of Brain Dopamine Neuronal Projections in the Neonatal Rat

Thomas G. Heffner,
Lewis S. Seiden,
and Alfred Heller

Introduction

Brain neurons that contain the neurotransmitter dopamine (DA) influence a variety of behaviors in mammals (Seiden & Dykstra, 1977). The role of central DA neurons in the control of behavior in adult animals has been assessed by determining the behavioral effects of drugs, neurotoxins, or brain lesions that alter central DA neurotransmission. As an approach to studying the functional role of central DA neurons in developing animals, a number of investigators have examined the effects on behavioral development of intraventricular (ivt.) injections of 6-hydroxydopamine (6-HDA), a neu-

Copyright © 1984 by Academic Press, Inc.
All rights of reproduction in any form reserved.
ISBN 0-12-052901-7

rotoxin that can be used selectively to deplete brain DA (Breese & Traylor, 1970; Stricker & Zigmond, 1974). Depletion of brain DA by ivt. 6-HDA in adult animals causes few permanent alterations in locomotor function (Stricker & Zigmond, 1974; Zigmond & Stricker, 1974).

In contrast, DA-depleting 6-HDA injections in neonatal rats results in increased locomotor activity during subsequent development (Shaywitz, Yager, & Klopper, 1976; Erinoff, MacPhail, Heller, & Seiden, 1979). These results have suggested that central DA neurons have a special function in the ontogeny of locomotor behavior. This chapter describes the effect of brain DA depletion in neonatal rats on locomotor development, locomotor responses to psychoactive drugs, and the ability to acquire an operant response. These studies not only describe the consequences for behavioral development of neurochemically-defined brain lesions during early life, but may also provide information concerning the role of central DA neurons in the normal ontogeny of behavior.

Brain Dopamine and Locomotion

Anatomical studies have described several major DA neuronal projections in the mammalian brain (i.e., Moore & Bloom, 1978). Among these, the nigrostriatal and mesocortical projections have been most closely linked to motor function. Nigrostriatal DA neurons arise bilaterally in the substantia nigra of the midbrain and send axons to terminate primarily in the caudate putamen of the telencephalon. Brain lesions that destroy nigrostriatal DA neurons produce deficits in sensory–motor integration in animals (Marshall, Richardson, & Teitelbaum, 1974). Diseases that involve impairments in motor function in man, such as Parkinson's disease, Huntington's chorea and tardive dyskinesia, are believed to stem in part from impairment of nigrostriatal DA systems (Lloyd & Hornykiewicz, 1978; Tarsy & Baldessarini, 1977). Mesocortical DA neurons arise predominantly from more medial aspects of the midbrain ventral tegmentum and send axons to a variety of telencephalic areas, including the frontal cortex, septum, and nucleus accumbens. The release of DA from mesocortical neurons is believed to facilitate locomotion (Creese & Iversen, 1973; Kelly, 1977).

The development of brain catecholamines (CA) and the development of locomotor function correspond in time. The levels of CA in the rat brain increase rapidly during the first 2 weeks of life (Coyle, 1976). This period is characterized by similarly rapid increases in

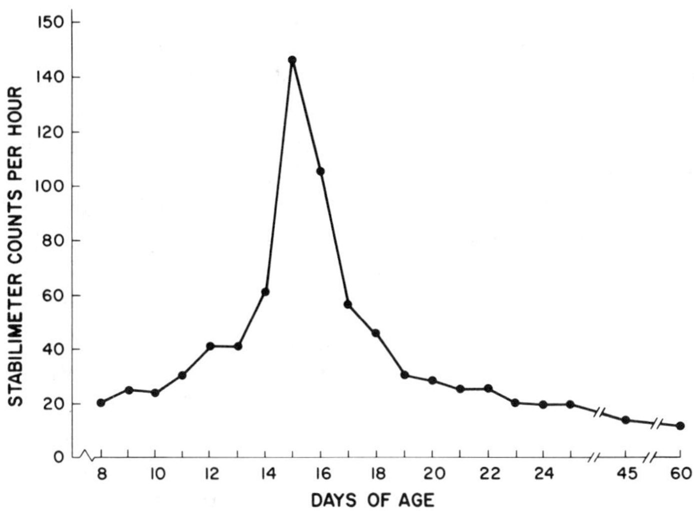

Figure 1. Development of locomotor activity in normal rats. Locomotion was determined for 1 hour daily.

neurochemical indexes of CA function, including active neuronal uptake of CA (Coyle, 1976), levels of CA synthesizing and degradative enzymes (Porcher & Heller, 1972), and CA receptor mediated events (Coyle, 1976; Pardo, Creese, Burt, & Snyder, 1977). Locomotor behavior also displays a characteristic developmental pattern in the rat (Figure 1). Limited locomotion is seen during the first week of life. During the end of the second week of life, however, a dramatic increase in locomotion occurs. Following this peak in activity, locomotion normally declines towards the low levels seen in adulthood (Bolles & Woods, 1964; Campbell, Lytle, & Fibiger, 1969; Erinoff, MacPhail, Heller, & Seiden, 1979). Based on these parallel changes in brain CAs and locomotor behavior during early life, as well as the ability of amphetamines to increase locomotion during this time, Campbell, Lytle, & Fibiger (1969) proposed that the increase in locomotion seen during the end of the second week of life was due to the onset of functioning of central CA projections.

The Effect of Neonatal Brain Dopamine Depletion on Locomotor Activity

In order to further examine the role of brain CA projections in locomotor activity in the developing rat, brain CA neurons were destroyed in neonatal rats by ivt. administration of 6-HDA. The 6-HDA was administered to rats at 3 and 6 days of age, following systemic injections of desmethylimipramine (DMI), a drug that prevents the uptake of 6-HDA by central norepinephrine (NE) neurons (Breese & Traylor, 1970). Control rats received ivt. injections of the 6-HDA vehicle solution at 3 and 6 days of age following DMI pretreatment. Locomotion was measured for 1 hour daily, during the light cycle with use of stabilimeter cages. These rectangular wire mesh cages tilt across central axles when the midline of the floor is crossed, resulting in the registration of an activity count.

Erinoff *et al.* (1979) showed that a DMI and 6-HDA (100 μg, ivt.) treatment given at 3 and 6 days of age produced large decreases in DA in the corpus striatum (−90%), with only minimal effects on brain NE, as determined when the rats reached adulthood. Brain DA depletion by 6-HDA in neonatal rats failed to alter locomotion prior to the normal peak in activity seen at 16 days of age. During the third and fourth weeks of life, locomotion declined in control rats; however, locomotion remained at high levels in 6-HDA-treated rats, and remained at higher-than-normal levels throughout the ninth week of life. These results suggest that loss of brain DA neurons results in locomotor hyperactivity in the developing rat. Additional studies revealed that DMI and 6-HDA treatment produced increased locomotor activity when administered on 11 and 14 days of age or on 20 and 23 days of age but not if DMI and 6-HDA were administered to adult rats (46 and 48 days of age). Each of these groups showed comparable losses of striatal DA (70–80%) with minimal effects on brain NE. These studies suggest that the age of the animal at the time of brain DA neuron destruction is an important determinant of the effect on locomotion.

The ability of brain DA depletion in neonatal rats to increase locomotion has also been reported by other investigators (Shaywitz *et al.*, 1976; Stoof, Dijkstra, & Hillegers, 1978). However, in these studies, the locomotor hyperactivity caused by neonatal 6-HDA administration was transient in nature, disappearing by the fourth or fifth week of life. In contrast, the studies conducted by Erinoff *et al.* (1979) demonstrated that the effects of 6-HDA on locomotion could be long lasting; increased locomotor activity was still evident during the ninth week of life. Other studies (Seiden & McGuire, unpublished observations), have revealed that locomotor hyperactivity following neonatal DMI and 6-HDA treatment was evident as long as 1 year after treatment.

Additional studies suggest that the duration of the locomotor effects of neonatal 6-HDA administration is related to the extent of

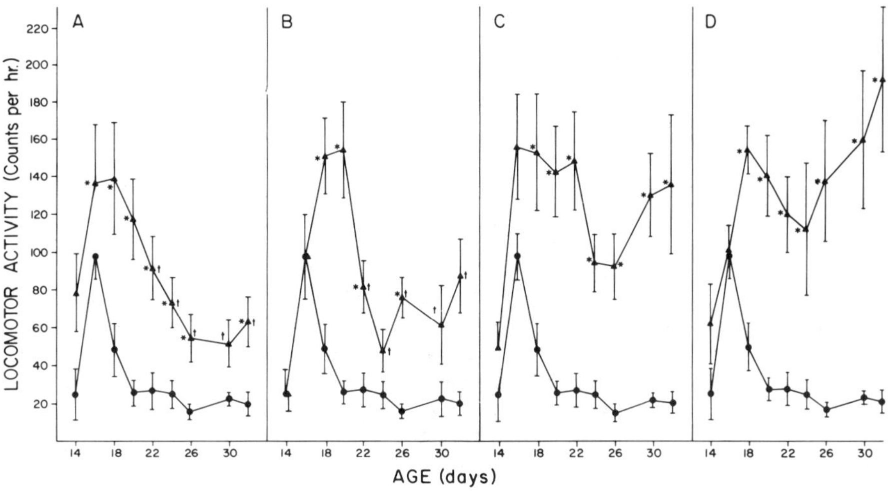

Figure 2. Locomotor activity of neonatal rats given DMI (i.p.) and 6-HDA (ivt.) at 3 and 6 days of age. a: ●, DMI-vehicle ($n = 7$); ▲, DMI-50 μg 6-HDA ($n = 7$); b: ●, DMI-vehicle ($n = 7$); ▲, DMI-70 μg 6-HDA ($n = 6$); c: ●, DMI-vehicle ($n = 7$); ▲, DMI-100 μg 6-HDA ($n = 8$); d: ●, DMI-vehicle ($n = 7$); ▲, DMI-200 μg 6-HDA ($n = 7$). Each point represents the mean ± S.E.M. $^*p < 0.05$, compared to DMI-vehicle group (t-test); $^\dagger p < 0.05$ compared to mean locomotor activity of same group at 18 days of age (Scheffe test). (From Miller *et al.*, 1981, reproduced with permission.)

brain DA depletion in neonatal life. We addressed the issue by administering different doses of 6-HDA to neonatal rats pretreated with DMI (Miller, Heffner, Kotake, & Seiden, 1981). For this experiment, groups of rats were given 6-HDA doses of 25, 35, 50, or 100 μg at both 3 and 6 days of age. During Days 18–32 of life, all groups displayed increased locomotor activity when compared to control rats treated with DMI plus the 6-HDA vehicle solution at 3 and 6 days of age (Figure 2). However, the magnitude of locomotor hyperactivity seen in the 6-HDA-treated groups during Days 26–32 of life was directly proportional to the dose of 6-HDA administered at 3 and 6 days of age. When retested in adulthood, only those rats treated with the highest 6-HDA dose (2 × 100 μg) in neonatal life continued to display locomotor hyperactivity (Figure 3). Determination of brain DA in rats given different doses of 6-HDA as neonates, revealed dose-related depletions of DA in the caudate putamen as well as in brain regions innervated by the mesocortical DA projection: amygdala, septum, frontal cortex, and olfactory tubercle (Table 1). Additional neurochemical determinations showed no effects of the neonatal DMI plus 6-HDA treatments on brain NE or serotonin. Treatment of adult rats

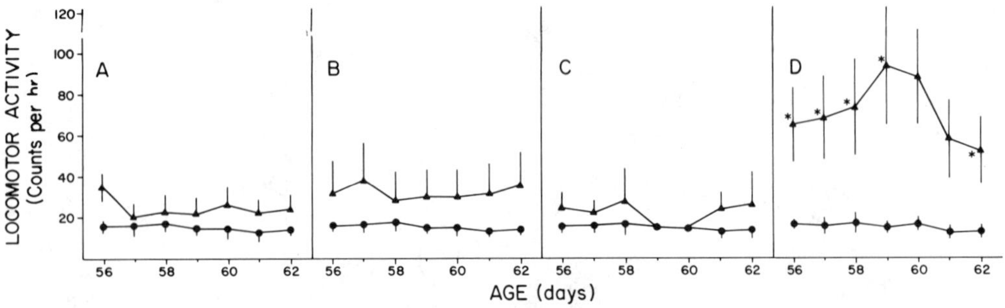

Figure 3. Locomotor activity of adult rats given DMI (i.p.) and 6-HDA (ivt.) at 3 and 6 days of age. a: ●, DMI-vehicle (n = 7); ▲, DMI-50 μg 6-HDA (n = 7); b: ●, DMI-vehicle (n = 7); ▲, DMI-70 μg 6-HDA (n = 6); c: ●, DMI-vehicle (n = 7); ▲, DMI-100 μg 6-HDA (n = 8); d: ●, DMI-vehicle (n = 7), ▲ = DMI-200 μg 6-HDA (n = 7). Each point represents the mean ± S.E.M. $^*p < 0.05$ compared to DMI-vehicle group (t-test). (From Miller *et al.*, 1981, reproduced with permission).

with doses of 6-HDA that produced depletions of DA in terminal fields of both nigrostriatal and mesocortical DA projections that were comparable to those seen in the neonatally treated groups (Table 1) failed to alter locomotor activity. The magnitude of locomotor hyperactivity seen in the neonatally treated rats during early life was found to be positively correlated with the extent of brain DA depletion produced (Miller *et al.*, 1981).

These results suggest that the magnitude and duration of locomotor hyperactivity produced by neonatal 6-HDA treatment are a function of the extent of loss of brain DA. Furthermore, the effect of brain DA depletion on locomotion appeared to be age dependent. In support of the notion that decreased DA activity during early life is associated with increased locomotor activity, additional studies demonstrate that temporary antagonism of central DA function induced by exposure to the DA receptor antagonist haloperidol during prenatal life or by administration of the DA synthesis inhibitor α-methyl-tyrosine during neonatal life, caused increased locomotion in neonatal rats (Miller & Seiden, 1983; O'Donnell & Seiden, 1980).

The studies with ivt. 6-HDA injections suggested that central DA neurons exert an important influence on the normal development of locomotion. In order to determine which central DA neuronal projection was involved in this role, we compared the effects on locomotor development of electrolytic lesions designed to destroy nigrostriatal or mesocortical DA neurons in neonatal rats (Heffner, Heller, Miller, Kotake, & Seiden, 1983). Nigrostriatal DA neurons were destroyed in

TABLE 1

Effect of Neonatal or Adult Treatment with DMI and 6-HDA on Dopamine Concentrations in Brain Regions[a]

Treatment	N	Caudate putamen	Amygdala	Septum	Frontal cortex	Olfactory tubercle
Neonatal						
DMI/vehicle	7	85.2 ± 7.8 —	0.82 ± 0.03 —	5.58 ± 0.02 —	0.54 ± 0.04 —	54.6 ± 2.0 —
DMI/50 μg 6-HDA	7	32.6 ± 9.9* —62	0.65 ± 0.09 —22	1.93 ± 0.76* —66	0.40 ± 0.07* —33	42.9 ± 6.1 —31
DMI/70 μg 6-HDA	6	14.5 ± 5.4* —83	0.56 ± 0.05* —32	1.11 ± 0.24* —80	0.31 ± 0.04* —48	45.6 ± 5.5* —35
DMI/100 μg 6-HDA	8	9.2 ± 2.3* —89	0.45 ± 0.04* —46	0.88 ± 0.25* —84	0.28 ± 0.04* —54	21.3 ± 2.8* —61
DMI/200 μg 6-HDA	7	1.7 ± 0.1* —98	0.26 ± 0.03* —68	0.52 ± 0.16* —91	0.19 ± 0.03* —68	11.8 ± 0.2* —78
Adult						
DMI/vehicle	7	100.6 ± 3.1 —	0.83 ± 0.05 —	5.40 ± 0.74 —	0.60 ± 0.05 —	68.8 ± 3.6 —
DMI/125 μg 6-HDA	8	42.2 ± 4.1* —58	0.50 ± 0.04* —40	0.69 ± 0.10* —88	0.46 ± 0.06* —33	29.3 ± 4.3* —57
DMI/200 μg 6-HDA	7	14.9 ± 5.1* —75	0.29 ± 0.04* —65	0.33 ± 0.05* —94	0.33 ± 0.03* —45	12.6 ± 2.0* —82
DMI/275 μg 6-HDA	8	5.5 ± 1.6* —95	0.25 ± 0.03* —70	0.33 ± 0.06* —94	0.26 ± 0.02* —57	7.1 ± 1.1* —90

[a]Values represent the mean ± S.E.M. in ng/mg protein. Values following dashes represent the decrease from respective DMI/Vehicle treatment group.

*$p < 0.05$, t-test.

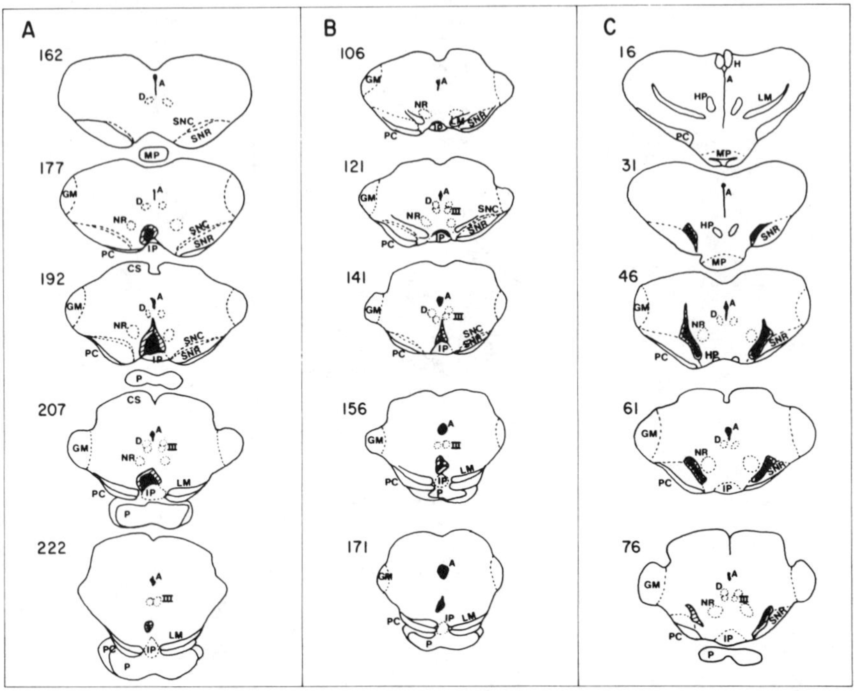

Figure 4. Projection tracings of brain sections showing brain lesions in representative animals from each of the three groups. Panel a: a typical lesion from the large VTA lesion group. Panel b: a typical lesion from the small VTA lesion group. Panel c: typical bilateral lesion from the SN group. Numbers at the upper left of each section denote the position within the serial sections, numbered rostrally to caudally. Darkened areas correspond to the cavity of the lesion; stippled areas correspond to the area around each lesion which was devoid of cells. A, Cerebral aqueduct; CS, Superior colliculus; D, Nucleus of Darkschewitz; GM, Medial geniculate body; HP, Habenulo-interpeduncular tract; IP, Interpeduncular nucleus; LM, Medial lemniscus; MP, Posterior mammillary nucleus; NR, Red Nucleus; P, Pons; PC, Cerebral peduncle; SNC, Substantia nigra pars compacta; SNR, Substantia nigra pars reticulata; III, Nucleus of the oculomotor nerve. Horizontal bars represent 1 mm. (From Heffner *et al.*, 1983; reproduced with permission).

4-day-old rats by bilateral electrolytic lesions in the substantia nigra (Figure 4c) using a specially designed head holder for the neonatal rat (Heller, Hutchens, Kirby, Karapas, & Fernandez, 1979). Mesocortical DA neurons were destroyed in two groups of 4-day-old rats by a single electrolytic lesion (produced by either 1 na or 0.5 na of current) in the medial ventral tegmental area (VTA, Figures 4a & 4b, respectively). Analysis of brain DA in adulthood revealed that the SN lesions caused a 68% reduction of DA in the corpus striatum but only mini-

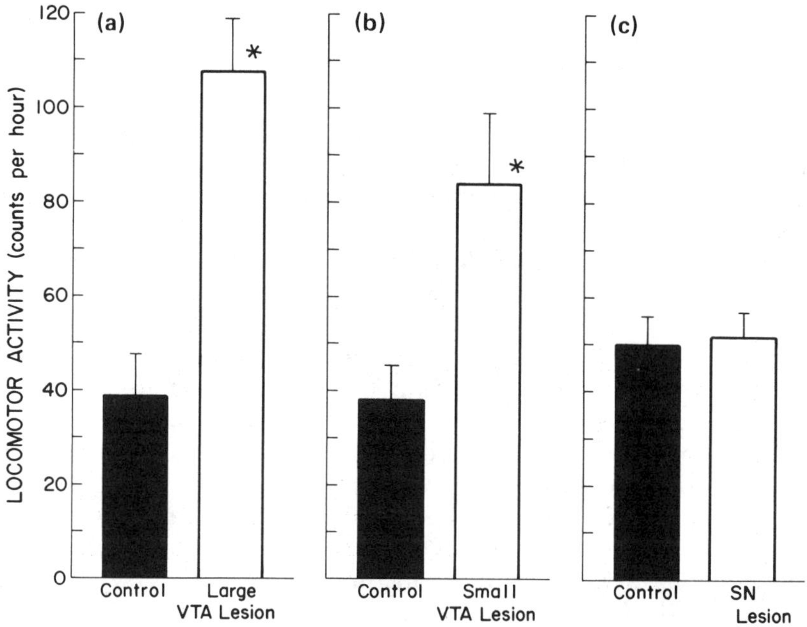

Figure 5. Locomotor activity of rats during 22–24 days of age following brain lesions at 4 days of age. a: open bar, large VTA lesion ($n = 9$); shaded bar, control ($n = 9$). b: open bar, small VTA lesion ($n = 10$); shaded bar, control ($n = 10$). c: open bar, SN lesion ($n = 12$); shaded bar, control ($n = 12$). Each bar represents the mean ± S.E.M. $^{*}p < 0.05$, compared to control group. (From Heffner *et al.*, 1983, reproduced with permission).

mal effects on DA levels in terminal fields of the mesocortical DA projection. In contrast, both the small and large VTA lesions caused 30–60% losses of DA in the septum, nucleus accumbens, and frontal cortex with minimal effects of DA in the corpus striatum. Locomotion was measured during Days 16–20 of life in SN- and VTA-lesioned groups and in sham-lesioned control rats. Rats with VTA lesions displayed locomotor hyperactivity during the third week of life (Figures 5a & 5b), whereas rats with SN lesions displayed normal levels of activity (Figure 5c). Although electrolytic lesions do not destroy DA neurons selectively, additional studies employing infusions of 6-HDA into the medial VTA of 4 day old rats demonstrated that the presumably more selective VTA neurotoxin infusions destroyed mesocortical DA neurons and caused locomotor hyperactivity in neonatal rats, similar to that seen with ivt. 6-HDA or electrolytic VTA lesions (Heller, Heffner, Kotake, Miller, & Seiden, 1981). Collectively, these results suggest that destruction of mesocortical DA neurons is responsible for the failure of neonatal rats with brain DA depletion to display the normal suppression of locomotion after the second week of life.

Previous results have suggested that mesocortical DA neurons exert important influences on locomotion in the adult rat (Kelly, 1977). LeMoal and colleagues have attributed the locomotor hyperactivity caused in adult rats by large bilateral lesions in the VTA to the destruction of mesocortical DA neurons (LeMoal, Stinus, Simon, Tassin, Thierry, Blanc, Glowinski, & Cardo, 1977; Tassin, Stinus, Simon, Blanc, Thierry, LeMoal, Cardo, & Glowinski, 1977). These authors have also demonstrated similar increases in locomotion in adult rats following infusions of 6-HDA into the VTA. It is therefore possible that mesocortical DA neurons exert an inhibitory influence on locomotion in both neonatal and adult life. However, several important differences appear to exist between the effects on locomotion of DA neuron destruction during neonatal and adult life. First, whereas global destruction of brain DA neurons by ivt. administration of 6-HDA in neonatal rats results in locomotor hyperactivity, ivt. 6-HDA injections fail to augment locomotion in adult rats, despite comparable depletion of DA in terminal fields of mesocortical DA projections in rats treated at different ages (see above). Second, although locomotor hyperactivity following lesions of the VTA in adult rats appears to be relatively permanent, the duration of locomotor hyperactivity following ivt. 6-HDA injections in neonatal rats is transient or permanent, depending on the extent of depletion of brain DA (see preceding). Third, whereas the locomotor stimulant effect of d-amphetamine is reduced following lesions of mesocortical DA neurons in adult life (Kelly, 1975), d-amphetamine produces a dose-dependent reduction of locomotor hyperactivity in rats depleted of brain DA in neonatal life (see succeeding). These different consequences of brain DA depletion in neonatal and adult rats suggest that some effects of brain DA neuron loss are age dependent.

Pharmacological Studies in Dopamine-Depleted Neonatal Rats

Because loss of brain DA in the neonatal rat was associated with locomotor hyperactivity, we sought to determine if this hyperactivity could be reduced by augmentation of residual DA neurotransmission

TABLE 2

Effect of D-Amphetamine on Locomotor Activity in Rats Given DMI-6-HDA or DMI-Vehicle Treatments at 3 and 6 Days of Age[a]

Group	*N*	Days of age			
		21	29	39	46
DMI-vehicle					
Saline	8	34.6 ± 4.0	34.1 ± 6.1	25.5 ± 2.4	23.2 ± 6.1
d-amphetamine (1 mg/kg)	8	299.9 ± 31.5*	179.3 ± 30.3*	121.3 ± 25.8*	142.0 ± 32.5*
DMI-6-HDA					
Saline	8	210.4 ± 23.2	325.8 ± 45.3	231.2 ± 39.1	151.0 ± 29.9
d-amphetamine (1 mg/kg)	8	104.1 ± 18.4*	99.0 ± 38.6*	68.7 ± 27.8*	19.7 ± 8.9*

[a]Values represent mean ± S.E.M. locomotor activity counts per hour.
*$p < 0.01$, compared to saline treatment, *t*-test.

TABLE 3

Effect of Drug Treatments on Locomotor Hyperactivity in Rats Given DMI-6-HDA at 3 and 6 Days of Age[a]

Treatment[b]	Locomotor activity (counts per hour)
Saline	215 ± 40
Saline-amphetamine (1 mg/kg)	33 ± 12*
Spiroperidol (0.1 mg/kg)-amphetamine (1 mg/kg)	41 ± 15
Methysergide (2 mg/kg)-amphetamine (1 mg/kg)	153 ± 42**
Propranolol (5 mg/kg)-amphetamine (1 mg/kg)	35 ± 13
Atropine (0.5 mg/kg)-amphetamine (1 mg/kg)	32 ± 10
Naloxone (10 mg/kg)-amphetamine (1 mg/kg)	31 ± 13
Quipazine (4 mg/kg)	63 ± 18*
Fenfluramine (3 mg/kg)	22 ± 10*

[a]Values represent the mean ± S.E.M. results from 6–8 rats tested during days 37–46 of age.

[b]Rats received drug pretreatments 30 min prior to amphetamine and received amphetamine, quipazine or fenfluramine 30 min prior to the 1 hour locomotor test.

*$p < 0.05$, compared to saline treatment. **$p < 0.05$, compared to saline-amphetamine treatment.

(Heffner & Seiden, 1982). For this purpose, we first examined the effects on locomotion of d-amphetamine, a drug that has been shown to increase locomotion in normal rats by increasing the release of DA from central neurons (Creese & Iversen, 1973). For this experiment, 6-HDA (100 μg) was administered (ivt.) to rats at 3 and 6 days of age following systemic DMI injections. This treatment caused large, selective depletions of DA in the brain, as determined in adulthood. Rats so treated displayed seven-fold increases in locomotor activity during Days 16 to 55 of life, in agreement with previous results. Throughout this period, administration of d-amphetamine (1 mg/kg, ip) significantly reduced locomotor hyperactivity in 6-HDA treated rats at 21, 29, 39, and 46 days of age while increasing locomotion in control rats (Table 2). This finding is in agreement with other studies on the effects of amphetamine in the DA-depleted neonatal rat (Shaywitz, Klopper, Yager, & Gordon, 1976; Sorenson, Vayer, & Goldberg, 1977). The effect of amphetamine was dose-related, with 2 mg/kg producing a maximal response.

In contrast to our original prediction, the ability of amphetamine to reduce locomotor hyperactivity in rats treated with 6-HDA in neonatal life did not appear to involve the release of DA from residual DA neurons. Diminished hyperactivity caused by amphetamine was not blocked by the DA antagonist spiroperidol (Table 3). Instead, the effect of amphetamine in 6-HDA-treated rats appeared to be mediated by central serotonin neurons, because pretreatment with the serotonin antagonist methysergide reduced the effect of amphetamine and because the serotonin agonists quipazine and fenfluramine reduced locomotor hyperactivity (Table 3). Drugs which should reduce the effects of amphetamine mediated by other neurotransmitters did not alter the hyperactivity-reducing effect of amphetamine (Table 3). Like amphetamine, methylphenidate reduced locomotor hyperactivity in rats depleted of brain DA in neonatal life. Our findings suggest that the ability of amphetamine to reduce hyperactivity stems from an augmentation of central serotonergic neurotransmission. As such, these findings are consistent with previous studies demonstrating that central catecholaminergic and serotonergic neurons exert opposing influences on locomotion in the rat (Green & Harvey, 1974; Hollister, Breese, Kuhn, Cooper, & Shanberg, 1976).

The Effect of Neonatal Brain Dopamine Depletion on the Acquisition of Operant Behavior

In addition to their role in the control of locomotion, central DA neurons also appear to contribute to the performance of conditioned behaviors maintained by positive or negative reinforcement. Loss of brain DA neurons in adult rats is accompanied by disruption of operant behavior (Cooper, Breese, Grant, & Howard, 1973). In addition, the turnover rate of DA in central neurons is enhanced during the performance of positively reinforced operant responding (Schoenfeld & Seiden, 1969; Heffner & Seiden, 1980). In order to determine the effects of neonatal loss of brain DA neurons on the ability to acquire an operant response, rats were administered 6-HDA and DMI at 3 and 6 days of age and acquisition of a positively reinforced operant response (lever-pressing for water) was determined during Days 30–42 of life (Heffner & Seiden, 1983). For these tests, a low dose of 6-HDA (2 $\times$ 35 μg) was employed. Hyperactivity abates by Day 30 of age after this treatment, thus enabling the determination of acquisition ability in the absence of potential confounding changes in motor function. The DMI and 6-HDA treatment caused a 60% decrease in brain DA without altering brain NE. Rats were deprived of water for 20 hours daily from Days 29 to 40 of life and were exposed for 1 hour daily to

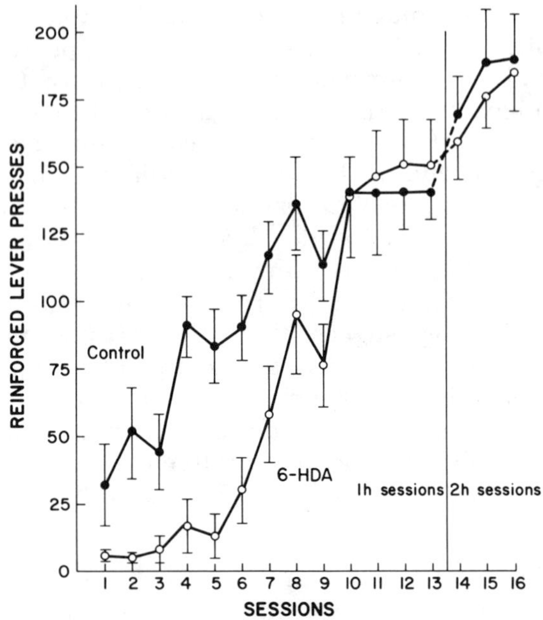

Figure 6. Effect of neonatal DMI + 6-HDA treatment on number of lever presses emitted during acquisition of operant behavior. Rats treated with DMI + 6-HDA (n = 13) or DMI + vehicle (n = 11) at 3 and 6 days of age were exposed to a FR-1 schedule of water reinforcement for 1 hour daily on Days 30–42 of life and for 2 hours daily on Days 43–45 of life. Values represent the mean ± SEM lever presses emitted. Data from the four DMI + 6-HDA-treated rats that failed to acquire the operant schedule are not included. (From Heffner & Seiden, 1983, reproduced with permission).

an operant schedule on which each lever press or the passage of 1 minute without pressing resulted in the brief presentation of water. Control rats rapidly acquired the operant schedule, reaching the performance level used as a criterion for acquisition (50 reinforced lever presses per hour) in 3.1 ± 0.5 sessions. In contrast, nearly one fourth of the DMI + 6-HDA-treated rats failed to acquire the response after 16 sessions and the remaining rats required more than twice as many sessions for acquisition (7.8 ± 0.7 sessions) (Figure 6). Once the 6-HDA-treated rats had acquired the response, however, they performed at normal levels and retained the response after a 10-day period during which they were not exposed to the schedule. These results suggest that loss of brain DA neurons during neonatal life results in impaired acquisition of conditioned behavior in later life. This effect is independent of changes in locomotor activity and appears to be independent of motor deficits because the animals were not hyperactive at the time of testing and were capable of performing the response following acquisition.

Summary

These studies demonstrate that the loss of brain DA neuronal projections during early life results in an inability to suppress locomotion normally during development. The magnitude and duration of locomotor hyperactivity is related to the extent of brain DA neuron loss and appears to be mediated by the destruction of mesocortical DA neurons. Amphetamine and methylphenidate are capable of reducing locomotor hyperactivity in rats depleted of brain dopamine in neonatal life, perhaps by augmenting central serotonergic neurotransmission. In addition to altering locomotor development, lesions of brain DA neurons in neonatal rats is associated with impaired acquisition of operant behavior in later life.

These results indicate that central DA neurons exert important influences on the normal development of behavior. In addition, the characteristics of the DA-depleted neonatal rat may bear a resemblance to some of the symptomology of attentional deficit disorder (ADD) in children (Shaywitz, Yager, & Klopper, 1976). Based on the ability of drugs used in the treatment of ADD to reduce locomotor hyperactivity in the DA-depleted neonatal rat, such animals may be useful for the evaluation of new drugs to reduce hyperactivity in children with ADD.

Acknowledgments

We thank Dr. C. Fernandez, F. Karapas, Dr. C. Kotake, Dr. F. Miller, and G. Vosmer for their participation in various aspects of these studies and B. X. Knight for preparation of the manuscript. This research was supported by grants from USPHS (NS-12324) and the Brain Research Foundation of Chicago, Illinois. L. Seiden is a recipient of a Research Scientist Award (MH-10562).

References

Bolles, R. C., & Woods, P. J. (1964). The ontogeny of behavior in the albino rat. *Animal Behavior, 12,* 427–441.

Breese, G. R., & Traylor, T. D. (1970). Effect of 6-hydroxydopamine on brain norepinephrine and dopamine: Evidence for selective degradation of catecholamine neurons. *Journal of Pharmacology and Experimental Therapeutics, 174,* 413–420.

Campbell, B. A., Lytle, L. D., & Fibiger, H. C. (1969). Ontogeny of adrenergic arousal and cholinergic inhibitory mechanisms in the rat. *Science, 166,* 635–637.

Cooper, B. R., Breese, G. R., Grant, L. D., & Howard, J. L. (1973). Effects of 6-hydroxydopamine treatments on active avoidance responding: Evidence for involvement of brain dopamine. *Journal of Pharmacology and Experimental Therapeutics, 185,* 358–370.

Coyle, J. T. (1976). Neurochemical aspects of the development of the dopaminergic innervation to the striatum. In M. Brazier and F. Cocani (Eds.), *Brain Dysfunction in Infantile Febrile Convulsions,* New York, Raven Press, 1976, pp. 25–39.

Creese, I., & Iversen, S. D. (1973). Blockade of amphetamine-induced motor stimulation and stereotypy in the adult rat following neonatal treatment with 6-hydroxydopamine. *Brain Research, 55,* 369–382.

Erinoff, L., MacPhail, R. C., Heller, A., & Seiden, L. S. (1979). Age-dependent effects of 6-hydroxydopamine on locomotor activity in the rat. *Brain Research, 164,* 195–205.

Green, T. K., & Harvey, J. A. (1974). Enhancement of amphetamine action after interruption of ascending serotonergic pathways. *Journal of Pharmacology and Experimental Therapeutics, 190,* 109–117.

Heffner, T. G., & Seiden, L. S. (1980). Synthesis of catecholamines from ^{3}H-tyrosine in brain during the performance of operant behavior. *Brain Research, 183,* 403–419.

Heffner, T. G., & Seiden, L. S. (1982). Possible involvement of serotonergic neurons in the reduction of locomotor hyperactivity caused by amphetamine in neonatal rats depleted of brain dopamine. *Brain Research, 244,* 81–90.

Heffner, T. G., & Seiden, L. S. (1983). Impaired acquisition of an operant response in young rats depleted of brain dopamine in neonatal life. *Psychopharmacology, 79,* 115–119.

Heffner, T. G., Heller, A., Miller, F. E., Kotake, C., & Seiden, L. S. (1983). Locomotor hyperactivity in neonatal rats following electrolytic lesions of mesocortical dopamine neurons. *Developmental Brain Research, 9,* 29–37.

Heller, A., Hutchens, J. O., Kirby, M. L., Karapas, F., & Fernandez, C. (1979). Stereotaxic electrode placement in the neonatal rat. *Journal of Neuroscience Methods, 1,* 41–76.

Heller, A., Heffner, T., Kotake, C., Miller, F., & Seiden, L. (1981). Locomotor hyperactivity in neonatal rats following lesions of mesocortical dopaminergic neurons. Society for Neuroscience Abstracts.

Hollister, A. S., Breese, G. R., Kuhn, C. M., Cooper, B. R., & Shanberg, S. M. (1976). An inhibitory role for brain serotonin-containing neurons in the locomotor effects of d-amphetamine. *Journal of Pharmacology and Experimental Therapeutics, 198,* 12–22.

Kelly, P. H. (1977). Drug-induced motor behavior. In L. L. Iversen, S. O. Iversen, & S. H. Snyder (Eds.), *Handbook of Psychopharmacology* (Vol. 8). New York: Plenum Press, pp. 295–331.

LeMoal, M., Stinus, L., Simon, H. J., Tassin, J. P., Thierry, A. M., Blanc, G., Glowinski, J., & Cardo, B. (1977). Behavioral effects of a lesion in the ventral mesencephalic tegmentum: evidence for involvement of A_{10} dopaminergic neurons. In E. Costa & G. L. Gessa (Eds.), *Nonstriatal Dopaminergic Neurons.* New York: Raven Press, pp. 237–245.

Lloyd, K. G., & Hornykiewicz, O. (1978). Catecholamines in regulation of motor function. In A. J. Friedhoff (Ed.) *Catecholamines and Behavior* (Vol. 1). New York: Raven Press, pp. 41–57.

Marshall, J., Richardson, J., & Teitelbaum, P. (1974). Nigrostriatal bundle damage and the lateral hypothalamic syndrome. *Journal of Comparative and Physiological Psychology, 87,* 808–830.

Miller, F. E., Heffner, T. G., Kotake, C., & Seiden, L. S. (1981). Magnitude and duration of hyperactivity following neonatal 6-hydroxydopamine is related to the extent of brain dopamine depletion. *Brain Research, 229,* 123–132.

Miller, F. E., & Seiden, L. S. (1983). Locomotor hyperactivity following chronic alpha-methyltyrosine administration in the neonatal rat. *Developmental Brain Research, 6,* 91–92.

Moore, R. Y., & Bloom, F. E. (1978). Central catecholamine neuron systems: anatomy and physiology of the dopamine systems. *Annual Review of Neurosciences, 1,* 129–169.

O'Donnell, J. M., & Seiden, L. S. (1980). Effect of prenatal haloperidol treatment on the ontogeny of locomotor activity in rat pups. *Society for Neuroscience Abstracts.*

Pardo, J. V., Creese, I., Burt, D. R., & Snyder, S. H. (1977). Ontogenesis of dopamine receptor binding in the corpus striatum of the rat. *Brain Research, 125,* 376–382.

Porcher, W., & Heller, A. (1972). Regional development of catecholamine biosynthesis in rat brain. *Journal of Neurochemistry, 19,* 1917–1930.

Schoenfeld, R. I., & Seiden, L. S. (1969). Effect of alpha-methyltyrosine on operant behavior and brain catecholamine levels. *Journal of Pharmacology and Experimental Therapeutics, 167,* 319–327.

Seiden, L. S., & Dykstra, L. (1977). Psychopharmacology: A Biochemical and Behavioral Approach, New York: Van Nostrand Reinhold.

Shaywitz, B. A., Klopper, J. H., Yager, R. D., & Gordon, J. W. (1976). Paradoxical response to amphetamine in developing rats treated with 6-hydroxydopamine. *Nature (Lond.), 261,* 153–155.

Shaywitz, B. A., Yager, R. D., & Klopper, J. H. (1976). Selective brain dopamine depletion in developing rats: an experimental model of minimal brain dysfunction. *Science, 191,* 305–308.

Sorenson, C. A., Vayer, J. S., & Goldberg, C. S. (1977). Amphetamine reduction of motor activity in rats after neonatal administration of 6-hydroxydopamine. *Biological Psychiatry, 12,* 133–137.

Stricker, E. M., & Zigmond, M. J. (1974). Effects on homeostasis of ivt. injection of 6-hydroxydopamine in rats. *Journal of Comparative and Physiological Psychology,* 1974, *86,* 973–994.

Stoof, J. C., Dijkstra, H., & Hillegers, J. P. M. (1978). Changes in the behavioral response to a novel environment following lesioning of the central dopaminergic system in rat pups. *Psychopharmacology, 57,* 163–166.

Tarsy, D., & Baldessarini, R. J. (1977). The pathophysiologic basis of tardive dyskinesia. *Biological Psychiatry, 12,* 431–450.

Tassin, J. P., Stinus, L., Simon, H., Blanc, G., Thierry, A. M., LeMoal, M., Cardo, B., & Glowinski, J. (1977). Distribution of dopaminergic terminals in rat cerebral cortex; role of dopaminergic mesocortical system in ventral tegmental area syndrome. In E. Costa and G. L. Gessa (Eds.) *Nonstriatal Dopaminergic Neurons.* New York: Raven Press, pp. 21–28.

Zigmond, M. J., & Stricker, E. M. (1974). Ingestive behavior following damage to central dopamine neurons: Implication for homeostasis and recovery of function. In E. Usdin (Ed.), *Neuropsychopharmacology of Monoamines and Their Regulatory Enzymes.* New York: Raven Press, pp. 385–401.

6

Early Brain Damage and Attentional Deficit Disorder: An Animal Model*

Lisa A. Raskin, Bennett A. Shaywitz, Sally E. Shaywitz, Donald J. Cohen, and George M. Anderson

Background

The Clinical Syndrome

Attentional deficit disorder (ADD) is a predominant behavior of childhood that affects between 3 and 20% of the school-age population (see Schwartz & Johnson, 1981). The symptoms of ADD typically become apparent before 7 years of age and continue through adoles-

* Supported in part by USPH grants from Mental Health Clinical Research Center 1P50 MH-30929; Children's Clinical Center Grant RR00125; Berger Foundation and the State of Connecticut.

Copyright © 1984 by Academic Press, Inc.
All rights of reproduction in any form reserved.
ISBN 0-12-052901-7

cence, affecting boys much more frequently than girls (American Psychiatric Association, 1980). Although there is some controversy regarding whether or not ADD exists as a unique syndrome, many clinicians agree that ADD children exhibit a similar constellation of symptoms even though the behavioral profiles of individual children may vary considerably (Rapoport & Zametkin, 1980). According to the American Psychiatric Association (1980), cardinal signs of ADD include impulsivity, an inability to sustain attention, and distractability; the existence of these symptoms in conjunction with age-inappropriate hyperactivity leads to the diagnosis of ADD plus hyperactivity (ADD + H). Children who suffer from ADD or ADD + H often exhibit learning impairments and show poor academic performance, which can be influenced to some extent by situational variables such as classroom structure and teaching style (see Keogh & Barkett, 1980).

ADD had historically been referred to as "minimal brain damage" or "minimal brain dysfunction"; however, the difficulty in determining a precise, consistent aberration in the central nervous system of clinical populations contributed to a change in diagnostic classification (see Schwartz & Johnson, 1981; Shaywitz, Cohen & Shaywitz, 1979). Despite the fact that no organic etiology for this disorder has yet been identified, there is provocative evidence from a variety of methodological approaches that justifies continued investigation into the biological bases of ADD (see Shaywitz & Shaywitz, in press; Rapoport & Ferguson, 1981, for review).

Consistent with the view that biological factors may influence attentional deficits, many investigators have examined the role that monoaminergic neurotransmitter systems play in mediating ADD and ADD + H. Early reports proposing such a relationship were merely suggestive and not indicative of monoaminergically mediated attentional or motor deficits. For example, following the great pandemic of Economo's encephalitis in the early part of this century, many children were diagnosed as having hyperactivity and attentional problems (see Shaywitz, Shaywitz, Cohen, & Young, in press), whereas adults were diagnosed as having Parkinson's disease. Given the relationship between parkinsonism and dopamine (DA) deficiency, Wender (1971) has suggested that the behavioral problems in children who suffered from this pandemic might also reflect dopaminergic deficits. Although this connection is intriguing, it must remain speculative, given that the virus of Economo's encephalitis was never isolated (Shaywitz *et al.*, in press).

Considerable interest in the monoaminergic mediation of attentional deficits also stemmed from the therapeutic effect of psychomotor stimulants on clinically diagnosed children. Since the initial report by Bradley in 1937, an impressive number of investigations have shown that drugs which increase central nervous system monoamines, such as dextro-amphetamine, methylphenidate, and magnesium pemoline, effectively ameliorate disturbances in attention and activity (See Whalen & Henker, 1980, for review). Although ADD children are impulsive and unable to sustain their attention, they appear calmer, less active, and more attentive following administration of psychomotor stimulants, a drug effect that has been considered paradoxical. However, the finding that ADD symptoms are improved following administration of drugs that stimulate monoamine systems does not necessarily indicate that such symptoms originate from monoaminergic deficiencies; aspirin improves symptoms of rheumatic fever, but clearly rheumatic fever does not result from a deficiency in aspirin. Accepting the suggestion of a relationship between aberrations in monoamine function and both attentional processes and motor behavior, investigators have attempted to determine more systematic means of assessing the role these neurotransmitters play in the expression of ADD.

One approach has been to use clinical studies that measure monoamine metabolite levels in the blood or urine of ADD children as a possible index of neurotransmitter function. An accumulation of evidence shows that levels of norepinephrine metabolites are altered in the urine of ADD children (see Hunt, Cohen, Shaywitz, & Shaywitz, 1982 for review); however, measuring levels of metabolites in urine or blood can yield inconsistent results. Other clinical studies have reported lowered levels of DA metabolites in the cerebrospinal fluid (CSF) of ADD children following probenecid loading, a technique that prevents egress of metabolites from the CSF (Shaywitz, Cohen, & Bowers, 1980). The advantage of measuring metabolite levels in the CSF is that they better reflect central nervous system (CNS) function; in contrast, urinary and blood levels indicate both peripheral and central metabolism (Shaywitz & Shaywitz, in press).

Although the investigation into a biology of ADD might ideally be achieved through clinical studies, such studies are severely limited by ethical, technical, and practical constraints. Hence many investigators turn to the use of animal models that parallel the symptomatology of the disorder. The advantages of an animal model are obvious: Environmental variables can be systematically manipulated, neurotransmitter levels can be measured, and the behavioral effects of therapeutic agents can be determined. Any investigator who is sensitive to the psychosocial complexities that determine a human behavior disorder will not attempt to extrapolate results from animal studies to the human condition. However, the value of an animal model may come from a parallel with some components of the human syndrome that may generate hypotheses for practical clinical investigations. Although a number of animal models have been employed in the production of hyperactivity, that which was developed by Shaywitz and his associates (Shaywitz, Yager, & Klopper 1976; Shaywitz, Yager, Klopper, & Gordon, 1976) appears to satisfy the criterion for ADD and is discussed in the following section. This model suggests that neonatal damage to the central catecholamine systems (CA) results in behaviors that seem to parallel ADD and ADD + H.

An Animal Model

The preweanling rat serves as an excellent model for studying developmental disorders because, like the human infant, it is altricial and is born with an immature CNS that undergoes dramatic changes postnatally (Rosenblatt, 1979). It is useful to study the rat as a model for disorders of motor activity because the young rat goes through a period during normal development, between the 2nd and 3rd week of life, when it is hyperactive in comparison to adult conspecifics (Campbell, Lytle, & Fibiger, 1969).

By studying the rat one can determine both the extent to which postnatal insult to the rapidly maturing CNS influences the normal ontogenetic pattern of locomotor activity and the sensitivity of aberrations in activity to environmental manipulation. In addition, one can determine if neonatal insult leads to learning impairments, and if so, one can assess the permanence of such impairments.

Shaywitz and his colleagues (Shaywitz, Yager, & Klopper, 1976; Shaywitz, Klopper, Yager, & Gordon, 1976) have presented an abundance of data showing that early damage to CNS CA systems produces animals that show severe deficits in activity and learning throughout development. When DA is selectively damaged early in life, the rat exhibits a constellation of symptoms that are strikingly similar to those observed in the clinical diagnosis ADD + H. Approximately 1 week following neonatal DA depletion, animals become significantly more active than their littermate controls. The developmental time course of their activity is the same as that of normal animals, showing peak activity levels between the 2nd and 3rd week of life. Activity levels remain slightly higher than controls during development and normalize in adulthood (Shaywitz, Yager & Klopper, 1976). In addition, DA-depleted pups fail to habituate to a novel environment and spend more time than control animals in generalized activity such as grooming, gnawing, rearing, and ambulation (Shaywitz, Gordon, Klopper, Zelterman, 1977). Following neonatal damage to DA systems, profound deficits in learning are also observed; these learning impairments appear prior to weaning and persist throughout adulthood (Shaywitz, Yager & Klopper, 1976). Interestingly, the disappearance of motor deficits coupled with a prolongation of learning problems throughout adulthood has also been reported for ADD children and is referred to by the American Psychiatric Association (1980) as *ADD-residual type.*

Behavioral aberrations that result from neonatal DA depletion in the rat have been shown to be influenced by external factors. Psychomotor stimulants such as amphetamine or methylphenidate reportedly reverse the hyperactivity and learning deficits that have resulted from early damage to DA systems (Shaywitz, Klopper, & Gordon, 1978; Shaywitz, Klopper, Yager, & Gordon, 1976). This finding is particularly intriguing in light of the reported therapeutic effects of stimulant drugs on ADD children (Bradley, 1937). Environmental cues have also been shown to influence activity levels of the DA-depleted pup. If an anesthetized conspecific is placed in the test chamber with the DA-deficient pup, heightened activity levels are completely eliminated; however, the presence of other familiar cues are not sufficient to suppress lesion-induced hyperactivity (Teicher, Shaywitz, Kootz, & Cohen, 1981). Rearing conditions can also modify the expression of hyperactive behavior and learning impairments in the DA-depleted rat. Rearing pups that have been injected with 6-hydroxydopamine (6-HDA) in a litter solely comprising neurotoxin-treated pups actually exacerbates developmental behavior impairments, whereas rearing lesioned pups with normal littermates attenuates their deficits (Pearson, Teicher, Shaywitz, Cohen, Young, & Anderson, 1980). The finding that the behavior of DA-depleted pups can be influenced by environmental variables parallels the many reports that show that ADD behaviors in children are extremely affected by situational or environmental factors (see Paternite & Loney, 1980 for review).

Following neonatal insult to the central DA system, a specific behavioral profile that has been likened to the behaviors observed in children with ADD+H emerges. Studies suggest that selective depletion of norepinephrine (NE) systems produces severe learning impairments with no concomitant change in activity, which leads to a proposal that this constellation of behaviors more closely resembles the clinical diagnoses of ADD (without hyperactivity) (Raskin, Shaywitz, Anderson, Cohen, & Teicher, 1983; Shaywitz, Kretschmar, Levitt, Teicher, Anderson, Young, & Cohen, 1983). The following section elaborates on the animal experiments that assess the behavioral effects of neonatal damage to DA and NE systems, with particular emphasis on changes in motor activity and performance deficits. In addition, it presents research on the paradoxical response of DA-depleted animals to stimulant medication.

Animal Research

Behavioral Results of Early Damage to CA Systems

In the adult rat, lesions of ascending CA systems with 6-HDA produce significant disruption in activity (Evetts, Uretsky, Iversen, & Iversen, 1970); however, an unusual finding is that a similar lesion, performed neonatally, increases levels of activity during development. This phenomenon has been reported and replicated by many investigators (Fobes & Olds, 1981; Pappas, Gallivan, Dugas, Saari, & Ings, 1980), and research continues to identify the contribution of early damage to DA and NE systems in mediating lesion-induced hyperactivity during ontogeny (Shaywitz, Teicher, Cohen, Anderson, Young, & Levitt, in press).

There is compelling evidence that 6-HDA-induced hyperactivity in the young rat is a function of damage to DA rather than NE systems. When 6-HDA is injected directly into the brain of neonatal rats, significant destruction of CA pathways is effected. Pretreating the animals with desmethylimipramine (DMI) spares the destruction of NE-containing terminals and leads to specific depletion of DA systems (Miller, Heffner, Kotake, & Seiden, 1981; Shaywitz *et al.*, 1978). Preferential depletion of NE systems is best produced by parenteral injections of 6-HDA (either subcutaneous or intraperitoneal) during the first few days of life. Following this procedure, no elevations in locomotor activity have been observed during development (Pappas & Sobrian, 1972; Shaywitz *et al.*, 1983). Reports of increased activity levels following NE depletion are problematic due to the relatively short observation period used to measure activity in these experiments (McLean, Kostrzewa, & May 1976; Morgan, McLean, & Kostrzewa, 1979). On the other hand, selective lesions of DA systems early in life have repeatedly been shown to produce increases in locomotor activity throughout lengthy observation periods (Shaywitz *et al.*, 1977). In addition, the magnitude of DA depletion is positively correlated with the persistence of activity throughout development (Miller *et al.*, 1981). In studies in which depletion levels are around 60%, motor activity in the DA-lesioned pup returns to normal in adulthood (Shaywitz, Yager, & Klopper, 1976). More substantial lesions that eliminate about 98% of all CNS DA however, result in rats that remain hyperactive throughout adulthood (Miller *et al.*, 1981). Inasmuch as the heightened activity levels of ADD + H children typically return to normal during adulthood, those procedures that produce moderate rather than severe DA deficiencies lead to an activity pattern that more closely parallels that of the clinical syndrome. Moreover, clinical studies indicate that markers of DA function are moderately, and not severely, impaired in ADD children (Shaywitz *et al.*, 1980).

Following neonatal insult to DA systems, the young rat exhibits an increase in locomotion, accompanied by elevated levels of general activities such as grooming, sniffing, rearing, and crawling. Interestingly, although the levels of general activity are elevated, the duration of specific categories of active behavior are significantly shorter in the A-deficient animal than in controls. Thieme, Dijkstra, and Stoof (1980) report that animals display shorter bouts of grooming and upward sniffing following DA lesions and propose that such a disruption in behavior may parallel the deficits that ADD children have in maintaining their attention toward specific tasks. Although the link between attention in children and stereotyped motor behaviors in rats is tenuous, this study helps to further characterize the motor deficits that result from early damage to DA systems in the rat. The underlying mechanism that leads to an increase in activity following DA depletion, as well as the precise DA pathway that mediates this effect, is under investigation and is reviewed in Chapter 5.

So far, this discussion has focused on components of the animal model that parallel disorders of motor activity observed in ADD + H children. Hyperactivity, although problematic, is only one of the constellation of symptoms required for a diagnoses of ADD + H. As mentioned earlier, ADD + H children show profound deficits in attention that often lead to disabilities in learning (Keogh & Barkett, 1980). Ideally, an animal model for this disorder should directly assess those components of attention that are disrupted in children, such as vigilance, sustained as well as selective attention, and distractibility. Although a variety of paradigms have been used to measure attention in the rat (Mason & Fibiger, 1979; Oke & Adams, 1978), none has achieved widespread acceptance. Because of the difficulties in measuring a multidimensional process such as attention in laboratory animals, and because learning disabilities are a prominent consequence of ADD, the work by Shaywitz and his collaborators has focused on identifying changes in learning abilities that occur following neonatal damage to CA.

Neonatally DA-lesioned animals show impairments in habituation in both novel (Thieme *et al.,* 1980) and familiar environments (Teicher *et al.,* 1981). Severe deficits are also observed when DA-depleted pups are tested in one- or two-way avoidance paradigms (Shaywitz *et al.,* 1976, 1978), a finding that cannot be explained by a difference in shock threshold between lesioned and control animals (Shaywitz, personal communication). A study by Weldon, Wool, Teicher, Shaywitz, Cohen and Anderson, (1982) attempted to dissociate motor impairments from performance deficits when DA-depleted pups are tested in active avoidance paradigms. In this experiment both control and DA-depleted pups were trained to perform a conditioned appetitive response at 5 days of age. An intraoral burst of milk solution was paired with a novel (and slightly aversive) odor. After 2 days, pups were tested for a preference to the conditioned odor. Control pups, having acquired the response, showed a preference for the previously novel odor, whereas DA-depleted animals, although not anosmic, did not. The reversal of performance deficits when DA-depleted pups were given systemic injections of the DA agonist apomorphine prior to conditioning suggests that deficits were due to an aberration in DA systems. Most important, this study showed that decrements in performance following DA depletion occurred at an age that precedes the emergence of lesion-induced hyperactivity (Pappas *et al.,* 1980; Shaywitz *et al.,* 1978), suggesting a dissociation of the motor and learning deficits produced by the lesion.

Alterations in performance have been observed in the neonatally NE-depleted pup on a variety of learning paradigms both during ontogeny and in adulthood (Mason & Fibiger, 1979; Raskin *et al.,* 1983). Studies that have reported no change in learning abilities following neonatal NE depletion have used either procedures that resulted in low depletion levels (Shaywitz *et al.,* in press) or learning paradigms in which testing procedures were not rigorous (Pappas & Sobrian, 1972). Although many studies have confirmed performance deficits in NE-depleted animals, such alterations have been interpreted as a reflection of a variety of phenomena such as a decrease in response inhibition (Peterson & Laverty, 1976), an increase in anxiety (Gray, Davis, Feldon, Rawlins, & Owen, 1981), and a decrease in selective attention (Mason & Fibiger, 1979). Although these interpretations need not be mutually exclusive, research is needed to determine the extent to which performance impairments observed in the NE-depleted pup reflect specific deficits in attention.

The finding that damage to NE systems leads to learning deficits without concomitant changes in motor activity is particularly intriguing in that it suggests that selective lesions of DA and NE systems during infancy produce a unique constellation of behaviors. It is tempting to speculate that children who suffer from ADD without hyperactivity have deficits in NE systems whereas children with ADD + H suffer from abnormalities in DA systems. Although this speculation may be premature, it does suggest a strategy for investigators who study the neural correlates of ADD through clinical research. Investigations in which the protocol consists of measuring neurotransmitter metabolite levels in the blood, urine, or CSF of ADD children have yielded inconsistent results (see Hunt *et al.*, 1982). This may reflect either differences in methodology between experiments or the heterogeneity of subject populations. Investigators should insure that their clinical populations are homogeneous for either ADD or ADD + H, inasmuch as the etiology of these disorders may differ.

Paradoxical Effect of Amphetamine

Early investigations of Shaywitz and his associates revealed that DA-depleted pups, although hyperactive in comparison to controls, became significantly less active following treatment with either amphetamine or methylphenidate—an effect that was directly opposite the activity-inducing effect of amphetamine observed in normal untreated animals (Shaywitz, Klopper, Yager, & Gordon, 1976; Shaywitz *et al.*, 1978). That a similar paradoxical effect reportedly occurred in the treatment of ADD children with psychomotor stimulants (Bradley, 1937) makes this component of the animal model an enticing parallel to the clinical syndrome.

Although a paradoxical calming effect of stimulants in DA-depleted animals was observed, the precise mechanism underlying this phenomenon was not determined. In keeping with a dual transmitter hypothesis (Antelman & Caggiula, 1977), Shaywitz and his associates proposed the following interaction of NE and DA systems: In the normal animal, NE facilitates locomotor activity (Campbell *et al.*, 1969) and DA may modulate and restrain NE systems. In the 6-HDA-injected pup, the absence of DA removes constraints from NE and locomotor activity is unchecked. After at least 2 weeks of denervation, DA receptors in the young rat become supersensitive (Lipton, McGrough, & Shaywitz, 1980); thus when amphetamine is injected, DA is released from remaining terminals onto supersensitive receptors. Such activation of the DA system leads to the inhibition of locomotor activity.

Since the original report by Shaywitz and his associates, this phenomenon has been successfully replicated (Heffner & Seiden, 1982; Sorenson, Vayer, & Goldberg, 1977). Reports of unsuccessful replications are difficult to interpret due to the vast differences in methodology between the reports of other investigators and those of Shaywitz and his associates (Eastgate, Wright, & Werry, 1978; Thieme *et al.*, 1980). For example, Pappas *et al.* (1980), who failed to observe activity-reducing effects of amphetamine in DA-depleted animals, did not test animals between 19 and 26 days of age, the ages at which the paradoxical response was previously observed. In addition, their injection protocol differed considerably (Shaywitz, Klopper, Yager & Gordon, 1976; Shaywitz *et al.*, 1978). Other investigations that have failed to reproduce this phenomenon have either reported DA depletion levels that are considerably lower than those reported by Shaywitz (Concannon & Schechter, 1982) or have not reported depletion values at all (Eastgate *et al.*, 1978). One report noted the critical importance that high levels of depletion have for producing a paradoxical amphetamine effect (Heffner & Seiden, 1982). The work of Thieme *et al.* (1980) showed that 6-HDA-injected pups were hyperactive during development and showed shorter bout lengths of behaviors such as locomotion, sniffing, and grooming. Although behavior was observed at the same ages as those reported by Shaywitz, and depletion levels were comparable, administration of amphetamine further decreased bout length of behavior and did not reverse lesion-induced hyperactivity. An activity-reducing effect of the stimulant was not observed in this study. However, there was a tendency for amphetamine to have less effect in increasing activity and decreasing bout length in 6-HDA-injected animals than in controls, a finding which is implicit in the data yet not explicitly discussed by the authors. This finding is consistent with that reported by Eastgate *et al.* (1978), which showed that methylphenidate-induced activity was significantly lower in 6-HDA-treated pups than in controls.

Heffner and Seiden (1982) both replicated the activity-reducing effect of stimulants in DA-depleted animals and proposed an alternative underlying mechanism of action. This report found that amphetamine injections reduced lesion-induced hyperactivity, and that at certain ages the effect of amphetamine was dose dependent. Furthermore, the activity-reducing effect of amphetamine in 6-HDA-treated pups was specifically blocked by serotonin antagonists but not by noradrenergic, dopaminergic, cholinergic, or opiate antagonists. Thus, in keeping with the reports that serotonergic systems inhibit catecholaminergic-induced locomotor activity (Mabry & Campbell, 1973), these authors offered a new proposal for the paradoxical effect of amphetamine. If DA is sufficiently depleted, then the stimulating effect of amphetamine on serotonergic systems is expressed, which thereby leads to a decrease in locomotor activity. Under this proposal, researchers who report DA depletion levels of approximately 55% (Concannon & Schechter, 1982) would not be expected to observe this phenomenon. Further support for this proposal comes from the finding that serotonergic agonists decrease activity in DA-depleted animals but not in controls (Heffner & Seiden, 1982). The finding that DA-receptor blockers do not reverse the paradoxical effects of amphetamine conflicts with the originally proposed mechanism of this phenomenon (Shaywitz, Klopper, Yager & Gordon, 1976). Although there is evidence that DA receptors are supersensitive following 6-HDA-induced denervation (Lipton *et al.*, 1980), their function in stimulating the paradoxical effect of amphetamine still remains unclear. Thus research shows that stimulant-induced hyperactivity is either attenuated (Eastgate *et al.*, 1978; Thieme *et al.*, 1980) or reversed (Heffner & Seiden, 1982; Shaywitz, Klopper, Yager & Gordon, 1976) in DA-depleted rats. The observation of an activity-reducing effect of stimulants in DA-depleted animals depends upon depletion levels as well as on the age of the subjects.

Recent epidemiologic advances in the development of criteria to define ADD more precisely suggest that the paradoxical response to stimulants is neither a reliable nor a necessary diagnostic criterion. Clinical studies support such a notion. Thus although clinical experience indicated that ADD children responded differentially to stimulant medication, it is only recently that this issue has been examined critically. Rapoport and her colleagues have been able to compare stimulant-induced behavior of ADD children, normal boys, and men and have found few differences in the responses of these groups.

Amphetamine increased performance on cognitive tasks, while decreasing motor behavior, and the magnitude and direction of this effect did not differ between the groups (see Rapoport & Zametkin for review, 1980). Although this finding is compelling, firm conclusions regarding a paradoxical drug effect cannot be made in the absence of dose response curves for amphetamine-induced behavior. It is possible that although the responses of clinically diagnosed children are consistent with those of normal children and adults at a particular drug dose, their responsivity to a range of drug dosages may differ (C. A. Sorenson, personal communication). In addition, the "normal" boys that participated in the Rapoport studies may not in fact represent a normal comparison group, because their IQ scores fell within the range of gifted children. Shaywitz and McGraw (1982) have reported that gifted children share some characteristics of ADD children, and one such characteristic is hyperactivity.

Directions for Future Research

The animal model presented here suggests that early brain damage to developing CA systems results in behaviors that parallel the childhood disorder ADD. Neonatal lesions of DA systems produce young rats that show increased motor activity and decreases in performance, symptoms that parallel ADD + H, whereas selective lesions of NE systems produce learning deficits with no concomitant change in activity, a behavioral profile more reminiscent of ADD. The validity of this model will become more apparent as future work determines the extent to which the performance deficits of DA- and NE-depleted rats truly reflects problems in attention. Although these animals exhibit severe impairments on learning paradigms, the etiology of these deficits is not clear. We are working to further characterize and specify the nature of the deficits that result from neonatal DA depletion (Pearson, Raskin, Shaywitz, Anderson, & Cohen, 1983).

In addition, this model posits some research strategies for clinical study of the childhood disorder. First, it is clear that identification of a consistent change in neurotransmitter metabolism must be performed in clinical populations that are as homogeneous as possible, given that the symptoms of ADD and ADD + H may have different neural mediation. Secondly, the finding that serotonergic mechanisms play a role in the paradoxical amphetamine effect in DA-depleted rats suggests that serotonin may influence the behaviors in

ADD children (Heffner & Seiden, 1982). However, to date no studies have found a consistent change in serotonergic system function that correlates with the performance-enhancing effect of amphetamine in ADD children (Hunt *et al.*, 1982). Furthermore, the notion that stimulant drugs are in fact paradoxical, and therefore the notion that this drug effect is a necessary condition for the validity of an animal model, has been challenged.

Shaywitz and his associates have devised a technique for measuring CSF monoamine metabolites in rats following DA and NE depletion and have found high correlations between changes in neurotransmitter metabolite levels in the brain and CSF of rats. Measurement of CSF in animals may provide an interface between human and animal studies (Shaywitz & Shaywitz, in press).

References

American Psychiatric Association (1980). *Diagnostic and statistical manual of mental disorders* (3rd ed.). Washington, D.C.

Antelman, S. M., & Caggiula, A. R. (1977). Norepinephrine-dopamine interactions and behavior. *Science, 195,* 646–653.

Bradley, C. (1937). The behavior of children receiving benzedrine. *American Journal of Psychiatry, 94,* 557.

Campbell, B. A., Lytle, L. D., & Fibiger, H. C. (1969). The ontogeny of adrenergic arousal and cholinergic inhibitory mechanisms in the rat. *Science, 166,* 637–638.

Concannon, J. T., & Schechter, M. D. (1982). Failure of amphetamine isomers to decrease hyperactivity in developing rats. *Pharmacology, Biochemistry, & Behavior, 17,* 5–9.

Eastgate, S. M., Wright, J. J., & Werry, J. S., (1978). Behavioral effects of methylphenidate in 6-hydroxydopamine-treated neonatal rats. *Psychopharmacology, 58,* 157–158.

Everts, K. D., Uretsky, N. J., Iversen, L. L., & Iversen, S. D. (1970). Effects of 6-hydroxydopamine on CNS catecholamines, spontaneous motor activity and amphetamine induced hyperactivity in rats. *Nature, 225,* 961–962.

Fobes, J. L., & Olds, M. E. (1981). Effects of neonatal 6-Hydroxydopamine treatment on catecholamine levels and behavior during development and adulthood. *Psychopharmacology, 73,* 27–30.

Gray, J. A., Davis, N., Feldon, J., Rawlins, N. P., & Owen, S. R. (1981). Animal models of anxiety. *Progress in Neuro-Psychopharmacology, 5,* 143–157.

Heffner, T. G., & Seiden, L. S. (1982). Possible involvement of serotoninergic neurons in the reduction of locomotor hyperactivity caused by amphetamine in neonatal rats depleted of brain dopamine. *Brain Research, 224,* 81–90.

Hunt, R. D., Cohen, D. J., Saywitz, S. E., & Shaywitz, B. A. (1982). Strategies for study of the neurochemistry of attention disorder in children. *Schizophrenia Bulletin, 8,* 236–252.

Keogh, B. K., & Barkett, C. J. (1980). An educational analysis of hyperactive children's achievement problems. In C. K. Whalen & B. Henker (Eds.), *Hyperactive children*. New York: Academic Press.

Lipton, S. V., McGrough, J. P., & Shaywitz, B. A. (1980). Effects of apomorphine on escape performance and activity in developing rat pups treated with 6-Hydroxydopamine (6-OHDA). *Pharmacology, Biochemistry and Behavior, 13,* 371–377.

Mabry, P. D., & Campbell, B. A. (1973). Serotonergic inhibition of catecholamine-induced behavioral arousal. *Brain Research, 49,* 381–391.

McLean, J. H., Kostrzewa, R. M., & May, J. G. (1976). Behavioral and biochemical effects of neonatal treatment of rats with 6-hydroxydopa. *Pharmacology, Biochemistry and Behavior, 4,* 601–607.

Mason, S. T., & Fibiger, H. C. (1979). Current concepts: 1. Anxiety: The locus coeruleus disconnection. *Life Sciences, 25,* 2141–2147.

Miller, F. E., Heffner, T. G., Kotake, C., & Seiden, L. S. (1981). Magnitude and duration of hyperactivity following neonatal 6-hydroxydopamine is related to the extent of brain dopamine depletion. *Brain Research, 229,* 123–132.

Morgan, D. N., McLean, J. H., & Kostrzewa, R. M. (1979). Effects of 6-hydroxydopamine and 6-hydroxydopa on development of behavior. *Pharmacology, Biochemistry and Behavior, 11,* 309–312.

Oke, A. F., & Adams, R. N. (1978). Selective attention dysfunctions in adult rats neonatally treated with 6-hydroxydopamine. *Pharmacology, Biochemistry & Behavior, 9,* 429–432.

Pappas, B. A., Gallivan, J. V., Dugas, T., Saari, M., & Ings, R. (1980). Intraventricular 6-hydroxydopamine in the newborn rat and locomotor responses to drugs in infancy: No support for the dopamine depletion model of minimal brain dysfunction. *Psychopharmacology, 70,* 41–46.

Pappas, B. A., & Sobrian, S. K. (1972). Neonatal sympathectomy for 6-hydroxydopamine in the rat: No effects on behavior but changes in endogenous brain norepinephrine. *Life Sciences, 11,* 653–659.

Paternite, C. E., & Loney, J. (1980). Childhood hyperkinesis: Relationships between symptomatology and home environment. In C. K. Whalen & B. Henker (Eds.), *Hyperactive children*. New York: Academic Press.

Pearson, D. E., Raskin, L. A., Shaywitz, B. A., Anderson, G. M., & Cohen, D. J. (1983). Radial arm maze performance in rats following neonatal 6-hydroxydopamine depletion. Manuscript submitted for publication.

Pearson, D. E., Teicher, M. H., Shaywitz, B. A., Cohen, D. J., Young, J. G., & Anderson, G. M. (1980). Environmental influences on body weight and behavior in developing rats after neonatal 6-hydroxydopamine. *Science, 209,* 715–717.

Peterson, D. W., & Laverty, R. (1976). Operant behavioral and neurochemical effects after neonatal 6-hydroxydopamine treatment. *Psychopharmacology, 50,* 55–60.

Rapoport, J. L., & Ferguson, H. B. (1981). Biological validation of the hyperkinetic syndrome. *Developmental Medicine and Child Neurology, 23,* 667–682.

Rapoport, J. L., & Zametkin, A. (1980). Attention deficit disorder. *Child Psychiatry: Contributions to Diagnosis, Treatment, and Research, 3,* 425–441.

Raskin, L. A., Shaywitz, B. A., Anderson, G. M., Cohen, D. J., Teicher, M. H., & Linakis, J. (1983). Differential effects of selective dopamine, norepinephrine, or catecholamine depletion on activity and learning in the developing rat. *Pharmacology, Biochemistry & Behavior 19,* 743–749.

Rosenblatt, J. S. (1979). The sensorimotor and motivational bases of early behavioral development of selected altricial mammals. In N. E. Spear & B. A. Campbell (Eds.), *Ontogeny of learning and memory*. New Jersey: Erlbaum.

Schwartz, S., & Johnson, J. H. (1981). *Psychopathology of childhood.* New York: Pergamon.

Shaywitz, B. A., Cohen, D. J., & Bowers, M. B. (1980). Cerebrospinal fluid monoamine metabolites in neurological disorders of childhood. In J. H. Wood (Ed.), *Neurobiology of cerebrospinal fluid.* New York: Plenum.

Shaywitz, B. A., Cohen, D. J., & Shaywitz, S. E. (1979). New diagnostic terminology for minimal brain dysfunction. *Journal of Pediatrics, 95,* 734–736.

Shaywitz, B. A., Gordon, J. W., Klopper, J. H., & Zelterman, D. A. (1977). The effect of 6-hydroxydopamine on habituation of activity in the developing rat pup. *Pharmacology, Biochemistry, & Behavior, 6,* 391–396.

Shaywitz, B. A., Klopper, J. H., & Gordon, J. W. (1978). Methylphenidate in 6-hydroxydopamine-treated developing rat pups. *Archives of Neurology, 35,* 463–469.

Shaywitz, B. A., Klopper, J. H., Yager, R. D. & Gordon, J. W. Paradoxical response to amphetamine in developing rats treated with 6-hydroxydopamine (1976). *Nature, 261,* 153–155.

Shaywitz, B. A., Kretschmar, C. S., Levitt, P., Teicher, M. H., Anderson, G. M., Young, J. G., & Cohen, D. J. (1983). *Selective damage to noradrenergic systems in the developing rat pup affects escape and avoidance performance but does not influence activity.* Manuscript submitted for publication.

Shaywitz, B. A., Teicher, M. H., Cohen, D. J., Anderson, G. M., Young, T. G., & Levitt, P. (in press). Dopaminergic but not noradrenergic mediation of hyperactivity and performance deficits in the developing rat pup. *Psychopharmacology.*

Shaywitz, B. A., Yager, R. D., & Klopper, J. H. (1976). Selective brain dopamine depletion in developing rats: An experimental model of minimal brain dysfunction. *Science, 191,* 305–308.

Shaywitz, S. E., & McGraw, K. (1982). Gifted and learning disabled: Shared behavior characteristics of gifted and learning disabled children. *Pediatric Research, 16,* 93a.

Shaywitz, S. E., & Shaywitz, B. A. (in press). Biological influences in attentional disorders. In M. D. Levine *et al.* (Ed.), *Developmental behavioral pediatrics.* Philadelphia, PA: Saunders.

Shaywitz, S. E., Shaywitz, B. A., Cohen, D. J., & Young, J. G. (in press). Monoaminergic mechanisms in hyperactivity. In M. Rutter (Ed.), *Behavioral syndromes of brain dysfunction in childhood.* New York: Guilford.

Sorenson, C. A., Vayer, J. S., & Goldberg, C. S. (1977). Amphetamine reduction of motor activity in rats after neonatal administration of 6-hydroxydopamine. *Biological Psychiatry, 12,* 133–137.

Teicher, M. H., Shaywitz, B. A., Kootz, H. L., and Cohen, D. J. (1981). Differential effects of maternal and sibling presence on hyperactivity of 6-hydroxydopamine-treated developing rats. *Journal of Comparative and Physiological Psychology, 95,* 134–145.

Thieme, R. E., Dijkstra, H., & Stoof, J. C. (1980). An evaluation of the young DA lesioned rat as an animal model for MBD. *Psychopharmacology, 67,* 165–169.

Weldon, D. A., Wool, R. S., Teicher, M. H., Shaywitz, B. A., Cohen, D. J., & Anderson, G. M. (1982). Effects of apomorphine on appetitive conditioning in 6-hydroxydopamine treated rat pups. *Pharmacology, Biochemistry and Behavior, 17,* 1281–1284.

Wender, P. M. (1971). *Minimal brain dysfunction in children.* New York: Wiley.

Whalen, C. K., & Henker, B. (1980). The social ecology of psychostimulant treatment: A model for conceptual and empirical analysis. In C. K. Whalen & B. Henker (Eds.), *Hyperactive children.* New York: Academic Press.

7

Recovery or Malformation after Fetal Radiation and Other Injuries*

Samuel P. Hicks,
Constance J. D'Amato,
and Roy A. Glover

Introduction

The regeneration of lost parts, the regulation of development and growth, the healing of wounds, and the grotesque distortions that these processes may undergo have long been a part of mythology, literature, and scientific observation. Prometheus, for giving fire from heaven to mortals, had his liver devoured by a vulture each day and regenerated a new one each night (Wessells, 1977). In the real world the capacity of the salamander to regenerate an amputated limb into a completely functional new one, even in adult life, is spectacular

*This work was supported by USPHS grant NS10531 and a University of Michigan Biomedical Research Council grant 2S07RR05383-22.

Copyright © 1984 by Academic Press, Inc.
All rights of reproduction in any form reserved.
ISBN 0-12-052901-7

(Nicholas, 1955). Anything like this degree of restoration in mature mammals, including man, has not been seen, perhaps because we do not know how to control the circumstances that would allow it. Probably no less spectacular in its way was the demonstration that amphibian embryos at early stages could recover from severe experimental injuries and mature normally or nearly normally as illustrated by the classic experiments of Harrison (1947). Of comparable interest to mammalologists were findings that rat and mouse fetuses that were severely injured by radiation can match some of the recovery feats of the amphibians (Hicks, 1954, 1958; Hicks, Brown, & D'Amato, 1957). We have shown that rats whose developing brains, spinal cords, and some other tissues were devastated by radiation at as late a stage as 35 somite pairs recovered by regulative regeneration so successfully as to be sometimes indistinguishable from normal rats in adult stages (D'Amato, 1982; D'Amato & Hicks, 1980).

Regulation, Morphogenetic Fields, and Recovery from Injury

Regulation includes all of the developmental processes that assure that the genetic blueprints are translated into a bee, a whale, or a human. The meaning of the word *regulate* in embryology is essentially its general meaning: to govern, direct according to rule, to fix the rate, time, degree or amount of something by adjusting or rectifying. Experimental embryologists have been most concerned with the rectifying activities of regulation, the "wholeness-restoring" capacity of the embryo in which an undamaged part of an embryo restores a damaged part (Cooke, 1980). It has been shown that as the neural plate formed, it developed "presumptive" regions, the removal of which prevented the formation of specific parts of the adult nervous system. But if a certain number of cells in one of these presumptive regions remained, they still had the regulative capacity to form the part of the nervous system that the whole region would have formed at that stage. Such cells were said to have the properties of a *morphogenetic field,* the smallest unit of tissue that could reproduce a whole organ or a substantial part of it. If insufficient cells remained, malformation or frank deficit resulted. Harrison (1947) showed that when one lateral half of the presumptive hindbrain was removed in amphibian embryos, the other half proliferated to restore it, and some of the animals that had been operated on matured with hindbrains that were structurally and functionally virtually normal. However, when both sides were removed, normal development failed. Little is known about the mechanisms of regulation and early development—how primitive regulating cells remaining after injury communicate with and contact each other as they regenerate losses and become integrated into the rest of the growing organism. Attempts to quantitate the influences from morphogenetic field centers as they govern development of surrounding cells have led to estimates that the influences may reach as far as 50 cell widths, a long distance in a tiny embryo (Wolpert, 1981). The nature of these influences is almost wholly unknown, but they are probably mediated by the three ways in which cells appear to communicate: (1) by exchange of molecules through special membrane channels in their junctions (gap junctions), (2) by release of molecules that reach receptors on other cells (humoral communication), and (3) by interaction between a pair of molecules on two adjacent cell membranes, sometimes via a helper glycoprotein (Loewenstein, 1980). Glover (Glover, D'Amato & Hicks, 1984) discovered in rat fetuses another significant form of communication, the extension of a short cytoplasmic process of one neuroepithelial cell into a coated vesicle in another (as described later). This may herald a significant mechanism for macromolecular change.

Cell Contacts and Junctions in the Neural Plate and Tube

Observations of the normally developing neural tube in lower vertebrates have shown that gap junctions may arise from tight junctions or appear de novo. Many detailed studies of the properties of these junctions have been made (Hertzberg, Lawrence & Gilula, 1981; Larsen, 1977). In one study of a mammal (mouse), during closure of the neural tube from forebrain to hindbrain, the first cells to come in contact over the midbrain were ectodermal, whereas at other levels they were neuroepithelial. In neither case was any elaborate junction formed until closure had occurred. The process was not a simple zipper-like operation (Geelen & Langman, 1979).

Interactions between the Epithelium (Neuroepithelium) and the Extracellular Matrix, including the Basement Membrane

Interest in how various epithelia interact with the extracellular matrix (ECM) including the basement membrane (BM) has grown rapidly, and neuroepithelial interaction promises to be one of the most exciting areas in normal and abnormal development of the nervous system. From the work of Hay (Cohen & Hay, 1971; Hay, 1978, 1981, 1982) it may be inferred that the BM that lies under embryonic epithelia and surrounds muscle is a cell exoskeleton composed of a dense, collagenous mat probably attached to the plasmalemma. It contains an inner and outer layer of glycosaminoglycan particles. BM are substrates for mesenchymal cells that migrate around embryonic epithelial tissues. By means of BM, epithelial cells influence the polymerization of underlying collagen fibrils. BM serve to filter ions and other molecules, controlling intracellular environments, and by the ECM molecules that they contain they interact with epithelia influencing their synthetic functions. The BM includes the *basal lamina,* a dense mat of ECM seen by electron microscopy, and other elements of the ECM.

When epithelium such as that of the embryonic chick cornea is deprived in vitro of its BM, the basal cytoplasm rapidly forms blebs. If it is provided with a basal lamina (lens capsule), alive or dead, it smooths out in a few hours and assumes a normal appearance. When epithelial cells are placed on an orthogonal lattice of collagen fibrils (dermis), they sit on it with their basal surfaces opposed to it; in contrast, mesenchymal cells invade such a matrix. The basal surface of epithelial cells is quite different from their lateral and apical surfaces. Both epithelial and mesenchymal cells contribute molecules such as those of collagen to the ECM including the BM. The neuroepithelium of the neural tube of the early chick embryo was shown to incorporate [^{3}H] proline, which was secreted in the form of collagen molecules that were demonstrated a short time later in the basal lamina and striated fibrils (Cohen & Hay, 1971). The secreted collagen and other substances may be inductors of those somites that appear at these early stages.

The developing cornea has also been used to demonstrate some interactions between the embryonic cell surface and cytoskeleton and the ECM. Among these actions, which were demonstrated in in vitro experiments, collagens I–IV, proteoglycans, fibronectin, and laminin, a glycoprotein of the lamina densa, all stimulated the epithelium to introduce more collagen and other substances into the ECM. These actions were heralded by the formation of organized cortical mats of basal cytoskeletal material in the epithelium. It is clear that the interface between embryonic epithelium, including neuroepithelium, and the ECM is a dynamic region, and it may be imagined that development can be disturbed in many ways here (Hay, 1982). As is seen in our current work (following) an altered BM has been implicated in abnormal development of the neural tube in in our experimental animals.

Radiation as an Experimental Tool in Studying Mammalian Regulation and Malformation

The degree of reproducibility of the malformative processes in rats that can be initiated by single exposures to 150–200 and occasionally 300 R, from induction of the neural plate to early infancy, when the retina and cerebellum are still developing, has not been approached by other teratogenic agents. This dose range produces the optimal combination of malformation and survival in the offspring. As the timetable in Figure 1 summarizes, there are other outcomes, including those from lower and higher doses. Experiments using dose levels that produce malformed offspring with little or no liklihood of postnatal survival may also yield valuable information.

Radiation can injure cells nonlethally in many ways, altering their reproduction, chromosomes, differentiation, and mature functions, and can also kill them outright. Rapid cell killing, chiefly of primitive proliferative and early differentiating cells in G_1 and G_2 phases, whether they be in the nervous system, mesenchyme, somites, or elsewhere, is the principle factor initiating the malformative processes in the 150–200-R range. This has been shown by [^{3}H] thymidine histologic autoradiography (to monitor stages in the mitotic and differentiation cycles) and by other observations. In a typical morphogenetic study we surgically removed by caesarean sections two or three fetuses from the same litter at a succession of stages during gestation, allowing some of the litter to be born and studied up to adult stages. From several litters it is possible to reconstruct the stepwise morphogenesis of malformations, recovery, or death.

We demonstrated that the fetal mammal's capacity for regulative recovery rivaled that of the amphibian (Hicks, 1954; Hicks, Brown &

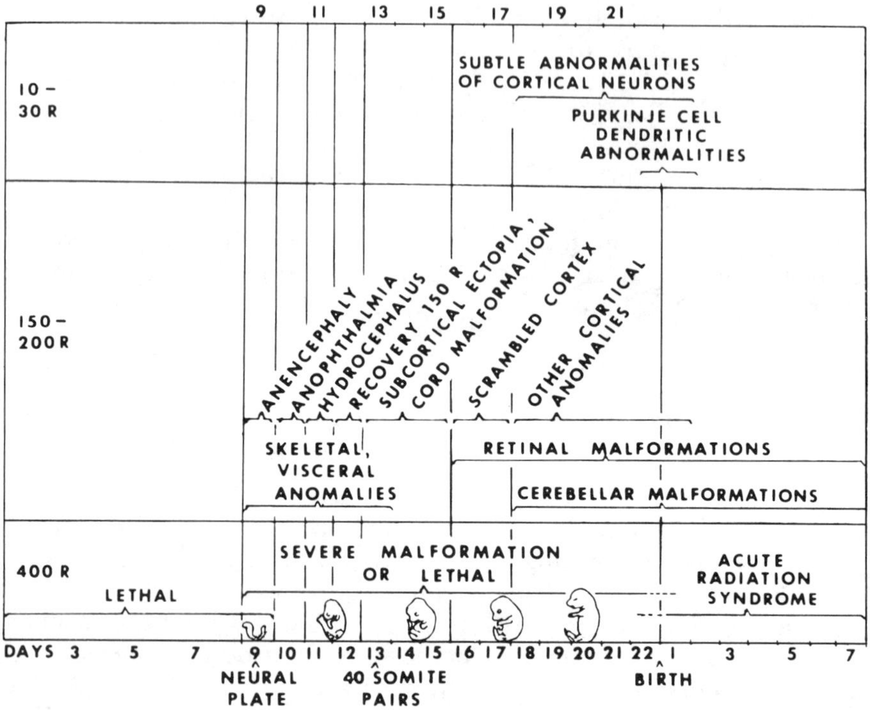

Figure 1. Timetable of effects of X-rays on rats at different stages of early life (From Hicks and D'Amato, American Journal of Forensic Medicine and Pathology, *1*, 309–317, 1980, with permission of the publisher).

D'Amato, 1957; D'Amato, 1982). In 10th-day fetal rats at about the 10–12 somite pair stage, there are rising neural folds and the spinal cord is already a neural tube. The primitive proliferative cells mentioned earlier, including especially those of the nervous system, dense mesenchyme, and parts of the somites, were decimated by 150 R. Mitotic activity, which was temporarily halted by the radiation, resumed after 2 or 3 hours, and by 24 hours proliferation of the residual primitive cells had already substantially restituted the losses. A majority of the dead cells had disappeared. In the spinal cord, those dead cells remaining had been pushed toward the periphery by the proliferating cells adjacent to the lumen. By 2 to 3 days after 150 R the fetuses were usually approaching the normal appearance for those stages; at birth and in adulthood the animals appeared normal, except that occasionally the eyes were small. If the radiation was given earlier on the 10th day, around 4 to 6 somite pairs, regulation again seemed to be very successful after 150 R, occurring everywhere that primitive cells were destroyed except where the optic vesicles would appear. The resulting adult animals had virtually no eyeballs or very rudimentary eye structures (anophthalmia) (Figure 1). When 150 R was given late on the 9th day at a stage comparable to Harrison's amphibian neural-plate stage, regulation by surviving presumptive forebrain cells and various cells of the dorsal head region failed. The animals that lived until birth showed what is best summed up as anencephaly, with the rest of the body being essentially normal except for an undifferentiated pituitary gland. Larger doses of radiation at this stage brought about death of the fetus (Hicks & D'Amato, 1966, 1978, 1980; Hicks, D'Amato, & Lowe, 1959).

Current Studies of Successful and Failed Regulation in Developing Rats

Introduction

To determine how a relatively few residual primitive neural cells left behind after radiation injury can regulate recovery, and how interactions between the neuroepithelium and the ECM and BM may contribute, we have set up five experiments.

The first two compare the effects of 150 and 200 R on the 12th fetal day, 35 somite pairs: After 150 R, as noted earlier, regulation may be virtually perfect, but after 200 R regulation fails, and encephalocele, a defective mantle, and other defects lead to death at birth.

In the second pair of experiments the effects of 150 and 225 R are observed on the 11th fetal day when regulation is successful after 150 R except for eye defects but 225 R leads to prenatal stenosis of the aqueduct with hydrocephalus. This is caused by an overgrowth of the midbrain–thalamus junction (MTJ) (D'Amato & Hicks, 1981b). This condition initiated by 225 R causes death of the rat at birth.

The fifth experiment involves a mutant rat in which the same kind of stenosis of the aqueduct and hydrocephalus occurs but it is compatible with survival to adulthood (D'Amato & Hicks, 1981a). This naturally occurring failure of regulation is associated with a defect in the neuroepithelial BM (Glover, D'Amato, & Hicks, 1983a). It is of interest that a form of prenatal aqueduct stenosis with hydrocephalus, that closely resembles that in 225 R irradiated fetuses and the mutant fetuses, has been produced by depriving pregnant rats of

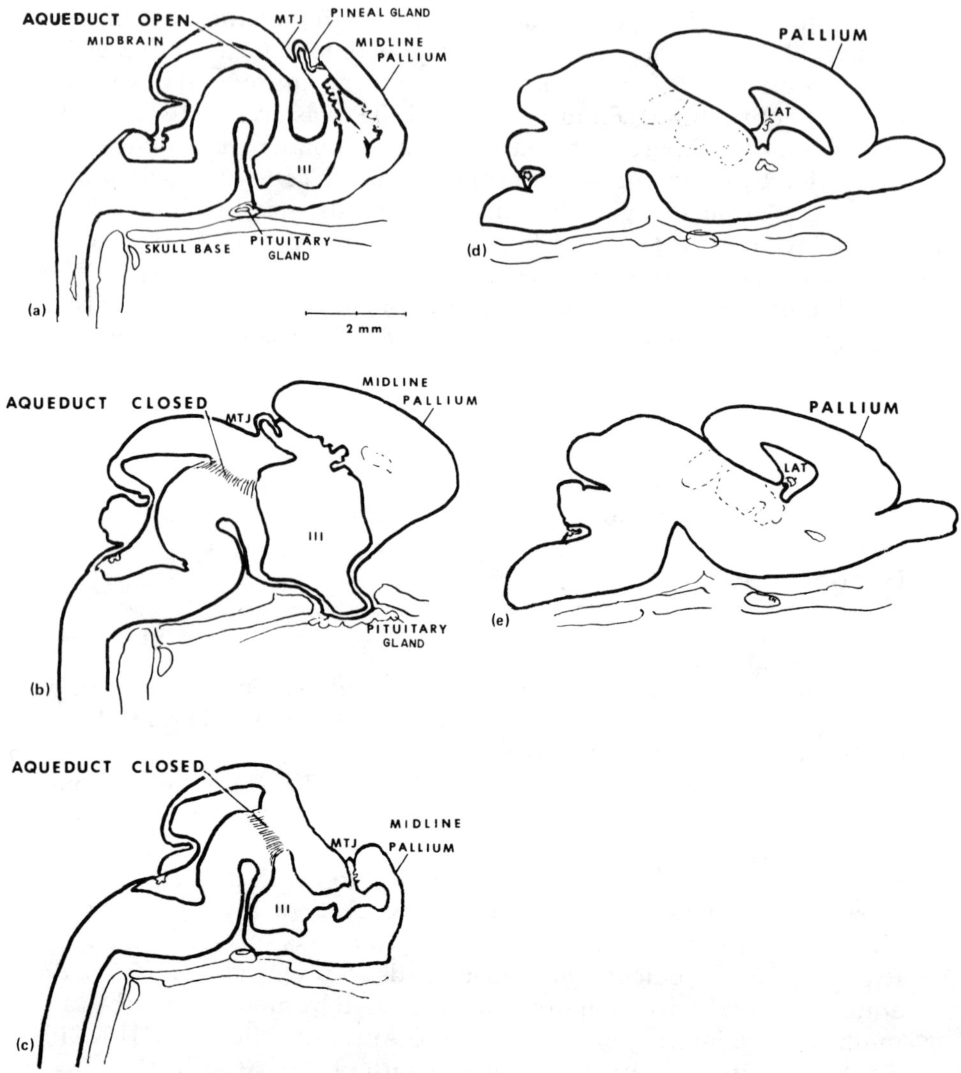

Figure 2. Sagittal views of the brains of normal, irradiated, and mutant fetal rats made by direct tracings of microscopic sections. (a) is a midline view of a normal 19th-day fetal brain with open aqueduct and normal MTJ. III indicates third ventricle. (b) is a midline view of a 21st-day fetal rat that may be compared with the 19th-day normal. It was exposed to 225 R on the 11th fetal day. The aqueduct is closed by the overgrowth and lengthening of the MTJ region. Pituitary gland and floor of third ventricle are abnormally placed compared with the normal fetus. More lateral views, not shown, reveal greatly enlarged lateral ventricles. (c) is a midline view of a 19th-day fetal mutant rat. The aqueduct is closed by overgrowth and lengthening of the MTJ region.

vitamin B_{12} or giving them folic acid analogs (Newberne & O'Dell, 1961; Stempak, 1965).

We give a brief account of these animals as the experiments have advanced so far. Figure 2 (a–e) summarizes some of the results that follow.

Irradiation on the 12th Fetal Day

During the 12th fetal day our rats progress from about 25 to 35 somite pairs. At this stage the animal has early developing cerebral hemispheres and beginning limb buds, the lungs and liver have appeared, and the heart is beating red blood. The wall of the cerebral hemisphere or vesicle is composed entirely of primitive proliferative neural cells that are likened to pseudostratified epithelium and also called fetal neuroepithelium or matrix cells, among others. Synthesis phase usually occurs when the nuclei of the cells are farthest from the lumen, and mitosis usually occurs after those nuclei move within their cellular cytoplasm close to the ventricular lumen.

Examination of a succession of stages from the time of exposure to 150 R revealed the following light-microscopic findings. In the dorsal pallium of the cerebral hemispheres, the optic vesicles, the diencephalon and dorsal midbrain, the lower brainstem and spinal cord, the mesenchyme, and the dermatomes of the somites from more than one half to three quarters of the primitive cells had been killed and were disintegrating several hours after irradiation. Dead cells were principally in the outer two thirds of the cerebral vesicle but were also fairly often close to the ventricular surface, especially where the continuity of the ventricular lining was briefly disrupted. Some dead cells escaped into the ventricle. A few phagocytes occurred for the first time several hours after irradiation on the 12th day, but they seemed to contribute almost nothing to the total dissolution of the dead cells. After 24 hours the residual primitive cells had largely replaced the losses, and most of the dead cells had disappeared. The

---

More lateral views, not shown, reveal greatly enlarged lateral ventricles. (d) is a sagittal view, lateral to the midline, of a normal 21st-day fetal rat. LAT indicates lateral ventricle, dotted lines indicate certain thalamic regions. (e) is a comparable view of the 21st-day fetal rat exposed to 150 R on the 12th fetal day. The brain as a whole is slightly smaller than that of the normal. This could be due to less than perfect regulative recovery after irradiation, or it could be that the fetus was slightly younger than the normal at the time of removal for study.

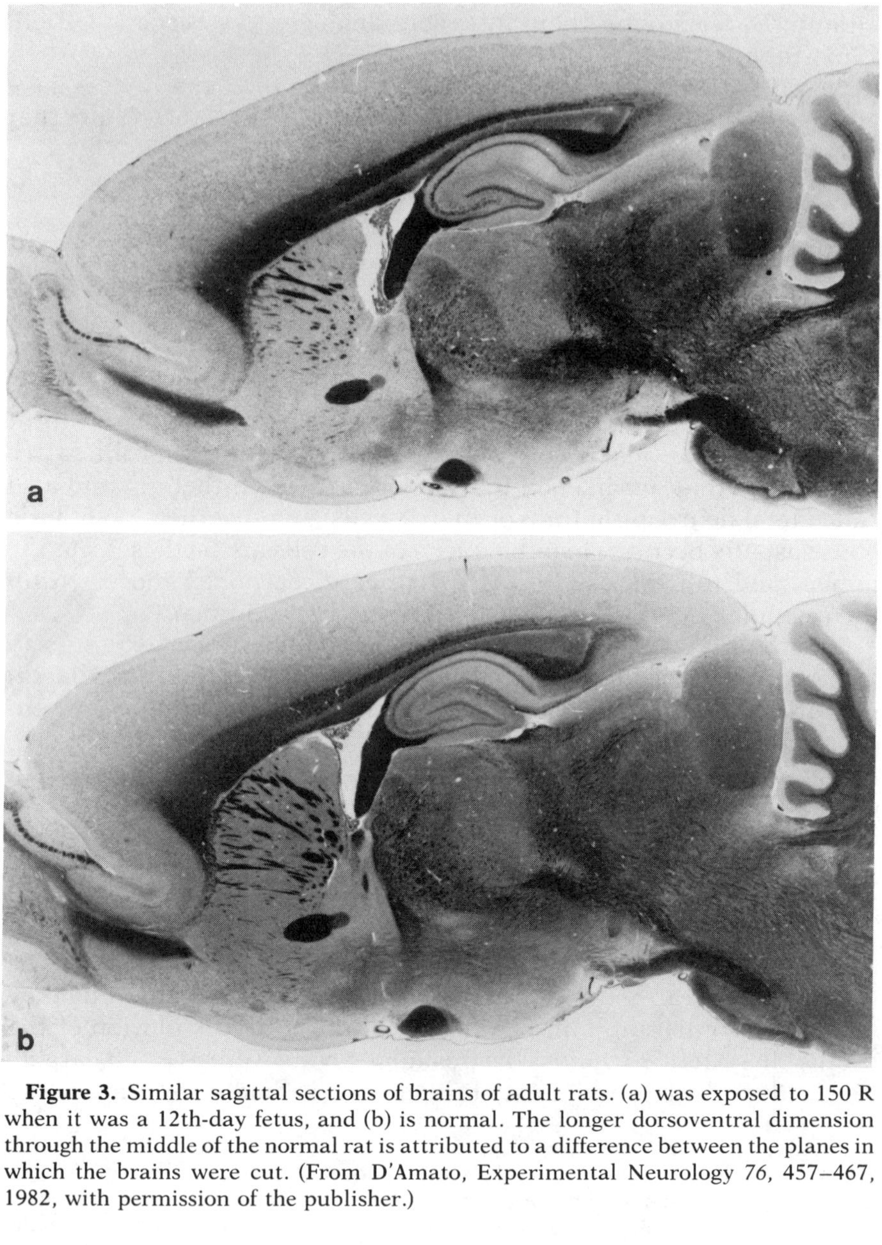

Figure 3. Similar sagittal sections of brains of adult rats. (a) was exposed to 150 R when it was a 12th-day fetus, and (b) is normal. The longer dorsoventral dimension through the middle of the normal rat is attributed to a difference between the planes in which the brains were cut. (From D'Amato, Experimental Neurology *76*, 457–467, 1982, with permission of the publisher.)

few phagocytes persisted. The nuclei and cytoplasmic surfaces of the proliferative cell populations were more sharply defined by light microscopy than they are in normal brains. By 48 hours the animals were well on their way to normal development, and at 72 hours it was essentially impossible to distinguish the irradiated fetuses from normal fetuses. Dead cells and phagocytes had disappeared by 72 hours.

Also examined were 10 mature animals that had been irradiated with 150 R on the 12th fetal day. Some were indistinguishable from normal animals, both grossly and by examination of serial histologic sections of the brain (Figure 3). Of the 10, 3 showed a slight deficiency of the medial occipital part of the cerebral hemispheres, which was made evident by an abnormal slight exposure of the midbrain. Retrograde labeling of corticospinal neurons with horseradish peroxidase showed that in some animals the apical dendrites were very rarely bifurcated, a curious and unexplained finding. Slow-motion movies of some of these adults showed normal ordinary and certain skilled forms of locomotion, such as jumping various distances from one platform to another or traversing narrow paths. The most serious defect, found in 3 of the 10, was maldevelopment of the eyes; 1 of the 3 in which this occurred was a runt, but its brain was grossly normal (D'Amato & Hicks, 1980).

Twelfth-day fetal rats exposed to 200 R developed a posterior dorsal encephalocele that involved the roof of the third ventricle and the epithalamic region at its junction with the midbrain, and there was subcutaneous accumulation of leaked cerebrospinal fluid. The lateral ventricles were enlarged, the result of much reduced development of the mantle. This syndrome caused death at the time of birth.

Irradiation on the 11th Fetal Day

The rat fetus at the 11th fetal day shows the earliest cerebral vesicles, sometimes with the anterior neuropore just closing, the optic vesicles just beginning to form retinas, and anterior limb buds. During the 11th day the fetus advances from about 14 to 22 somite pairs. Results of the experiments, principally using light microscopy, are as follows. Destruction of cells after exposure to 150 R was generally comparable to that in 10th- and 12th-day fetuses, involving both neuroepithelium and mesenchyme in the dorsal MTJ. No phagocytes appeared at this stage. At 24 to 48 hours it appeared that regulation might be quite successful, although the eyes almost always showed some maldevelopment and occasionally there was a slight dorsal protrusion of the roof of the third ventricle close to the pineal gland in later fetal stages. Adults commonly but not always showed defects of the eyes and occasionally slight narrowing of the face. No hydrocephalus and no abnormality of the MTJ has been seen in fetal animals among a number of litters irradiated at different times during the 24-hour span of the 11th fetal day, except for the occasional, minute protrusion of the dorsal third ventricle.

At this point we are close to the threshold of failure of regulation of the MTJ region: this is indicated by (1) the occasional slight disturbance of third ventricle roof development, (2) the occurrence of hydrocephalus with postnatal survival by irradiation on the 11th fetal day with 150 R in other strains of rats, and (3) the production of overgrowth of the MTJ and consequent stenosis of the aqueduct with hydrocephalus by irradiation on the 11th day with 175 or 185 R (Hicks, Brown & D'Amato, 1957; Hicks & D'Amato, 1963; Glover, D'Amato & Hicks, 1983b). Many of these higher-dose offspring died at birth, and although hydrocephalus was frequent among them, others did not develop it and survived postnatally. Two animals grew to adulthood with enlarged heads and showed marked hydrocephalus of the lateral ventricles, with a paper-thin dorsal mantle, enlarged third ventricle, and stenosis of the aqueduct. Radiation-induced hydrocephalics are fragile, as we observed in earlier studies.

When 225 R was given on the 11th fetal day, hydrocephalus regularly developed, and the underlying cause was narrowing of the aqueduct. The condition was lethal at birth. The basic steps in the morphogenesis are as follows. The initial necrosis of cells is heavier after this dose than after 150 R. There is substantial repair at first, but by about the 14th fetal day the MTJ is a little thicker than normal, and by 16 days it is definitely thicker, with some increase of fibers of the posterior commissure and the commissure of the superior colliculus. Minute neuroepithelial ectopias of the dorsal MTJ region, similar to those to be described in the mutant, are sometimes seen 24 and 48 hours after 225 R on the 11th fetal day. By about 19 to 21 days the thickening of the MTJ, including the posterior epithalamic region, is quite marked, either substantially narrowing or closing the aqueduct. With closing, dilation of the lateral and third ventricles ensues. In all of the 225-R animals, the pituitary gland came to lodge in the roof of the nasal cavity, because of a developmental defect in the sphenoid bone. We have not seen the pituitary anomaly in the 175–185-R rats (D'Amato & Hicks, 1981b; Glover, D'Amato, & Hicks, 1983b).

Genetic Prenatal Aqueduct Stenosis with Hydrocephalus

We have studied for some time the developmental effects of a homozygous recessive mutation that arose spontaneously in our line of long brother–sister-mated Wistar albino rats. The gene is also kept in a related hooded line. The constant gene marker is a slight sparsity of hair that is recognized soon after birth; the aqueduct stenosis–hydrocephalus syndrome is variably expressed. The morphogenetic sequence leading to the aqueduct malformation as seen light-microscopically is as follows. On the 11th fetal day, foci of minute indentations of the ventricular lining cells appear in the MTJ region. Ectopic foci of neuroepithelial cells appear on the external surface of the MTJ region. These ectopias sometimes form a lumen. By the 14th fetal day there is a well-developed thickening and indentation of the region of the MTJ, with excessive numbers of posterior and collicular commissural fibers. Although there is lengthening and thickening of the MTJ region in both the radiation-induced and gene-induced syndromes, this indentation is peculiar to the mutant. The thickening and to some extent the indentation of the MTJ region continues to increase until the aqueduct is occluded or greatly narrowed, usually about the 18th or 19th fetal day. Hydrocephalus with enlargement of the lateral and third ventricles follow closure of the aqueduct. This is usually obvious at birth, but sometimes it either develops more slowly or is so minimally expressed (with partial aqueduct stenosis) as to be evident only at autopsy. Some homozygous animals, especially from heterozygote matings, show none of the hydrocephalic feature of the syndrome. The eyes are commonly but not always defective. The minute ectopias of the MTJ are rarely seen as microscopic, mature ectopic brain tissue in mature rats (D'Amato & Hicks, 1981a).

Electron Microscopic Studies of Normal, 11th-Fetal-Day Irradiated, and Mutant Rats

Electron microscope (EM) examinations have been made on the MTJ region of normal 11th-, 12th-, and 13th-day rat fetuses, on fetuses irradiated with 150 or 225 R on the 11th day and surgically removed $5\frac{1}{2}$ or 24 hours afterwards, and on mutant fetuses removed on the 11th or 12th fetal day. Junctional contacts have been observed between neuroepithelial cells of the neural tube wall in all fetuses examined, normal and abnormal. One type of junction appears as defined points of focal contact between adjacent cell membranes. These contacts are observed at many points along the apicobasal extent of the cells but appear to be less numerous at the base of the tube wall. Many of these junctions resemble the gap junctions described by other investigators in earlier stages of various species. Another morphologic surface feature between cells in primitive proliferative populations that has not been described previously occurs in early fetuses: a short cytoplasmic process extending from one neural tube cell into a large, coated vesicle at the surface of its neighbor. The process appears to contain a core of fine filaments and tubules, and it ends in a small saclike dilation. These specialized surface structures have been seen in all the normal and abnormal fetuses processed so far (Glover, D'Amato & Hicks, 1984). It is still unclear, however, what function these particular structures might perform. One might speculate that they are involved in the transfer of macromolecules from one differentiating cell to another. Such transfer might occur both through the uptake of surface molecules and possibly, and even more interestingly, through the ingestion of small pieces of cell cytoplasm. Some micrographs appear to show internalized coated vesicles containing a dense inclusion in their centers. It is well known that coated vesicles, which participate in intracytoplasmic transfer of material, might also be involved in the internalization of surface macromolecules that could influence cell differentiation.

The luminal surface of the neural tube in all fetuses examined so far shows specialized tight junctions that appear to seal the developing neurocoele from the intercellular environment of the tube wall. These junctions are thought to be important because of the role they might play in determining and directing the movement of migrating cells and also because of their control of freedom of passage of material from the neurocoele into the neural tube itself. The effect of luminal fluid on differentiation and cell proliferation presents an interesting problem in light of the fact that we have been able to see definitive breaks in the luminal lining in the mutant animals and in the irradiated animals a few hours after exposure. Altogether, the various kinds of cell contact seen have not differed qualitatively between normal and abnormal animals.

The basal surface of the neuroepithelium of all control fetuses and 150-R irradiated fetuses (Figure 4) have revealed a definitive, continuous BL separating the neuroepithelium from the underlying mesenchyme.

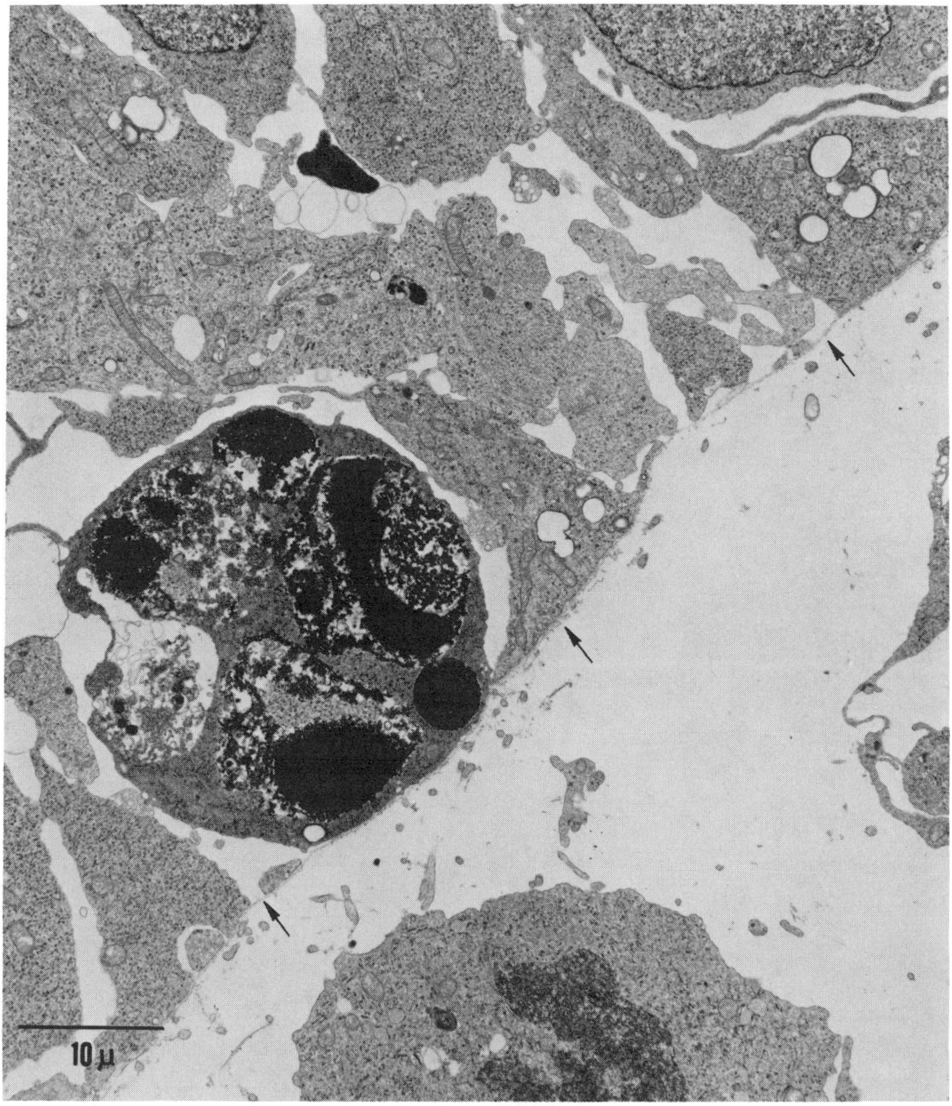

Figure 4. Eleventh-day fetus, 24 hours following irradiation with 150 R, midbrain–thalamic junction. Reduced from × 2750. The arrows indicate a continuous basement membrane between the neuroepithelium and the mesenchymal compartment. Note that this interface is regular in its organization in spite of the level of radiation exposure. A dead cell can be seen resting on the basement membrane.

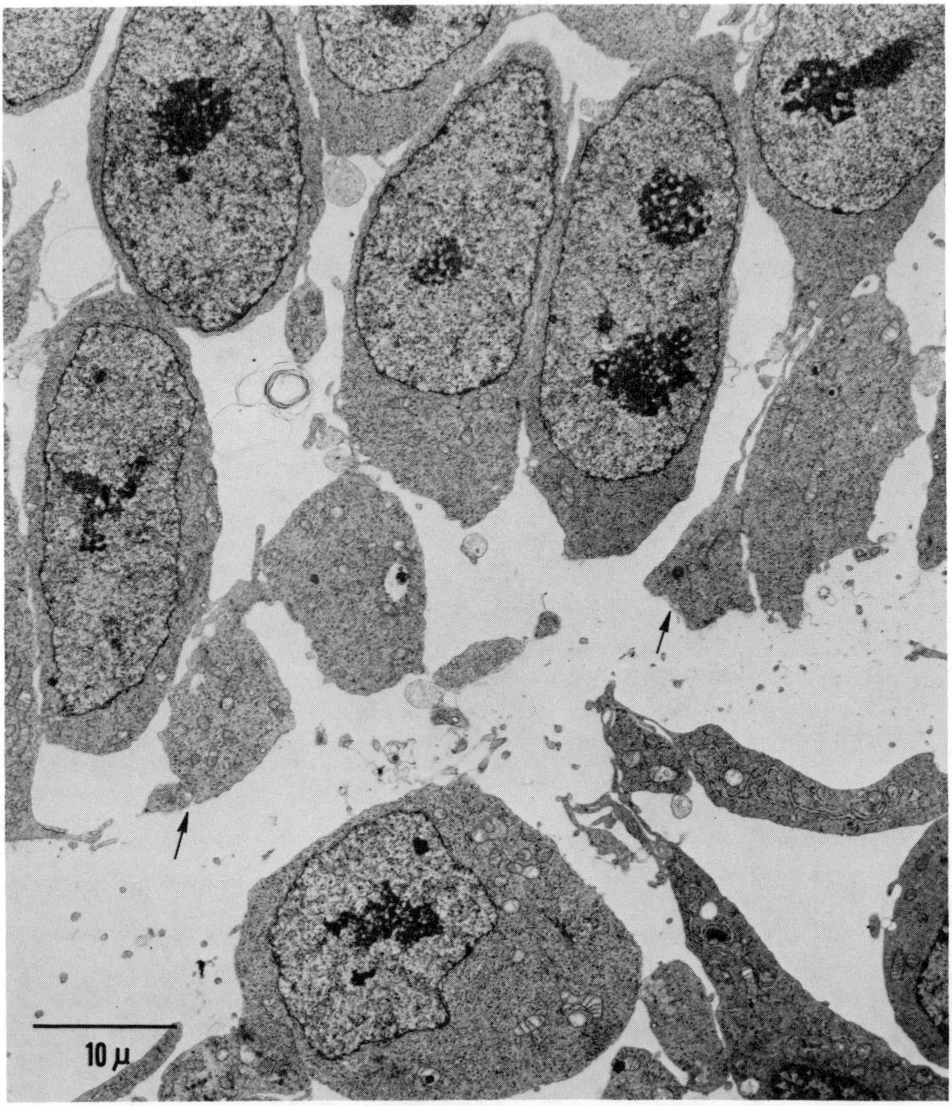

Figure 5. Eleventh-day mutant hydrocephalic fetus, midbrain–thalamus junction. Reduced from × 2750. The arrows indicate small segments of intact basement membrane that are separated by major discontinuities, thus allowing contact and mixing of cells between the neuroepithelium and mesenchyme. Note that this interface is very irregular and exhibits a lack of organization.

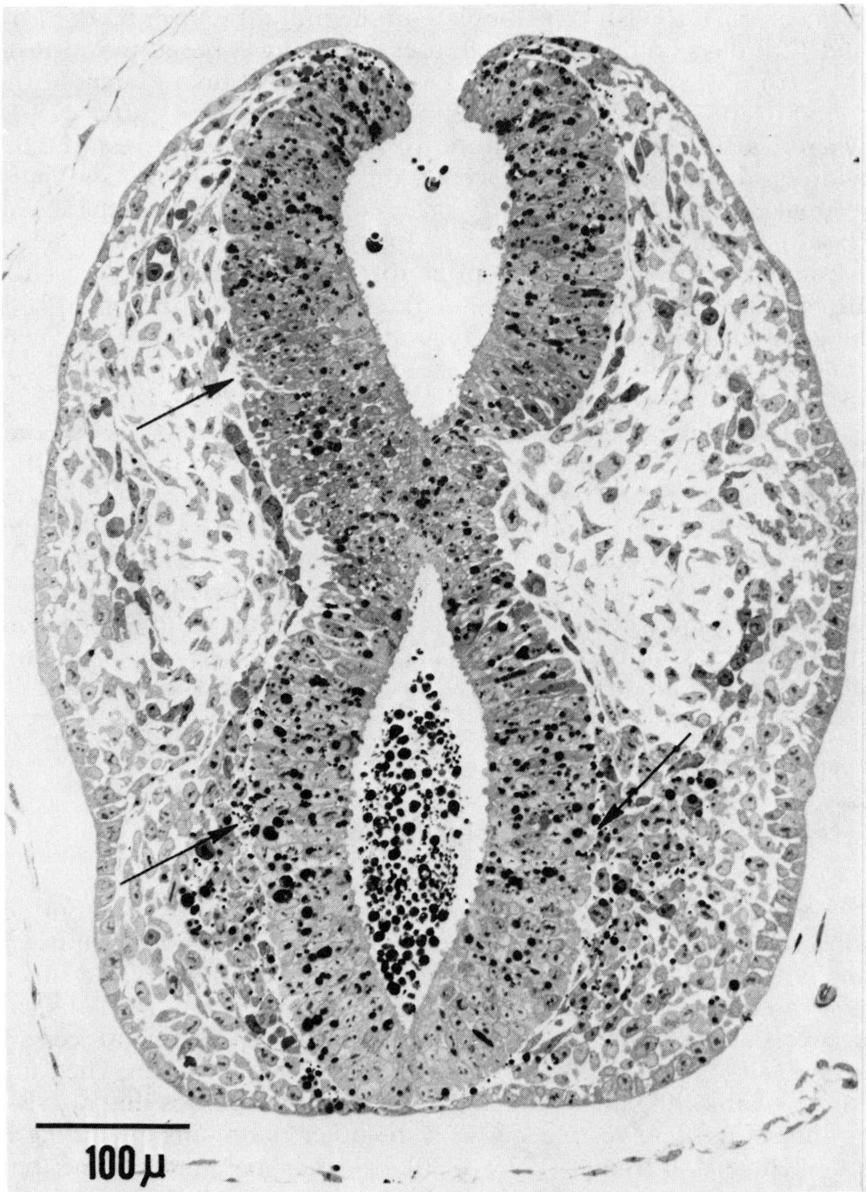

Figure 6. Eleventh-day fetus, $5\frac{1}{2}$ hours following irradiation with 225 R, midbrain–thalamus junction. Reduced from 200 ×. This 2-µ section shows extensive irradiation damage to the neuroepithelium with extensive cellular debris in the developing neurocoele. The arrows indicate focal irregularities along the base of the neural tube, where there often appears to be access of mesenchymal cells to the tube wall.

In contrast, the BL is incomplete in the mutant fetuses on the 11th and 12th days, and in normal fetuses that were exposed to 225 R on the 11th day and examined by EM $5\frac{1}{2}$, 24, or 48 hours later. In the mutant fetuses and in those examined 24 or 48 hours after 225 R, when regeneration had substantially, albeit abnormally, restored the neuroepithelium, the interface of the neuroepithelium and mesenchyme is no longer linearly ordered, but irregular and ragged. Basal neuroepithelial cells show cytoplasmic blebs (Figure 5). There is contact between the neuroepithelium and mesenchyme where the BL is absent (Glover, *et al.* 1983a, b). Thick sections from the MTJ $5\frac{1}{2}$ hours after 225 R show focal irregularities along the base of the neural tube, where there often appears to be access of mesenchymal cells to the tube wall (Figure 6).

In normal rat embryos it appears that blood vessels and accompanying mesenchymal elements first invade the parts of the wall of the neural tube under study between the 12th and 13th fetal days. Light-microscopic examination of thick sections on the 13th day show areas of penetration of vascular and cellular elements between cells of the basal layer of the neural tube. Occasional phagocytes within the tube wall can also be seen at this time. Study of electron micrographs confirms the presence both of these occasional phagocytes and of blood vessels between developing neuroepithelial cells in these normal animals.

Concluding Remarks

Regenerative processes that lead to spectacular recovery from destructive injury are commonly thought to be the preserve of submammalian vertebrates and simpler organisms. The studies of the effects of irradiation in the 150 R range show that the early rat fetus can recover remarkably well from devastating cell-killing at certain stages, rivalling the amphibian embryos (Harrison, 1947). The same kind of cell-killing and some of the reparative responses that are seen in the rat are known to occur in some other mammals, including in man (Hicks & D'Amato, 1978, 1980). It is reasonable to assume that, as a class, we mammals have evolved with a substantial capacity as fetuses to repair injuries to our primitive cell populations. Some viruses and many drugs and chemicals, as well as radiation, can destroy these primitive cells, but not necessarily as extensively as in the 150-R rat experiments. It is likely that many of us developed in the range we call normal because our regulative regenerative powers were successful in overcoming the effects of one of these lesser injuries.

Many of our radiation experiments have been designed to push the regulative responses of the fetuses to the limit, and as a consequence we have observed some animals that have nearly completely recovered, when others exhibit relatively minor defects (compared to extensive malformations after higher doses). The 12th-day and 11th-day fetuses exposed to 150 R are illustrative. By this approach we have begun to analyze some of the mechanisms by which regulation fails or succeeds. We have previously indicated that cell-killing is a prime initiator of the responses that the fetus puts forth to restore itself following injury, whether the outcome is recovery or malformation. The regenerative response is the fetus's attempt to restore its losses. However, little is known about how cell-killing initiates those responses. Our finding that alteration of the BL between the neuroepithelium and mesenchyme of the MTJ is associated with failure to regulate successfully after radiation injury indicates that integrity of this structure is a critical factor for normal development and successful regeneration. Just how cell-killing may relate to loss of integrity of the BL is not clear, however. More cells are killed after 11th-day fetuses are exposed to 225 R, following which the BL breaks down, than after 150 R, when it does not. It is possible that the fewer neuroepithelial cells remaining after 225 R, compared with those after 150 R, affects this cell-population's ability to produce or maintain the BL. However it is also possible that the higher dose of radiation directly affects the BL. In the case of the mutant there is a similar BL defect in the MTJ illustrating that cell-killing is not necessary for this condition to occur. The three situations represented by (1) the normal fetuses exposed to 225 R or (2) normal fetuses exposed to 150 R, or (3) the mutant fetuses, provide promising in vivo models of BL functions that may help answer questions about why fetal recovery succeeds or fails.

References

Cohen, A. M., & Hay, E. D. (1971). Secretion of collagen by embryonic neuroepithelium at the time of spinal cord-somite interaction. *Developmental Biology, 26,* 578–605.

Cooke, J. (1980). Early organization of the central nervous system: Form and pattern. *Current Topics in Developmental Biology, 15,* 373–407.

D'Amato, C. J. (1982). Regeneration and recovery in the fetal nervous system after radiation injury. *Experimental Neurology, 76,* 457–467.

D'Amato, C. J., & Hicks, S. P. (1980). Development of the motor system: Effects of radiation on developing corticospinal neurons and locomotor function. *Experimental Neurology, 70,* 1–23.

D'Amato, C. J., & Hicks, S. P. (1981a). Prenatal genetic aqueduct stenosis causing hydrocephalus. American Association of Neuropathologists Annual Meeting. *Journal Neuropathology Experimental Neurology, 40,* 358.

D'Amato, C. J., & Hicks, S. P. (1981b). Hydrocephalus produced by prenatal irradiation. Society for Neuroscience Annual Meeting. *Neuroscience Abstracts, 7,* 467.

Geelen, J. A. G., & Langman, J. (1979). Ultrastructural observations on closure of the neural tube in the mouse. *Anatomy & Embryology, 156,* 73–88.

Glover, R. A., D'Amato, C. J., & Hicks, S. P. (1983a). Basement membrane–neuroepithelial interrelations in the etiology of genetic aqueductal stenosis with hydrocephalus. American Academy Neurology, Annual Meeting, *Neurology. 33,* 221.

Glover, R. A., D'Amato, C. J., & Hicks, S. P. (1983b). Malformation (hydrocephalus) following x-irradiation: neuroepithelial-mesenchymal basal lamina relations. Society for Neuroscience Annual Meeting. *Neuroscience Abstracts 9,* 595.

Glover, R. A., D'Amato, C. J. & Hicks, S. P. (1984). A new cell surface relationship between neuroepithelial cells during rat neural tube development. *Experimental Neurology, 83,* 199–203.

Harrison, R. G. (1947). Wound healing and reconstitution of the central nervous system of the amphibian embryo after removal of parts of the neural plate. *Journal Experimental Zoology, 106,* 27–84.

Hay, E. D. (1978). Role of basement membranes in development and differentiation. In N. A. Kefalides (Ed.), *Biology and chemistry of basement membranes* (pp. 119–136). New York, Academic Press.

Hay, E. D. (1981). Extracellular matrix. *Journal Cell Biology, 91,* 205–223.

Hay, E. D. (1982). Interaction of embryonic cell surface and cytoskeleton with extracellular matrix. *American Journal Anatomy, 165,* 1–12.

Hertzberg, E. L., Lawrence, T. S., & Gilula, N. B. (1981). Gap junctional communication. *Annual Review Physiology, 43,* 479–491.

Hicks, S. P. (1952). Some effects of ionizing radiation and metabolic inhibition on the developing nervous system. *Journal Pediatrics 40,* 489–513.

Hicks, S. P. (1954). Mechanisms of radiation anencephaly, anophthalmia, and pituitary anomalies. Repair in the mammalian embryo. *Archives Pathology, 54,* 363–378.

Hicks, S. P. (1958). Radiation as an experimental tool in mammalian developmental neurology. *Physiological Reviews, 38,* 337–356.

Hicks, S. P., Brown, B. L., & D'Amato, C. J. (1957). Regeneration and malformation in the nervous system, eye, and mesenchyme of the mammalian embryo after radiation injury. *American Journal of Pathology, 33,* 459–481.

Hicks, S. P. & D'Amato, C. J. (1963). Effects of radiation on the developing embryo and fetus. In J. V. Meigs & S. H. Sturgis (Eds.), *Progress in Gynecology, 4* (pp. 58–74). New York: Grune & Stratton.

Hicks, S. P., & D'Amato, C. J. (1966). Effects of ionizing radiation on mammalian development. In D. H. M. Woollam (Ed.), *Advances in teratology* (Vol. 1, pp. 195–250). London: Logos.

Hicks, S. P., & D'Amato, C. J. (1978). Effects of ionizing radiations on developing brain and behavior. In G. Gottlieb (Ed.), *Studies on the development of behavior and the nervous system: Early influences* (pp. 35–72). New York: Academic Press.

Hicks, S. P., & D'Amato, C. J. (1980). Effects of radiation on development, especially the nervous system. *Journal Forensic Medicine & Pathology, 1*, 309–317.

Hicks, S. P., D'Amato, C. J., & Lowe, M. J. (1959). The development of the mammalian nervous system. I. Malformations of the brain, especially the cerebral cortex, induced in rats by radiation. II. Some mechanisms of the malformations of the cortex. *Journal Comparative Neurology, 113*, 435–469.

Larsen, W. J. (1977). Structural diversity of gap junctions. A review. *Tissue and Cell, 9*, 373–394.

Loewenstein, W. R. (1980). Symposium on molecular and morphologic aspects of cell–cell communication. Introductory remarks to the symposium. *In Vitro 16*, 1007–1009.

Newberne, P. M. & O'Dell, B. L. (1961). Vitamin B_{12} deficiency and hydrocephalus. In W. S. Fields & M. M. Desmond (Eds.), *Disorders of the developing nervous system* (pp. 123–143). Springfield, IL: Thomas.

Nicholas, J. S. (1955). Regeneration in vertebrates. In B. H. Willier, P. A. Weiss, & V. Hamburger (Eds.), *Analysis of development* (pp. 674–698). Philadelphia: Saunders.

Stempak, J. G. (1965). Etiology of antenatal hydrocephalus induced by folic acid deficiency in the albino rat. *Anatomic Record, 151*, 287–295.

Wessells, N. K. (1977). *Tissue Interactions and Development* (p 168), Menlo Park, CA: Benjamin/Cummings.

Wolpert, L. (1981). Positional information and pattern formation. *Philosophical Transactions Royal Society London B, 295*, 441–450.

III

Short- and Long-Term Neurological Effects of Brain Damage in Children

8

The Neurological Outcome of Perinatal Asphyxia

Katherine L. Kreusser
and Joseph J. Volpe

Introduction

Hypoxic–ischemic brain injury produced by perinatal asphyxia is the most important neurological problem of the perinatal period. It is the most frequent cause of neurological morbidity in the fullterm infant, and in conjunction with intraventricular hemorrhage it results in most of the major neurological morbidity in the premature infant (Volpe, 1981). The neurological morbidity that occurs as a result of neonatal hypoxic–ischemic encephalopathy accounts for a large percentage of the nonprogressive neurological deficits seen in children. The deficits of concern are, principally, mental retardation, seizures, and a number of motor deficits including spasticity, choreoathetosis, and ataxia.

In this chapter, we review the clinical aspects of neonatal hypoxic–ischemic encephalopathy and the long-term outcome of infants who

EARLY BRAIN DAMAGE, Volume 1
Research Orientations and Clinical Observations

Copyright © 1984 by Academic Press, Inc.
All rights of reproduction in any form reserved.
ISBN 0-12-052901-7

sustain this injury. In order to better explain the clinical aspects, we review the major neuropathological lesions, particularly as they relate to neurological features, prognosis, and management.

Neuropathological Features

The neuropathological features of neonatal hypoxic–ischemic encephalopathy vary considerably with the gestational age of the infant. Recognition of the basic lesions provides a useful framework for discussion of the clinical aspects. Brain swelling and brain necrosis are reviewed in addition to the distinct neuropathological varieties of neonatal hypoxic–ischemic encephalopathy.

Brain Swelling

Whether significant brain swelling occurs in neonatal hypoxic–ischemic encephalopathy in the absence of a major degree of tissue necrosis remains a controversial issue. Certainly, significant brain swelling is unusual in infants born prior to 36 weeks gestation. This may be explained on the basis of the observation that glial proliferation is not a prominent feature in the human cerebrum until the third trimester of gestation and beyond and glia are important sites for brain swelling in association with hypoxic–ischemic brain injury. When swelling does occur in mature infants, the severity of the swelling appears to be related to the severity of concomitant tissue necrosis. Experimental studies in nonhuman primates have failed to resolve this issue (Brann & Myers, 1975; Levy, Brierley, Silverman, & Plum, 1975).

Selective Neuronal Necrosis

Selective neuronal necrosis is the most common variety of injury observed in neonatal hypoxic–ischemic encephalopathy. It consists of necrosis of neurons in a characteristic though often widespread distribution. The injury often coexists with other manifestations of neonatal hypoxic–ischemic encephalopathy and is virtually always present when other specific hypoxic–ischemic lesions are present. As the extent and distribution of neuronal injury in living newborns cannot be determined precisely, the frequency of this injury in survivors of perinatal asphyxia is not known.

CELLULAR ASPECTS

In the neuron, cytoplasmic vacuolation occurs within 5 to 30 minutes of the onset of hypoxia (Levy *et al.*, 1975). The mitochondrion is the primary initial subcellular site of injury, as might be predicted from its function in oxidative phosphorylation and energy production. Early neuronal changes include eosinophilia of neuronal cytoplasm, loss of endoplasmic reticulum and pyknosis or fragmentation of nuclei. The identification of these neuronal changes will be affected by both the gestational age of the infant and the duration of survival after the asphyxial insult. The early changes are followed in several days by signs of cell necrosis, with the appearance of microglia and later, hypertrophic astrocytes.

REGIONAL ASPECTS

Sites of predilection for selective neuronal necrosis are numerous and widespread. Neurons of the cerebral cortex are particularly vulnerable, with the pyramidal cells of the hippocampus being especially prone to injury. Severe insults may lead to injury of neurons of the visual cortex and of the motor and sensory cortices. Neurons of deep cortical layers, particularly in the depths of sulci, are often affected (Takashima, Armstrong, & Becker, 1978). Particularly severe neuronal injury is consistently observed in border zones between major cerebral arteries.

In the diencephalon, thalamic and hypothalmic neurons as well as those of the lateral geniculate bodies are vulnerable to hypoxic–ischemic insult. Of the basal ganglia, neurons of the caudate, putamen, and globus pallidus are injured most often.

Involvement of the brainstem is particularly characteristic of hypoxic–ischemic encephalopathy in the newborn (Leech & Alvord, 1977). In the midbrain, the inferior colliculus appears to be most vulnerable. Neurons of the oculomotor and trochlear nuclei, substantia nigra, and reticular formation are also susceptible. In the pons, motor nuclei of n. V and n. VII, the reticular formation, the cochlear nuclei, and the pontine nuclei are frequently involved (Brierley, Meldrum, & Brown, 1973). Involvement of the pontine nuclei in conjunction with involvement of the neurons of the subicular portion of the hippocampus has led to the description of a particular pattern of neuronal injury, pontosubicular neuronal necrosis, which may be characteristic of the premature infant who experiences perinatal hypoxia and acidosis, followed by hyperoxia (Barmada, Moossy, & Painter, 1980; Friede, 1972).

In the medulla, dorsal motor nuclei of the vagus, nucleus ambiguus, inferior olivary nuclei, and cuneate and gracile nuclei are particularly vulnerable.

The cerebellum is also vulnerable to hypoxic–ischemic insults, and the Purkinje cells are the most vulnerable of the cerebellar neurons. Additionally, neurons of the dentate nuclei may be susceptible to injury in the newborn period.

PATHOGENESIS

Hypoxemia and related metabolic effects may be the critical factor in the production of selective neuronal necrosis. This suggestion is supported by the fact that the injury is not strictly in vascular distributions and by the experimental observation that selective neuronal necrosis may be produced by decreasing oxygen tension in cultured cerebellar explants (Kim, 1975). Disturbed calcium homeostasis, excessive intracellular lactate accumulation, and the toxicity of neurotransmitters released from damaged neurons may also be crucial in determining the extent of neuronal necrosis (Raichle, 1983; Siesjö, 1981). The precise reasons for the topographic patterns of selective neuronal necrosis are not known. The sequence of events *after* correction of oxygen deprivation may be critical.

Status Marmoratus

Status marmoratus is a striking lesion of the basal ganglia. It is the least common of the major neuropathological varieties of neonatal hypoxic–ischemic encephalopathy and is distinctly more common in term than in premature infants. Although the injury occurs in the perinatal period, the lesion itself is not seen in its fully developed form until the latter part of the 1st year of life.

CELLULAR ASPECTS

The three major features of status marmoratus are neuronal loss, gliosis, and hypermyelination (Malamud, 1950). Hypermyelination is an apparent increase in amount of an abnormal distribution of myelinated fibers within the affected nuclear structures, particularly the caudate and putamen. The abnormal myelin pattern lends a marbled appearance to the basal ganglia, hence the descriptive name *l'état marbré*. The abnormal myelinated fibers have been demonstrated by electron microscopy to be astrocytic processes.

REGIONAL ASPECTS

While the caudate and putamen are most consistently and severely affected, the globus pallidus and thalamus are similarly involved. In addition, cerebral cortical involvement occurs in approximately 60% of cases, usually taking the form of ulegyria. Ulegyria is a smooth scar involving one or more gyri and is characterized by loss of cortical neurons, gliosis, and abnormal myelination.

PATHOGENESIS

The pathogenesis of status marmoratus is unclear. Hypoxemia presumably plays a critical role, but contributory factors may include acidosis, hypotension, or changes in regional cerebral blood flow.

Parasagittal Cerebral Injury

Parasagittal cerebral injuries are lesions of the cerebral cortex and subcortical white matter with a characteristic distribution involving the parasagittal, superomedial aspects of the cerebral convexities.

CELLULAR AND REGIONAL ASPECTS

Parasagittal cerebral injuries are bilateral and usually involve the posterior aspects of the cerebral hemispheres more than the anterior aspects (Volpe, 1979). The areas of necrosis are in the order zones at the terminal fields of the anterior, middle, and posterior cerebral arteries and extend to large regions of the vulnerable parietal–occipital cortex (Volpe and Pasternak, 1977). The injury is characterized by necrosis of the cortex and the immediately subjacent white matter. Parasagittal cerebral injury is characteristic of the fullterm infant with intrauterine asphyxia and probably does not occur to any great extent in the premature infant because most interarterial meningeal anastomoses do not dissipate until the third trimester of gestation.

PATHOGENESIS

The sites of parasagittal cerebral injury are border zones or watershed zones between the end fields of major cerebral arteries, and such zones are most susceptible to a decrease in cerebral perfusion pressure. Brierley and co-workers (Brierley, Brown, Excell, & Meldrum, 1969) have demonstrated that this lesion can be produced in primates by profound systemic hypotension without hypoxemia, supporting the importance of *ischemia* in the production of the lesion. Brann and Myers (1975) have demonstrated that prolonged partial asphyxia of the monkey fetus may lead to areas of softening in the paracentral and posterior parietal–preoccipital junction areas, a location of damage virtually identical to that seen in the asphyxiated term infant. In human infants, impaired vascular autoregulation leads to pressure-passive cerebral blood flow (Lou, Lassen, & Friis-Hansen, 1979), rendering the infant extremely vulnerable to diminutions in systemic blood pressure. An additional predisposing factor to injury at the cortical-white matter junction in the depths of the sulci is the existence of a relatively avascular border zone in the distribution of the penetrating branches of the meningeal arteries (Takashima, *et al.*, 1978).

Periventricular Leukomalacia

Periventricular leukomalacia is necrosis of white matter adjacent to the external angles of the lateral ventricles and involves particularly the centrum semiovale and the acoustic and optic radiations. This lesion is observed most often in premature infants with evidence of cardiorespiratory disease and postnatal survival of more than a few days. Analysis of clinical data has led to the conclusion that periventricular leukomalacia is a result of inadequate cerebral perfusion secondary to impaired cardiac function.

CELLULAR AND REGIONAL ASPECTS

The pathological features of periventricular leukomalacia consist of foci of necrosis around the anterior and posterior ends of the lateral ventricles, in the centrum semiovale adjacent to the bodies of the lateral ventricles, in the optic radiations adjacent to the occipital horns, and in the acoustic radiations adjacent to the temporal horns (Banker and Larroche, 1962). Lesions may extend further into the cerebral white matter. The most common sites are at the level of the occipital radiation at the trigone of the lateral ventricles and at the level of the cerebral white matter around the foramen of Monro. These sites are border zones between penetrating branches of major cerebral arteries (DeReuck, Chattha, & Richardson, 1972).

Coagulation necrosis, which may be seen within 6 to 12 hours after an acute hypoxic–ischemic insult, is followed over the next 24 to 48 hours by infiltration by microglia, proliferation of hypertrophic astrocytes, and endothelial hyperplasia. A not uncommon complication of periventricular leukomalacia is hemorrhage into the lesion. This may occur in up to 25% of patients. Tissue loss may be extensive with periventricular leukomalacia, and severe destruction may result in multicystic encephalomalacia or porencephaly.

PATHOGENESIS

Periventricular leukomalacia is the principal ischemic lesion of the premature infant. Impaired vascular autoregulation, incompletely developed periventricular vasculature, and the existence of periventricular arterial border zones are probably all contributory to the occurrence of this lesion in premature infants (Leviton & Gilles, 1981; Lou, Skov, & Pedersen, 1979; Shuman & Selednik, 1980; Young, Hernandez, & Yagel, 1982). The relative sparing of the cerebral cortex and subcortical white matter appears to be a result of the many meningeal interarterial anastamoses between the anterior, middle, and posterior cerebral arteries, which do not dissipate until approximately 40 weeks gestation. White matter damage may result, additionally, as a consequence of the limited capacity of cerebral white matter to maximally vasodilate in response to hypercapnia and lactic acidosis (Cavazzuti & Duffy, 1982).

Focal and Multifocal Ischemic Brain Necrosis

Focal and multifocal ischemic brain necrosis is necrosis that occurs within the specific distribution of major cerebral vessels. Such focal and multifocal necrosis of the brain, which occurs in the prenatal and perinatal periods, could be associated with the dissolution of brain substance and the formation of cavities. Porencephaly is the presence of a single unilateral cavity within the cerebral hemisphere that may or may not communicate with the lateral ventricle. Hydranencephaly is characterized by massive bilateral lesions in which most or all of both cerebral hemispheres is reduced to fluid-filled sacs of cerebrospinal fluid. Multicystic encephalomalacia is characterized by multiple cavitated foci of cerebral necrosis, usually bilateral. Although these lesions can be produced by any major destructive insult occurring from approximately 6 months of gestation to the early postnatal period, we emphasize the ischemic causes of focal and multifocal brain destruction.

REGIONAL ASPECTS

Porencephaly and hydranencephaly are usually distributed within vascular territories. In a large majority of cases the distribution of the middle cerebral artery is affected. Documentation of vascular occlusion or vascular maldevelopment has been limited by the usually long interval between the occurrence of the insult and neuropathological examination. Few well-documented cases of vascular maldevelopment and arterial occlusion by embolus or thrombus have been recorded (Barmade, Moossy, & Shuman, 1979).

PATHOGENESIS

The factors that determine the propensity of the immature brain to undergo dissolution and cavitation with necrosis during this time are the relatively high water content of unmyelinated tissue, the relative paucity of myelinated fibers, and the deficient astroglial response to injury (Volpe, 1981).

Generalized circulatory insufficiency with impaired perfusion of the brain, occurring either in utero or in the neonatal period, accounts for a large proportion of these cavitated lesions. Porencephaly may occur with associated polymicrogyria in the border zones of major cerebral arteries, and this combination suggests a generalized hypoxic–ischemic disturbance at approximately the 6th month of gestation (Volpe, 1981). Insults occurring in the neonatal period, including infarction in the distribution of the middle cerebral artery and periventricular leukomalacia, are, of course, not associated with such cerebral dysgenetic lesions. Differentiation of an occult thromboembolic event from a focal vascular response to generalized circulatory disturbance has not been possible.

Clinical Aspects

The clinical settings in which neonatal hypoxic–ischemic injuries occur have in common diminished oxygen supplied to the brain. This deprivation of oxygen may occur either by hypoxemia (diminished oxygen in the cerebral blood supply) or ischemia (diminished amount of blood perfusing the brain). The major causes of serious hypoxemia in the perinatal period are (1) intrauterine asphyxia, with disturbed gas exchange across the placenta and associated respiratory failure at the time of birth, (2) postnatal respiratory insufficiency due to severe respiratory distress syndrome or recurrent apnea, and (3) severe right-to-left shunt as a result of cardiac disease or persistent fetal circulation. The major causes of serious ischemia are (1) intrauterine asphyxia, with cardiac insufficiency both in utero and at the time of birth, (2) postnatal cardiac insufficiency due to severe congenital heart disease or recurrent apnea, and (3) postnatal cardiovascular collapse as a result of sepsis (Volpe, 1981). Undoubtedly, intrauterine asphyxia is of prime importance in the genesis of hypoxic–ischemic encephalopathy. It occurs in approximately 90% of infants with this syndrome (Volpe, 1981). Postnatal insults alone account for only about 10% of infants with evidence of hypoxic–ischemic encephalopathy (Brown, Purvis, Forfar, & Cockburn, 1974; Volpe, 1981).

The clinical features of neonatal hypoxic–ischemic encephalopathy in the first 12 hours after the insult are those of bilateral cerebral hemispheric disturbance (Brown *et al.*, 1974; Volpe, 1976). The infant is deeply stuporous or in a coma, and periodic breathing may be observed. Dysconjugate eye movements may be seen, but rarely are signs of distinct brainstem disturbance observed. Pupillary responses to light are intact and spontaneous eye movements are full. The infants are usually diffusely hypotonic and demonstrate minimal spontaneous or elicited movement. Seizures occur in approximately 50% of the infants by 6 to 12 hours after birth. These seizures may be generalized tonic seizures, particularly in premature infants, multifocal clonic seizures, especially in fullterm infants, or any of a variety of "subtle seizures." Subtle seizures are characterized by (1) tonic horizontal deviation of eyes, (2) eyelid blinking or fluttering, (3) oral–buccal–lingual movements, (4) swimming or rowing movements of the limbs, and (5) apneic spells, usually accompanied by one or more of the above.

By 12 to 24 hours, the infant's level of consciousness often appears to improve. The appearance of alertness, however, is not accompanied by visual fixation, habituation to sensory stimulation, or other evidence of higher cerebral function. Seizures may be difficult to control with anticonvulsant medication, and the occurrence of seizures by 24 hours of age has been correlated with poor outcome (Finer, Robertson, Richards, Pinnell, & Peters, 1981; Nelson & Ellenberg, 1981). Apnea, marked jitteriness, irritability, and weakness may be apparent during this period. Fullterm infants are more likely to exhibit proximal weakness, with the upper extremities more involved than the lower extremities, whereas premature infants are more likely to demonstrate primarily lower-extremity weakness.

Between 24 and 72 hours, the infant's level of consciousness may deteriorate to a deep stupor or a coma. Cessation of spontaneous respiration may occur and brainstem oculomotor disturbances may be apparent. The latter commonly include skew deviation, ocular bobbing, loss of extraocular movements to the doll's-eye maneuver and to cold caloric stimulation, and the development of fixed pupils. Signs of brain swelling and increased intracranial pressure, including bulging anterior fontanel and split cranial sutures, may appear in the fullterm infant. Infants who are to die with hypoxic–ischemic encephalopathy most often do so during this period.

Those infants who survive to 72 hours tend to improve slowly over the next several days to weeks. While the level of consciousness eventually returns to normal, a mild to moderate stupor usually persists for days to weeks. Disturbances of feeding are common and relate to abnormalities of sucking, swallowing, and tongue movements. Generalized hypotonia of limbs persist; hypertonia is uncommon in the early weeks after the insult. The patterns of weakness described earlier may become more apparent.

The rate of improvement of each of these features is variable, but those infants with the most rapid initial improvement appear to have the best long-term outlook. Indeed, those infants with an essentially normal neurological examination by 1 week of age have an excellent chance for normal outcome (Brown *et al.*, 1974; Finer *et al.*, 1981).

Diagnosis

Recognition of neonatal hypoxic–ischemic encephalopathy is dependent principally on a careful history and neurological examination. Details of the intrapartum and postpartum course are essential; hallmarks of intrauterine asphyxia include fetal heart-rate abnormalities, in utero passage of meconium, and depressed Apgar scores. Metabolic derangements such as hypoglycemia, hypoxemia, and hypocalcemia may exacerbate certain of the neurological features and may contribute to the severity of the neurological syndrome. The observation of hyperammonemia in infants with severe perinatal asphyxia is of interest, although the role of hyperammonemia in the genesis of the neurological syndrome has yet to be determined (Goldberg, Cabal, Sinatra, Plajstek, & Hodgman, 1979).

While detection of persistent abnormalities of the neurological exam is of the utmost importance, certain diagnostic studies may be of value in determining the long-term prognosis for infants who have sustained hypoxic–ischemic cerebral injury. These include electroencephalography, radionuclide brain scanning, computerized tomography, ultrasound scanning, and cortical-evoked responses and brainstem auditory-evoked potentials.

The value of electroencephalography in determining prognosis remains somewhat controversial. Most studies have concluded that a normal neonatal EEG is highly correlated with normal outcome (Rose & Lombroso, 1970), whereas markedly abnormal neonatal EEGs carry a more ominous prognosis for neurological sequelae (Rose & Lombroso, 1970; Sarnat & Sarnat, 1976; Watanabe, Miyazaki, Hara, & Hakamada, 1980). Several studies have found certain abnormalities of background activity (Holmes, Rowe, Hafford, Schmidt, Testa, & Zimmerman, 1982; Watanabe *et al.*, 1980), such as low voltage activity, burst suppression pattern, or electrocerebral inactivity, to correlate highly with neurological sequelae.

The radionuclide brain scan is particularly useful in demonstrating parasagittal cerebral injury (Volpe and Pasternak, 1977), but it may also be useful in defining other varieties of neonatal hypoxic–ischemic injury (O'Brien, Ash, & Gilday, 1979).

Computerized tomography (CAT) has become invaluable in many areas of child neurology and no less so in the neonatal period. Diffuse areas of hypodensity in the periventricular regions with extension into frontal and parietal–occipital gray matter appear to represent tissue injury and are highly correlated with neural developmental sequelae in term infants, whereas the absence of this abnormality suggests a good prognosis (Fitzhardinge, Flodmark, Fitz, & Ashby, 1981; Flodmark, Becker, Harwood-Nash, Fitzhardinge, Fitz, & Chuang, 1980). Such findings are of less certain value in preterm infants.

Ultrasound scanning has been utilized as an aid in assessing the severity of perinatal asphyxia. Abnormalities such as decreased ventricular size and homogenous and heterogenous increases in echodensity, suggesting infarction, can be recognized in the 1st week of life, whereas atrophy and cystic encephalomalacia may be recognized later. Long-term follow-up studies have not been made.

The value of measurement of brainstem auditory-evoked potentials (BAEPs) and visual-evoked potentials in newborn infants with hypoxic–ischemic encephalopathy is controversial. Serial examinations of infants who demonstrate abnormal BAEPs in the newborn period increase the prognostic value of this method of assessment (Stockard, Stockard, Kleinberg, & Westmoreland, 1983). The value of BAEPs in infants less than 32 weeks gestational age is undetermined.

Positron emission tomography (PET) is used at our institution to investigate the pathogenesis of neonatal hypoxic–ischemic encephalopathy. A study of 10 term infants with severe perinatal asphyxia demonstrated relative diminution in cerebral blood flow in parasagittal areas of the cerebral hemispheres bilaterally, suggesting ischemia as the dominant cause of that brain injury. (Volpe, Perlman, Herscovitch, Kreusser, & Raichle, 1983).

Clinicopathological Correlations

The neurological correlates of hypoxic–ischemic encephalopathy are less well described in the newborn period than in older children. Nevertheless, a number of probable relationships can be made on the basis of current information. This section reviews the major neurological sequelae in terms of the neuropathological lesions.

Selective Neuronal Necrosis

The neurological correlates of selective neuronal necrosis in the neonatal period are diverse. Derangements of level of consciousness can likely be attributed to bilateral cerebral hemisphere involvement and to involvement of the reticular activating system. Seizures result from cerebral cortical injury as well, although the tonic generalized seizures of the premature infant may emanate from subcortical nuclear structures in the thalamus or midbrain. Hypotonia probably relates to cerebral cortical or cerebellar cortical disturbance, and the oculomotor abnormalities are probably largely on the basis of brainstem cranial-nerve nuclear involvement.

The long-term neurological sequelae include intellectual retardation, a result of cerebral cortical injury, and a variety of motor derangements. The relation of cortical injury to spastic motor deficits is difficult to separate from the roles of ischemic parasagittal cerebral injury and periventricular leukomalacia; spastic quadriparesis and paraparesis are the most common of the motor disabilities (Brown *et al.*, 1974; Mulligan, Painter, O'Donoghue, MacDonald, Allen, & Taylor, 1980). Approximately 10% of infants with hypoxic–ischemic encephalopathy also develop seizure disorders, probably as a result of cerebral cortical injury. Disturbed sucking and swallowing may relate to nuclear injury or to upper motor-neuron injury. Attentional deficit disorders and hyperactivity observed later in less affected infants may relate to involvement of neurons of the reticular activating system. Visual and auditory disturbances may also result from involvement of neurons at the subcortical and cortical levels.

Status Marmoratus

The neurological correlates of status marmoratus in the neonatal period are unknown. Retrospective clinical data for those cases with adequate pathological documentation have not permitted identification of a neonatal syndrome that could be considered directly related to the injury of basal ganglia.

The long-term neurological sequelae, however, have been elucidated. Bilateral choreoathetosis is an extrapyramidal abnormality that seems clearly related to involvement of basal ganglia. Dystonia and resting tremors are less consistently observed. The onset of the extrapyramidal syndrome is usually not apparent until after the age of 1 year; the reason for this delay in the clinical presentation is not certain. Intellectual function is below average in all cases of pathologically proven status marmoratus, although living children with "athetoid cerebral palsy," many of whom presumably have varying degrees of status marmoratus, have less consistent impairment of intellectual function. The pathological substrate for the intellectual dysfunction may relate to the associated cerebral cortical injury or the concomitant thalamic injury.

Spastic quadriparesis is present in most cases of status marmoratus. Again, the pathological correlate of the quadriparesis is not clear, but it presumably relates to associated cortical or subcortical white-matter injury.

Parasagittal Cerebral Injury

The correlates of parasagittal cerebral injury in the neonatal period include weakness of the proximal limbs, more prominently in upper than in lower extremities, as is predicted from the topographic representation of the homunculus on the motor cortex. Other neonatal deficits referrable to parasagittal cerebral injury have not been defined.

The long-term sequelae of parasagittal cerebral injury are not clearly known, but they probably include at least some of the cases of spastic quadriparesis and hemiparesis which are observed on follow up. As the critical association areas of the parietal–occipital–temporal regions lie within the distribution of this injury, it is reasonable to suspect that disorders of learning, including dyslexia, may result from such injury. Our initial data support this suspicion.

Periventricular Leukomalacia

The neurological correlates of periventricular leukomalacia in the neonatal period have not been defined. Lower-extremity weakness and recurrent apnea have been observed in several infants with periventricular white-matter injury that has been documented by CAT scan. The affection of acoustic and optic radiations suggests that electrophysiological tests, including cortical and brainstem evoked responses, could be useful in determining prognosis in infants with periventricular leukomalacia.

The major long-term consequence of periventricular leukomalacia is spastic diplegia that is, spastic weakness of lower more than upper extremities. Again, the topography of the lesion explains the greater involvement of the lower extremities; periventricular cerebral white matter is traversed by descending fibers from the motor cortex, with lower-extremity fibers being closest to the frontal horns of the lateral ventricles. When lesions are more extensive, that is, involving the centrum semiovale and corona radiata, upper-extremity involvement and intellectual impairment can be expected as well.

The role of periventricular white-matter injury in the production of intellectual deficits has yet to be determined precisely, but visual, perceptive, and language dysfunctions have been attributed to this lesion (DeReuck *et al.*, 1972).

Although there has been a decline since 1970 in the incidence of spastic diplegia among survivors of premature birth, the lesion is still relatively common in many tertiary centers. We observe mild degrees of lower-extremity hypertonia, brisk, deep, tendon reflexes, and other signs of lower-extremity dysfunction in at least one half of our asphyxiated premature infants on follow up. Admittedly it is difficult to distinguish the sequelae of periventricular leukomalacia from those of periventricular hemorrhage or posthemorrhagic ventricular dilatation.

Focal and Multifocal Ischemic Brain Necrosis

The neurological correlates of focal and multifocal ischemic brain necrosis in the neonatal period are variable. Infants with major unilateral lesions usually exhibit slight but definite hemiparesis, with the upper extremity and the face more involved than the lower extremity. This pattern is compatible with injury in the distribution of the middle cerebral artery. The asymmetry of movement is best detected by observing the quantity and quality of spontaneous movements or of those elicited after gentle stimulation of the infant. The signs of major bilateral lesions vary with the severity of the lesion. Quadriparesis may be presaged by abnormal sensory–motor responses such as nonhabituating, short-latency, stereotyped responses to extremity stimulation.

The long-term neurological correlates of focal and multifocal ischemic brain necrosis, again, depend upon the extent of the injury. With unilateral lesions, spastic hemiparesis is typical. Focal lesions without cavitation, in the distribution of the middle cerebral artery, account for 50% of examples of "congenital hemiplegia" examined after the newborn period by CAT scan. Unilateral enlargement of the ventricular system, at times in communication with a porencephalic cyst, accounts for most of the remaining cases, as defined by CAT scan. Presumably, the congenital lesions that result in porencephalic cysts are more severe or occur earlier in brain development than the congenital lesions that do not cavitate. Intellectual function in porencephaly is usually abnormal and probably reflects bilateral cerebral disease.

The sequelae of major bilateral lesions, for example, hydranencephaly, are generally dire. Spastic quadriparesis, profound intellectual impairment, and failure to development of higher visual and auditory function are the rule.

Seizure disorders are common with both unilateral and bilateral lesions. Porencephaly may be associated with seizures that are so difficult to control that surgical extirpation of the lesion and the contiguous cortex can be necessary.

Conclusions

The likelihood of long-term neurological dysfunction in infants who were known to sustain perinatal hypoxic–ischemic insult but who did not develop a neonatal neurological syndrome is not known precisely. Few such patients have been followed prospectively to school age, but retrospective studies suggest that the incidence of neurological impairment in these children is small (Brown *et al.*, 1974).

The duration of neonatal neurological abnormalities is useful in identifying infants at greater risk for sequelae. Studies suggest that severely asphyxiated infants whose neurological abnormalities persist for less than 1–2 weeks have a good prognosis for normal long-term outcome (Sarnat & Sarnat, 1976). As mentioned previously, the electroencephalogram, radionuclide brain scan, and CAT scan may be particularly useful in determining prognosis. PET is currently being evaluated as a tool for assessing regional cerebral blood flow in asphyxiated infants and may further our understanding of the pathophysiology of neonatal hypoxic–ischemic encephalopathy.

References

Banker, B. Q., & Larroche, J-C. (1962). Periventricular leukomalacia of infancy. *Archives of Neurology, 7,* 386–410.

Barmada, M. A., Moossy, J., & Painter, M. (1980). Pontosubicular necrosis and hyperoxemia. *Pediatrics, 66,* 840–847.

Barmada, M. A., Moossy, J., & Shuman, R. M. (1979). Cerebral infarcts with arterial occlusion in neonates. *Annals of Neurology, 6,* 495–502.

Brann, A. W., & Myers, R. E. (1975). Central nervous system findings in the newborn monkey following severe in utero partial asphyxia. *Neurology, 25,* 327–338.

Brierly, J. B., Brown, A. W., Excell, B. J., & Meldrum, B. S. (1969). Brain damage in the rhesus monkey resulting from profound arterial hypotension. 1. Its nature, distribution and physiological correlates. *Brain Research, 13,* 68–100.

Brierly, J. D., Meldrum, B. S., & Brown, A. W. (1973). The threshold and neuropathology of cerebral "anoxic–ischemic" cell change. *Archives of Neurology, 29,* 367–374.

Brown, J. K., Purvis, R. J., Forfar, J. O., & Cockburn, F. (1974). Neurological aspects of perinatal asphyxia. *Developmental Medicine and Child Neurology, 16,* 567–580.

Cavazzuti, M., & Duffy, T. E. (1982). Regulation of local cerebral blood flow in normal and hypoxic newborn dogs. *Annals of Neurology, 11,* 247–257.

DeReuck, J., Chattha, A. S., & Richardson, E. P. (1972). Pathogenesis and evolution of periventricular leukomalacia in infancy. *Archives of Neurology, 27,* 229–236.

Finer, N. N., Robertson, C. M., Richards, R. T., Pinnell, L. E., & Peters, K. L. (1981). Hypoxic-ischemic encephalopathy in term neonates: Perinatal factors and outcome. *The Journal of Pediatrics, 98,* 112–117.

Fitzhardinge, P. M., Flodmark, O., Fitz, C. R., & Ashby, S. (1981). The prognostic value of computed tomography as an adjunct to assessment of the term infant with postasphyxial encephalopathy. *The Journal of Pediatrics, 99,* 777–781.

Flodmark, O., Becker, L. E., Harwood-Nash, D. C., Fitzhardinge, P. M., Fitz, C. R., & Chuang, S. H. (1980). Correlation between computed tomography and autopsy in premature and full-term neonates that have suffered perinatal asphyxia. *Radiology, 137,* 93–103.

Friede, R. L. (1972). Pontosubicular lesions in perinatal anoxia. *Archives of Pathology, 94,* 343–354.

Goldberg, R. N., Cabal, L. A., Sinatra, F. R., Plajstek, C. E., & Hodgman, J. E. (1979). Hyperammonemia associated with perinatal asphyxia. *Pediatrics, 64,* 336–341.

Holmes, G., Rowe, J., Hafford, J., Schmidt, R., Testa, M., & Zimmerman, A. (1982). Prognostic value of the electroencephalogram in neonatal asphyxia. *Electroencephalography and Clinical Neurophysiology, 53,* 60–72.

Kim, S. U. (1975). Brain hypoxia studied in mouse central nervous system cultures. I. Sequential cellular changes. *Laboratory Investigation, 33,* 658–669.

Leech, R. W., & Alvord, E. C. (1977). Anoxic–ischemic encephalopathy in the human neonatal period. *Archives of Neurology, 34,* 109–113.

Leviton, A., & Gilles, F. H. (1981). Periventricular leukomalacia. *Archives of Neurology, 38,* 398

Levy, D. E., Brierly, J. B., Silverman, D. G., & Plum, F. (1975). Brief hypoxia–ischemia initially damages cerebral neurons. *Archives of Neurology, 32,* 450–456.

Lou, H. C., Lassen, N. A., & Friis-Hansen, B. (1979). Impaired autoregulation of cerebral blood flow in the distressed newborn infant. *The Journal of Pediatrics, 94,* 118–121.

Lou, H. C., Skov, H., & Pedersen, H. (1979). Low cerebral blood flow: a risk factor in the neonate. *The Journal of Pediatrics, 95,* 606–609.

Malamud, N. (1950). Status marmoratus: A form of cerebral palsy following either birth injury or inflammation of the central nervous system. *The Journal of Pediatrics, 37,* 610–619.

Mulligan, J. C., Painter, M. J., O'Donoghue, P. A., MacDonald, H. M., Allen, A. C., & Taylor, P. M. (1980). Neonatal asphyxia. II. Neonatal mortality and long-term sequelae. *The Journal of Pediatrics, 96,* 903–907.

Nelson, K. B., & Ellenberg, J. H. (1981). Apgar scores as predictors of chronic neurologic disability. *Pediatrics, 68,* 36–44.

O'Brien, M. J., Ash, J. M., & Gilday, D. L. (1979). Radionuclide brain-scanning in perinatal hypoxia/ischemia. *Developmental Medicine and Child Neurology, 21,* 161–173.

Raichle, M. E. (1983). The pathophysiology of brain ischemia. *Annals of Neurology, 13,* 2–10.

Rose, A. L., & Lombroso, C. T. (1970). Neonatal seizure states. *Pediatrics, 45,* 404–425.

Sarnat, H. B., & Sarnat, M. S. (1976). Neonatal encephalopathy following fetal distress. *Archives of Neurology, 33,* 696–705.

Shuman, R. M., & Selednik, L. J. (1980). Periventricular leukomalacia: A one-year autopsy study. *Archives of Neurology, 37,* 231–235.

Siesjö, B. K. (1981). Cell damage in the brain: A speculative synthesis. *Journal of Cerebral Blood Flow and Metabolism, 1,* 155–185.

Stockard, J. E., Stockard, J. J., Kleinberg, F., & Westmoreland, B. F. (1983). Prognostic value of brainstem auditory evoked potentials in neonates. *Archives of Neurology, 40,* 360–365.

Takashima, S., Armstrong, D. L., & Becker, L. E. (1978). Subcortical leukomalacia: Relationship to development of the cerebral sulcus and its vascular supply. *Archives of Neurology, 35,* 470–472.

Volpe, J. J. (1976). Perinatal hypoxic–ischemic brain injury. *Pediatric Clinics of North America, 23,* 383–397.

Volpe, J. J. (1979). Cerebral blood flow in the newborn infant: Relation to hypoxic–ischemic brain injury and periventricular hemorrhage. *The Journal of Pediatrics, 94,* 170–173.

Volpe, J. J. (1981). *Neurology of the newborn* (pp. 141–238). Philadelphia: Saunders.

Volpe, J. J., & Pasternak, J. F. (1977). Parasagittal cerebral injury in neonatal hypoxic–ischemic encephalopathy: Clinical and neuroradiologic features. *The Journal of Pediatrics, 91,* 472–476.

Volpe, J. J., Perlman, J. M., Herscovitch, P., Kreusser, K. L., & Raichle, M. E. (1983). Positron emission tomography (PET) in the assessment of regional cerebral blood flow (CBF) in the asphyxiated newborn. *Annals of Neurology, 14,* 355–356.

Watanabe, K., Miyazaki, S., Hara, K., & Hakamada, S. (1980). Behavioral state cycles, background EEGs and prognosis of newborns with perinatal hypoxia. *Electroencephalography and Clinical Neurophysiology, 49,* 618–625.

Young, R. S. K., Hernandez, M. J., & Yagel, S. K. (1982). Selective reduction of blood flow to white matter during hypotension in newborn dogs: A possible mechanism of periventricular leukomalacia. *Annals of Neurology, 12,* 445–448.

9

Obstetrics, Neonatal Neurology, and Later Outcome

Bert C. L. Touwen
and Hendrik J. Huisjes

Introduction

Early Brain Damage

It is becoming more and more clear that "the act of birth marks no particular milestone in the development of the human brain" (Norman, 1963, p. 324). Proliferation and growth of cells continues, uninterrupted by birth (Dobbing & Sands, 1973). Behavioral patterns displayed by the newly born (Prechtl, 1977b) can be recognized in the fetus as early as the second trimester of gestation (De Vries, Visser, & Prechtl, 1982).

However, not only is normal development a continuous process, but also abnormalities in the nervous system may originate any time from conception until late in infancy. Many causes are operative in the prepartum period. Chromosomal anomalies transmitted by one of the

Copyright © 1984 by Academic Press, Inc.
All rights of reproduction in any form reserved.
ISBN 0-12-052901-7

parents, or, more often, arising de novo at conception, rarely leave the nervous system unharmed. More than 20% of congenital anomalies stemming from genetic or environmental sources involve the nervous system (Treffers, De Leeuw, Huidekoper, Gubler, Leschot, & Verjaal, 1981). The most important fetal infections, those caused by the TORCH agents (toxoplasma, "other", rubella virus, cytomegalovirus, and herpes simplex virus) have a preference for the brain, together causing up to 2 somewhat severe defects per 1000 live births (Johnson, 1977; Pettay, 1979). Intoxications, both common ones such as smoking and alcohol abuse and rare ones such as methyl mercury poisoning (Alvord & Sumi, 1977) lead intoxication, and perhaps treatment with coumarin derivatives (Hall, Pauli, & Wilson, 1979), affect the nervous system in particular. Deficiency of an essential element such as iodine may cause extremely serious neurological syndromes (Hetzel & Hay, 1979).

In most of the preceding instances the damage is done long before birth. Other injurious events, though starting during gestation, lead to a chain of events that may subsequently inflict damage during labor and delivery or during the neonatal period. Intrauterine growth retardation, although sparing the brain in comparison to many other organs, impairs its growth (Larroche & Korn, 1977). It doubles the incidence of intrapartum asphyxia in fullterms and increases it even more in preterms (Jurgens-van der Zee, *et al.*, 1979). In the small-for-dates newborn, hypoglycemia is a notorious complication. Because there is no fat in these hypoglycemic neonates, the necessary ketone bodies are not available to the brain (Brandt, 1981).

Although the causes of spontaneous preterm birth escape us to a large extent, its roots lie in a faulty development of pregnancy or of the fetus itself. The nervous system of premature infants is much more vulnerable than that of mature infants. The subependymal vessels are easily damaged by asphyxia or sudden changes in the cerebral architecture, and clotting factors are deficient in the newborn (Bowes, 1981); this often results in subarachnoid, periventricular, or intracerebellar hemorrhage (Volpe, 1977). In fact preterm birth is the most complex risk factor for the developing nervous system. Many preterm births are not spontaneous but are induced by the obstetrician because the intrauterine environment is considered even more hazardous for the fetus than the isolette. Indications for inducing birth are maternal diseases such as pregnancy-induced hypertension or diabetes mellitus, that affect the fetus or fetal jeopardy, such as intrauterine growth retardation. Spontaneous preterm birth after a relatively uncomplicated gestation carries the best prognosis, as far as later handicap is concerned (Drillien, 1972). In a case of preterm labor, many fetuses are born in breech presentation or are in danger of infection because of early rupture of the membranes.

Preferably, low-birthweight infants are treated in neonatal intensive care units. Since the 1950s, increasingly adequate treatment may (Alberman, Benson, & McDonald, 1982; Bavikotte, Bull, Bryson, Schreiner, Lemons, & Gresham, 1980; Stewart, Reynolds, & Lipscomb, 1981) or may not (Jones, Cummins, & Davies, 1979; Steiner, Sanders, Phillips, & Maddock, 1980; Kiely, Paneth, Stein, & Susser, 1981) have led to a lower mortality and handicap rate. There is no doubt, however, that intensive treatment has its particular hazards. Hyperoxia may not only cause retrolental fibroplasia, but also inhibit division of cells in the nervous system at least in the neonatal rat (Sokoloff, 1977). In one study mechanical ventilation was associated with a high incidence of neurodevelopmental sequelae (Rothberg, *et al.*, 1981). The possible effect on brain development of serious and often lethal complications in the neonatal period (e.g., bronchopulmonary dysplasia, sepsis, and necrotizing enterocolitis) is difficult to unravel from the consequences of pre- and perinatal injuries.

A Paradox

It is obvious that the basis for brain damage is most often laid during gestation (Knobloch, Malone, Ellison, Stevens, & Zdeb, 1982). Nevertheless, in many follow-up studies obstetrical data are accounted for only cursorily or not at all. The reason is that most of these follow-ups study low-birthweight infants and infant selection is based on having been treated in a neonatal intensive care center. More often than not, groups consist of both inborn and transferred infants, causing heterogeneity and variable accuracy of obstetrical data. Moreover, preterm and growth-retarded infants with birthweight over 1500 g are underrepresented among the transferred patients, as are those who experienced transient asphyxia or other complications at birth without apparent, immediate, pediatric consequences. In some follow-up studies of low-birthweight infants, prenatal variables, although considered important, are either not clearly defined (Knobloch *et al.*, 1982; Peacock & Hirata, 1981), or are limited to mode of delivery (Fairweather, 1981; Kumar, Anday, Sacks, Ting, & Delivoria-Papadopoulos, 1980).

Even when a more detailed analysis of prenatal data is provided, the relations with late sequelae are never impressive (Kitchen, *et al.*, 1980; Low, Galbraith, Muir, Killen, Pater, & Karchmar, 1982; Nelson & Broman, 1977; Niswander, Gordon, & Drage, 1975). Only for a few more commonly discussed variables is it possible to get an impression from the literature on their relation with late sequelae. Although most authors would probably agree that in low-birthweight infants (below 1500 g), being growth retarded or not does not affect later handicap rate (Driscoll, *et al.*, 1982; Fairweather, 1981; Knobloch, Malone, Ellison, Stevens, Zdeb, 1982; Lipper, Lee, Gartner, & Grellong, 1981; Stave & Ruvalo, 1980), there is no consensus at all on the relationship of birthweight and late sequelae. In some studies of low-birthweight children, an effect of gestational age is reported (Fairweather, 1981; Kitchen *et al.*, 1980). However, Nelson and Broman (1977), who analyzed risk factors in 90 children of all birthweights with severe handicaps, found that although immature, small infants were overrepresented, most of the severely handicapped children were born at term and with normal birthweights. The same authors found no relationship with more than 30 variables of pregnancy, and neither did De Souza and Richards (1978).

Even though the effects of asphyxia on the brain are well known (Brann & Dykes, 1977), the role of asphyxia in the causation of handicap in the newborn remains uncertain (Mitchell, 1981). There are few studies in which the subjects did not have additional conditions that may cause brain damage, such as growth retardation or prematurity. But even when asphyxia was the only adverse factor, the effects were contradictory (André, Vert, & Debruille, 1978; Low, Galbraith, Muir, Killen, Karchmar, & Campbell, 1978), probably due to differences in severity and duration of asphyxia. In the rhesus monkey, only severe hypoxia produces brain injury: The effect is a function of duration and severity (Adamsons & Myers, 1973).

There is more unanimity in the literature on the relative importance of events in the neonatal period for later handicap. Ventilatory problems are most frequently mentioned (Nelson & Broman, 1977; Peacock & Hirata, 1981; Rothberg *et al.*, 1981; Stewart, cited by Fairweather, 1981; Teberg, *et al.*, 1982). In this respect, it is interesting that most of the brain lesions found at autopsy in growth-retarded infants apparently are generated in the neonatal period (Larroche & Korn, 1977). This finding of a predominance of neonatal conditions over pre- and perinatal variables in the relationship with late sequelae is probably not an artifact caused by the design of the studies of low-birthweight infants. We found the same for neonatal neurological conditions in our own study of two birth cohorts (Touwen,

Huisjes, Jurgens-van der Zee, Bierman-van Eendenburg, Smrkovsky, & Olinga, 1980).

Thus we are confronted with a paradox:

1. Overwhelming evidence suggests that damage to the nervous system often starts during the prenatal period; but
2. Data indicate that permanent damage is more related to neonatal events than to prenatal complications.

One of the explanations that come to mind is the possibility of fallacious heuristic methods. Is there really no relationship between prenatal events and late sequelae, or is it just not found?

Retrospective studies are not really suspect, but neither are they the method of choice among epidemiologists to elucidate long-term relationships. Interviews with mothers of handicapped children reveal an extremely high incidence of babies who looked blue immediately after birth. Even when documented obstetrical data are used, their quality is often poor. This cannot be the main problem, however, because the studies mentioned before were all prospective.

Prospective studies have the advantage of independent variables with standard quality. A drawback, especially in longitudinal studies of long duration, is the attrition rate. This is invariably high when no special efforts are made to reduce it. Even when the withdrawal is caused, as is usually the case, by families moving out of the area, it is not to be taken lightly. If nothing is known of the subjects lost, the data of studies, especially of low-frequency abnormalities, may be distorted. In the more recently published studies, the attrition rate tends to be rather low, so this methodological problem probably had no great influence.

It is often stated that follow-up studies of hospital populations are inconclusive because they concentrate on a nonrepresentative sample of the population. That may be theoretically true, but it is improbable, again, that it explains the problem we are faced with. Handicap rates may vary with the population studied, but the internal relation with perinatal events should not.

It seems to us that biological factors merit a closer look. What is sought in longitudinal studies of the type under consideration here is the long-term effect of damage to a nervous system that is in an early phase of development. Several aspects must be discussed:

1. Recovery of the organism
2. Regression to the mean
3. Intercurrent variables.

In the following section we discuss these aspects using data from the Perinatal Project Groningen.

The Perinatal Project Groningen

The Perinatal Project Groningen was started in order to analyze the relationship between the obstetrical and the neonatal neurological condition. All infants born between July 1975 and July 1978 were extensively obstetrically documented and neonatally examined using Prechtl's specific neurological design for the fullterm newborn infant (Prechtl, 1977a). Prematurely born infants were examined at term age because no standardized examination technique is available for gestational ages prior to 40 weeks, and because in the absence of serious neonatal complications the rate of maturation of the central nervous system is comparable intra- and extrauterinely (Touwen, 1980).

The total group of infants was divided into two $1\frac{1}{2}$-year cohorts. Only singletons were considered. The first cohort consisted of 1507 infants, the second cohort of 1655 infants.

The obstetrical–neonatal neurological relationships were analyzed for each cohort separately; they turned out to be directly comparable (Huisjes, Touwen, Hoekstra, van Woerden-Blanksma, Bierman-van Eendenburg, Jurgens-van der Zee, Fidler, & Olinga, 1980). The neurologically deviant newborns were reexamined at ages 18 months and 4 years, together with a control group of normal newborns. The prematurely born infants and the infants who suffered intrauterine growth retardation were traced at the age of 6 years, and information about their medical status and behavioral performance was obtained. This part of the project is still in progress. In all instances a complete follow-up was achieved. (This simple statement does no justice to the amount of energy spent in tracing all infants.)

In the next section, data from the perinatal project are used to illustrate the discussion of the relevance of the pre- and perinatal conditions for later functioning of the nervous system. For details the reader is referred to earlier publications (Bierman-van Eendenburg, Jurgens-van der Zee, Olinga, Huisjes, & Touwen, 1981; Huisjes *et al.*, 1980; Jurgens-van der Zee *et al.*, 1979; Touwen, 1981; Touwen, Bierman-van Eendenburg, & Jurgens-van der Zee, 1977; Touwen, Huisjes, Lok-Meijer, & Olinga, 1982; Touwen *et al.*, 1980).

Obstetrics and Prenatal–Neonatal Relationships

Prenatal care consists of an evaluation of the quality of pregnancy in order to detect and treat disorders that may hamper the development of the fetus. In suggesting the evaluation of the significance of isolated events, this statement does not appreciate the complexity of the process of pregnancy and delivery. An example is preeclampsia, which is considered to be a major complication of pregnancy. It could be shown that the presence or even the severity of preeclampsia as such did not relate to the neurological condition of the newborn, but that the number of other accompanying unfavorable obstetric conditions turned the scales (Huisjes, Okken, Prechtl, & Touwen, 1975).

In the Perinatal Project Groningen, as the first of several heuristic approaches, three well-known obstetric diagnostic categories, preterm delivery, intrauterine growth retardation, and acidemia, were compared to neonatal neurological deviancy, which amounted to about 5% in each cohort ($n = 80$ and $n = 81$, respectively). These three categories can be considered the results of a number of complications. There appeared to be a two- to threefold increased risk of neurological morbidity in their presence ($p < .05$). However, only about half of the neurologically abnormal infants were preterm, growth retarded, or acidemic, and no significant relations were found with other, isolated variables.

To analyze this complex issue further, Prechtl's optimality concept (Prechtl, 1968) was applied. In this concept, *optimality* is defined as the best possible range of values of any variable describing the quality of pregnancy and delivery. The total number of those variables from a comprehensive and representative list that meet predefined optimal ranges gives a score of "obstetric optimality," thus quantifying the obstetric conditions. Because nonoptimal is obviously not the same as abnormal, a reduction of the optimality score cannot be identified with reduced normality. But a severely abnormal variable—that is, one lying far outside the optimal range—will be accompanied by a number of other nonoptimal variables. So the obstetric optimality score is self-weighting with regard to seriously abnormal obstetric conditions.

The optimality concept was applied to the obstetric data, using a list of 74 variables covering all aspects of the pre- and perinatal period, from social background to the condition of the newborn immediately after birth. In the same fashion it was used to quantify the

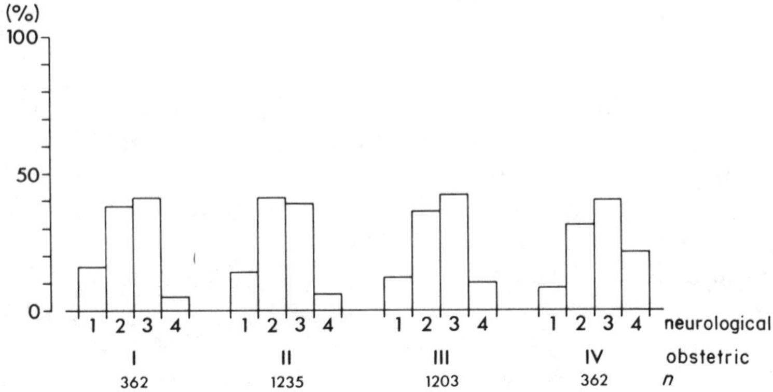

Figure 1. The distribution of four neurological optimality classes within each of four obstetric optimality classes. Obstetric optimality Class I = 74–66; II = 65–61; III = 60–55; IV ≤ 54 obstetric variables within the optimal range. Neurological optimality Class 1 = 60–59; 2 = 58–56; 3 = 55–50; 4 ≤ 49 neurological variables within the optimal range.

neonatal neurological condition by listing the neurological findings. For this purpose, 60 representative neurological items were used, for which an optimal range was defined. For convenience the obstetric and the neurological optimality-score distributions were divided into four classes each. Cut off points were set in the obstetric distributions at the upper and lower deciles and at the median. The neurologic optimality classes were formed on a clinical basis: a perfectly normal class, a definitely abnormal class, and two middle classes. Figure 1 shows the distribution of the neurological optimality classes within the obstetric optimality classes. The difference between the neurological distribution of obstetric Classes I and IV is statistically highly significant ($\chi^2 = 94.9$; $df = 9$; $p < .001$). Thus a large number of obstetric nonoptimal variables are related to a significantly higher proportion of neurological deviance.

Now, means are available to appraise the effect of single variables. An example is shown in Figure 2: the absence or presence of preeclampsia. In both subgroups—preeclamptic and nonpreeclamptic—the statistically significant relation between obstetric optimality and neurological optimality holds true, and although there seems to be an increase of neurological morbidity in the preeclamptic infants of the highest, that is, the most optimal obstetrical class, this increase is not statistically significant. However, the highest proportion of the preeclamptic group was found in the lowest obstetrical optimality class, that is, preeclampsia usually is accompanied by many other nonop-

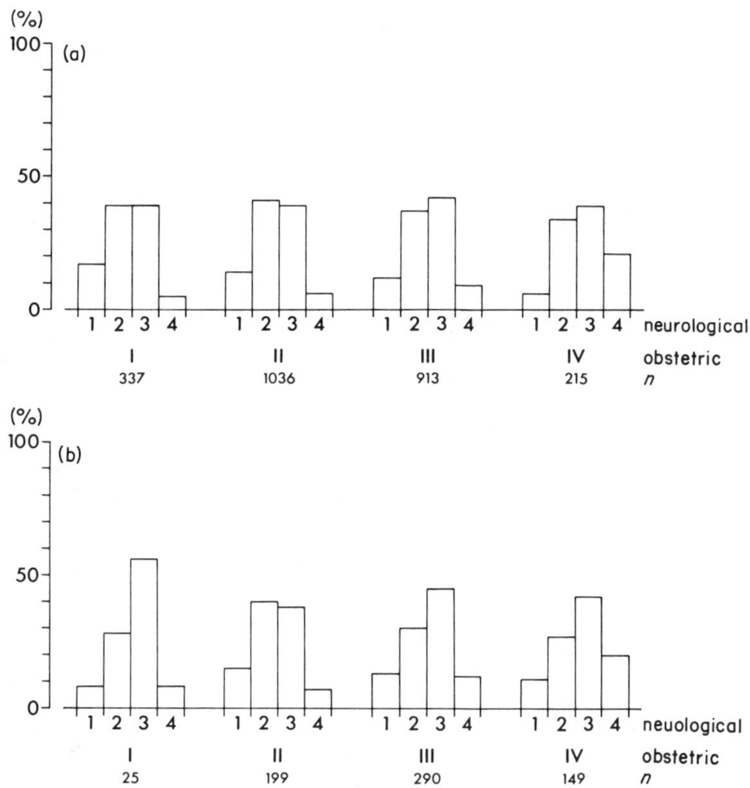

Figure 2. The distribution of the four neurological optimality classes within each of the four obstetric optimality classes in (a) 2501 nonpreeclamptic and in (b) 661 preeclamptic infants.

timal obstetric variables, all of which may contribute to the attack on the fetus. The same situation occurs with other variables such as nonobstetric diseases, preterm delivery in the reproductive history, vaginal bleeding, proteinuria, frequency of prenatal care, presentation at birth, or duration of the second stage: In the majority of these cases a nonoptimal value of the variable occurs in the infants of the lowest obstetric optimality class, which rules out the possibility of assessing the variable's particular contribution to neurological morbidity.

The conclusion therefore is that in the search for relationships between pre- and perinatal events and neonatal neurological morbidity, obstetrics must be appreciated in its complexity and not artificially analyzed. Relationships between neurological morbidity

TABLE 1

Obstetrical History Categories

Categories	Number of variables
1. Social background	13
2. Nonobstetric conditions during pregnancy	9
3. Obstetric past history	14
4. Obstetric aspects of present pregnancy	11
5. Diagnostic and therapeutic measures	8
6. Parturition	11
7. Neonatal condition immediately after birth	8
Total opimality score list	74

and isolated variables will be scarce in contrast to relationships with categories such as preterm delivery, intrauterine growth retardation, and acidemia, which by themselves are very complex conditions. The optimality score comprises the obstetric complexity fully, but at the expense of clinically recognizable diagnoses.

A further aid to analysis is the differentiation of the full obstetric optimality score into its parts, as shown in Table 1. Of the seven categories, it is obvious that Category 7 which describes the infant's condition immediately after birth, relates best to the neurological findings of a few days later. This category is directly derived from the infant. In the case of the neurologically deviant infants, the distribution of the optimality scores of this category showed a shift to the right, meaning a larger number of reduced optimality scores. The distributions of the other categories, which measure the infant's condition indirectly, via the mother's health, showed a comparable though slight shift to the right, with the exception of the first and third categories. However, scores computed for the first five categories taken together, thereby excluding the delivery process and the infant's condition immediately after birth, also showed a shift toward the right. Further analysis shows that low scores for individual infants in one category are not necessarily accompanied by low scores in another category. The opposite occurs as well, so that the effect of an unfavorable score in one category may be compensated in the total score by a favorable score in another category. It can be concluded that in many instances a disturbed pregnancy creates an increased risk of damage to the nervous system, whereas the perinatal events either further increase this risk or create it by themselves (see Michaelis, Rooschüz, & Dopher, 1980). This complex relationship is further confirmed by the fact that permanent damage to the brain, that is, neurological impairment that is still apparent at the age of 4 years, is found in infants with a wide scatter of obstetric scores, both for the first five categories and for the last two.

Thus it appears that relationships between pre- and perinatal events and neonatal neurological condition may be expected mainly in the case of complex variables such as preterm birth, intrauterine growth retardation, and acidemia, or when the complexity of the pre- and perinatal period is summarized as is done in the optimality score. The fact that the relationships are not very firm although statistically significant must be fully appreciated. For instance, it means that although in a Dutch teaching-hospital population (which may be called a negative selection as a consequence of the traditionally high (40%) proportion of home deliveries) the risk for neonatal neurological deviance increases two- or threefold in the presence of preterm birth, intrauterine growth retardation, or acidemia, 10 or at most 15% of the infants with these obstetric diagnoses are really found to be deviant. A decrease of obstetric optimality in combination with these obstetric diagnostic categories enhances the risk for neurological morbidity, as of course does the neonatal pediatric condition of the infant. Besides these factors, however, others hitherto insufficiently known, for example, genetic factors, must be involved. This becomes even clearer when long-term morbidity is considered.

Follow-up Studies

The 80 neurologically abnormal newborns of the first cohort were reexamined at the ages of 18 months and 4 years, as was a control group of 80 neurologically normal newborns (Figure 3). One originally abnormal infant had died at the age of 3 months from congenital anomalies. From the remaining 159 infants, all of whom could be traced, 5 were severely impaired at 18 months of age; all 5 belonged to the originally abnormal group. Another 10 infants showed minor neurological dysfunction, that is, nonhandicapping but evident neurological impairment. Of these 10 infants, 2 had been normal at birth; in both instances, interval complications were possibly involved. At the age of 4 years the number of severely impaired infants had increased to 8—all of them belonging to the neonatally abnormal group. The children responsible for this increase had been mildly abnormal at 18 months. The number of children with minor neurological dysfunction had increased to 16; 6 of them belonged to the

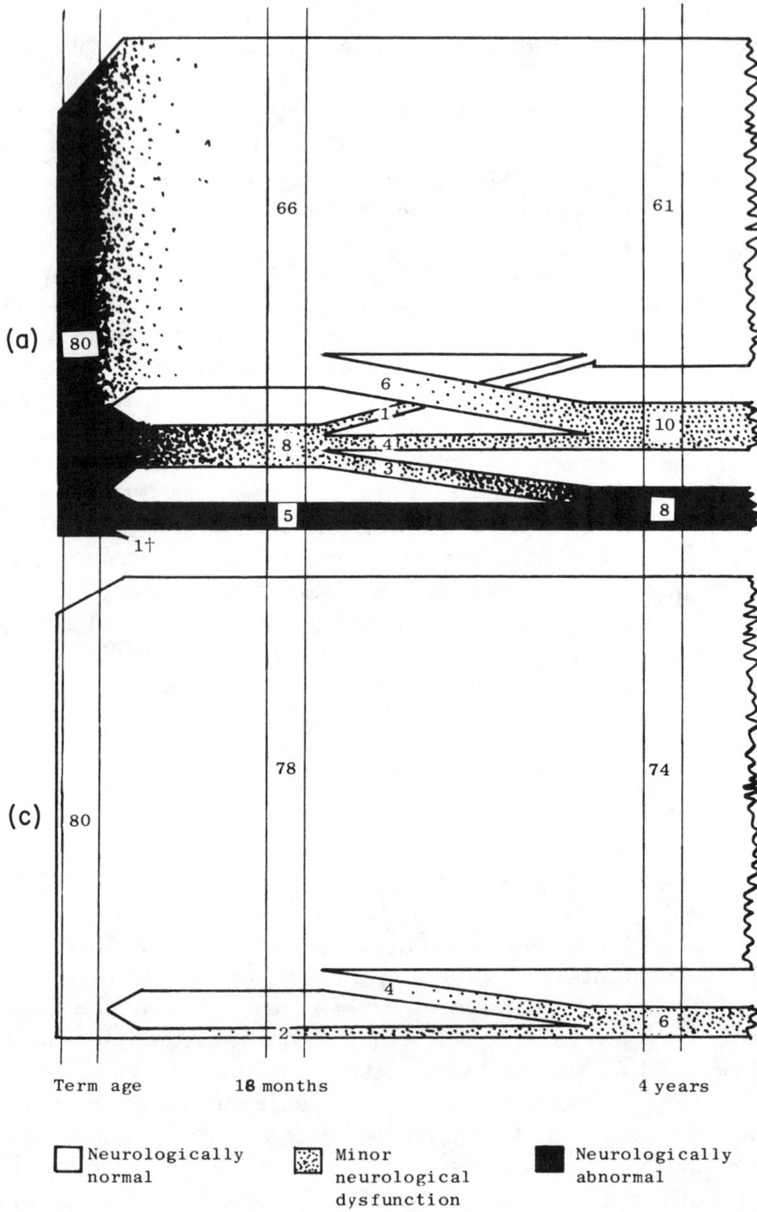

Figure 3. Schematic presentation of the neurological results. (a) study group of neurologically abnormal newborns; (c) control group selected on basis of neonatal neurological normality (No conclusion may be derived from this figure as to the time of transition from one diagnostic category to another.)

neonatally normal group, including the 2 mildly abnormal cases at 18 months. In only 1 child had no significant interval complications occurred. From the 10 mildly abnormal cases of the neonatally abnormal group, 4 had been mildly abnormal at 18 months. In 2 others interval complications had occurred. One child who had been mildly abnormal at 18 months of age was normal at 4 years.

A significant difference of the obstetrical condition, expressed in optimality scores, between the recovered and nonrecovered children could be found neither for the total score nor for the separate category scores, including Category 7. For the Apgar scores (representing the infants' condition in the first minutes after birth on basis of vital signs) a comparable lack of relationships has been found by Nelson and Ellenberg (1981). Of the 8 severely impaired infants, 6 belonged to one or more of the three obstetric diagnostic categories, but the majority of the infants in these categories had recovered.

The relationship with neonatal neurology is evident, however. Although the majority of the neonatally abnormal infants recovered, all severely abnormal ones and almost two-thirds of the mildly abnormal ones originated from the neonatally abnormal group. Expectedly, prognosis depended to a large extent on the neurological diagnosis. The apathy syndrome, hemisyndromes, and hypertonic syndromes appeared to have the worst prognosis; characteristically the infants with these syndromes tended to have low obstetric optimality scores including those for the pregnancy variables. Infants with a unilateral paresis of the VIth cranial nerve or a brachial plexus dysfunction (n = 11 and n = 2, respectively) showed a good prognosis. It is well known that neonatal peripheral nerve dysfunctions ususally recover. Not 1 of 13 neonates with the hyperexcitability syndrome showed neurological dysfunction at 4 years but the latency period of the frequently occurring choreiform sequelae may be long (Prechtl & Stemmer, 1962). The very pluriform etiology of hypotonia in the newborn period eliminates the possibility of an unequivocal prognosis for hypotonic infants. An eventful neonatal course occurred in none of the infants of the neonatally normal group, in about half of those of the neonatally abnormal group who remained abnormal, and in 15% of those of the neonatally abnormal group who recovered.

Interval complications—disorders that may influence brain development—occurred more often in the neonatally deviant group, and especially in the infants who remained abnormal. Interval complications occurring before the age of 18 months were most conspicuous in this respect. During the first 2 years the brain develops rapidly and may be more vulnerable; on the other hand, interval complications, possibly reflecting a genetically lower resistance against noxious adVents, may hamper recovery or even intensify the impairment.

Adverse factors such as a disturbed neonatal course, the presence of interval disorders, or a family history of neuropsychiatric disorders showed a cumulative effect, especially if the reduction of obstetric and neurological optimality was included.

We can conclude that the recovery from neonatal neurological dysfunction seems to depend on many biological factors, only one of which is the capacity of the brain to recover. The interplay of these factors is intricate, so that an evaluation of single factors, instead of for example, the interplay between brain dysfunction, interval disorders during the first years of life, and genetic factors, seems unreliable. In longitudinal studies the phenomenon called *regression to the mean* may play a role as well. Normal infants cannot become more normal, nor can abnormal infants become more abnormal. On the other hand, normal infants may become abnormal as a result of intercurrent disease, and abnormal infants may recover. Therefore, longitudinal relations may easily become blurred. But this does not imply that there is no relationship between neonatal and later neurological conditions.

Behavioral Sequelae

Finally, attention was paid to the relationship between obstetrics, neonatal neurological condition, and behavioral development. From the Perinatal Project Groningen three main points become apparent. First, the majority of infants with low obstetric optimality or even an evident obstetric diagnosis such as acidemia, preterm birth, or intrauterine growth retardation were neurologically normal at birth, at 18 months, and at 4 years. Until the latter age, behavioral development had been normal as well, that is, the parents did not complain about difficult behavior such as hyperactivity, temper tantrums, destructiveness, anxiety, or short concentration and attention span.

Second, the majority of infants who were neurologically deviant at birth were normal at 18 months and 4 years, neurologically as well as behaviorally. Relationships with, for example, acidemia (asphyxia during delivery, an ominous situation should one believe the popular literature on behavioral problems), which were present in the newborn period, had dissolved at the later ages. Third, however, the behavior of the children who were mildly abnormal at 4 years was slightly different, depending on the neonatal condition: the neonatally abnormal children more often showed extroverted acting-out behavior, whereas the neonatally normal children more often appeared shy or withdrawn. Of course the number of mildly abnormal children ($n = 16$) is too small to warrant pertinent conclusions, but findings bearing on the same issue have been reported by Nelson and Ellenberg (1982). Their findings contribute to the conception that environmental influences as well as the integrity of the brain and even the age at which an attack on the brain has taken place are involved in behavioral development.

Preliminary data of the follow-up examinations of preterm- and intrauterine growth-retarded infants also suggest such complex relationships. Although it seems that the preterm infants were at a disadvantage with regard to their neurological condition, at 6 years behavioral complaints were mainly offered for those in the group of original growth-retarded infants. Perhaps this may be seen as a long-term result of a lasting prenatal attack on the brain in the case of intrauterine growth retardation, in contrast to the consequences for the preterm infant of his too-early extrauterine existence, which are balanced by adequate neonatal intensive care.

Conclusion

Obstetrics is too complex for simple analyses, except in the case of extreme conditions. Obstetric–neurological relationships are found in the neonatal period; they dissolve hereafter, due to recovery that is very well possible in neurologically deviant infants. Obstetric situations are usually too complex to allow determination of specific conditions during pregnancy or during delivery as causes of deviance. In some cases, sudden, extreme situations arise during delivery, but in the majority of cases a heterogeneous group of nonoptimal conditions during pregnancy has already paved the way for difficulties in the perinatal period. Why most infants do recover, and some do not, cannot always be explained from particular diagnoses during pregnancy or delivery, not even from particular neonatal neurological diagnoses. Most likely, genetic factors play a role here. The neonatal neurological findings have more predictive value for the later outcome than the obstetric data.

A pre- or perinatal origin of neurological morbidity later in childhood is not refuted by the lack of statistical relations, however. For an efficient feedback on obstetric care, neonatal neurological evaluation appears to be the best strategy. For an evaluation of the risk for an abnormal neurological development, that is, for a selection of infants who should be followed up longitudinally, a combination of appraisal of the obstetric condition, the infant's condition immediately after birth, the neonatal course, and the neonatal neurological condition is the strategy of choice.

Acknowledgments

The Perinatal Project Groningen was supported by grants from the Praeventiefonds (no. 28.266) and the Prinses Beatrixfonds.

References

Adamsons, K., Myers, R. E. (1973). Perinatal asphyxia, causes, detection and neurologic sequelae. *Pediatric Clinics of North America, 20,* 465–480.

Alberman, E., Benson, J., & McDonald A. (1982). Cerebral palsy and severe educational subnormality in low-birth-weight children: A comparison of birth in 1951–1953 and 1970–1973. *Lancet, i,* 606–608.

Alvord, E. C., Sumi, S. M. (1977). Effects of drugs, narcotics and toxins on the chemical maturation of the infant brain. In S. R. Berenberg (Ed), *Brain, fetal and infant* (pp. 165–177). Nijhoff: Hague.

André, M. & Vert, P., & Debruille, Ch. (1978). Diagnostic et évolution de la souffrance cérébrale chez les nouveau-nés ayant presenté des signes d'hypoxie foetale. *Archives Françaises Pediatriques, 35,* 23–36.

Bavikotte, K., Bull, M. J., Bryson, C. O., Schreiner, R. L., Lemons, J. A., & Gresham, E. L. (1980). Dramatically improved outcome of extremely low birth weight infants. *Journal of the Indiana State Medical Association, 73,* 234–237.

Bierman-van Eendenburg, M. E. C., Jurgens-van der Zee, A. D., Olinga, A. A., Huisjes, H. J., & Touwen, B. C. L. (1981). Predictive value of neonatal neurological examination: A follow-up study at 18 months. *Developmental Medicine and Child Neurology, 23,* 296–305.

Bowes, W. A. (1981). Delivery of the very low birth weight infant. *Clinics in Perinatology, 8,* 183–195.

Brandt, I. (1981). Brain growth, fetal malnutrition, and clinical consequences. *Journal of Perinatal Medicine, 9,* 3–26.

Brann, A. W., & Dykes, F. D. (1977). The effects of intrauterine asphyxia on the full-term neonate. *Clinics in Perinatolgoy, 4,* 149–161.

De Souza, S. W., & Richards, B. (1978). Neurological sequelae in newborn babies after perinatal asphyxia. *Archives of Diseases in Childhood, 53,* 564–569.

De Vries, J. I. P., Visser, G. H. A., & Prechtl, H. F. R. (1982). The emergence of fetal behavior. I. qualitative aspects. *Early Human Development, 7,* 301–322.

Dobbing, J., & Sands, J. (1973). Quantitative growth and development of human brain. *Archives of Disease in Childhood, 48,* 757–767.

Drillien, C. M. (1972). Aetiology and outcome in low-birthweight infants. *Developmental Medicine and Child Neurology, 14,* 563–574.

Driscoll, J. M., Driscoll, Y. T., Steir, M. E., Stark, R. T., Dangman, B. C., Perez, A., Wung, J. -T., & Kritz, P. (1982). Mortality and morbidity in infants less than 1,001 grams birth weight. *Pediatrics, 69,* 21–26.

Fairweather, D. V. I. (1981). Obstetric management and follow-up of the very-low-birth-weight infant. *Journal of Reproductive Medicine, 26,* 387–392.

Hall, J. G., Pauli, R. M., Wilson, K. N. (1980). Maternal and fetal sequelae of anticoagulation during pregnancy. *American Journal of Medicine, 68,* 122–140.

Hetzel, B. S., & Hay, I. D. (1979). Thyroid function, iodine nutrition and fetal brain development. *Clinical Endocrinology, 11,* 445–460.

Huisjes, H. J., Okken, A., Prechtl, H. F. R., & Touwen, B. C. L. (1975). Neurological and paediatric findings in newborns of mothers with hypertensive disease in pregnancy. Perinatal medicine. *Proceedings of the 4th European Congress of Perinatal Medicine,* 407–416.

Huisjes, H. J., Touwen, B. C. L., Hoekstra, J., van Woerden-Blanksma, J. T., Bierman-van Eendenburg, M. E. C., Jurgens-van der Zee, A. D., Fidler, V. J., Olinga, A. A. (1980). Obstetrical–neonatal neurological relationship. A replication study. *European Journal of Obstetrics, Gynecology and Reproductive Biology, 10*(4), 247–256.

Johnson, R. T. (1977). Viral infections and brain development. In S. R. Berenberg (Ed.), *Brain, fetal and infant* (pp. 213–223). Nijhoff: Hague.

Jones, R. A. K., Cummins, M., & Davies, P. A. (1979). Infants of very low birthweight. *Lancet, i,* 1332–1335.

Jurgens-van der Zee, A. D., Bierman-van Eedenburg, M. E. C., Fidler, V. J., Olinga, A. A., Visch, J. H., Touwen, B. C. L., & Huisjes, H. J. (1979). Preterm birth, growth retardation and acidemia in relation to neurological abnormality of the newborn. *Early Human Development, 3,* 141–154.

Kiely, J. L., Paneth, N., Stein, Z., Susser, M. (1981). Cerebral palsy and newborn, *Developmental Medicine and Child Neurology, 23,* 533–538, 650–659.

Kitchen, W. H., Ryan, M. M., Rickards, A., McDougall, A. B., Billson, F. A., Keir, E. H., & Naylor, F. D. (1980). A longitudinal study of very low-birthweight infants. IV. An overview of performance at eight years of age. *Developmental Medicine and Child Neurology, 22,* 172–188.

Knobloch, H., Malone, A., Ellison, P. H., Stevens, F., & Zdeb, M. (1982). Considerations in evaluating changes in outcome for infants weighing less than 1,501 grams. *Pediatrics, 69,* 285–295.

Kumar, S. P., Anday, E. K., Sacks, L. M., Ting, R. Y., & Delivoria-Papadopoulos, M. (1980). Follow-up studies of low birth weight infants (1,250 grams or less) born and treated within a perinatal center. *Pediatrics, 66,* 438–444.

Larroche, J. C., & Korn, G. (1977). Brain damage in intrauterine growth retardation. In L. Gluck (Ed.), *Intrauterine asphyxia and the developing fetal brain.* Chicago/ London: Year Book Medical Publications.

Lipper, E., Lee, K., Gartner, L. M., & Grellong, B. (1981). Determinants of neurobehavioral outcome in low-birth-weight infants. *Pediatrics, 67,* 502–505.

Low, J. A., Galbraith, R. S., Muir, D., Killen, H., Karchmar, J., & Campbell, D. (1978). Intrauterine growth retardation: A preliminary report of long-term morbidity. *American Jouranl of Obstetrics and Gynecology, 130,* 534–545.

Low, J. A., Galbraith, R. S., Muir, D., Killen, H., Pater, B., & Karchmar, J. (1982).

Intrauterine growth retardation: a study of long-term morbidity. *American Journal of Obstetrics and Gynecology, 142,* 670–676.

Michaelis, R., Rooschüz, Dopher, R. (1980). Prenatal origin of congenital spastic hemiparesis. *Early Human Development, 4,* 243–255.

Mitchell, R. G. (1981). Antecedents of handicap. *Lancet, I,* 86–87.

Nelson, K. B., & Broman, S. H. (1977). Perinatal risk factors in children with serious motor and mental handicaps. *Annals of Neurology 2,* 371–377.

Nelson, K. B., & Ellenberg, J. H. (1981). Apgar scores as predictors of chronic neurologic disability. *Pediatrics, 68,* 36–44.

Nelson, K. B., & Ellenberg, J. H. (1982). Children who 'outgrew' cerebral palsy. *Pediatrics, 69,* 529–536.

Niswander, K. R., Gordon, M., Drage, J. S. (1975). The effect of intrauterine hypoxia on the child surviving to 4 years. *American Journal of Obstetrics and Gynecology, 121,* 892–899.

Norman, R. M. (1963). In W. Blackwood, H. McMenemey, A. Meyer, R. M. Norman, & D. S. Russell (Eds.), *Greenfield's neuropathology* (p. 324, 2nd ed.). Baltimore: Williams & Wilkins.

Peacock, W. G., & Hirata, T. (1981). Outcome in low-birth-weight infants (750–1,500 grams): A report on 164 cases managed at Children's Hospital, San Francisco, California. *American Journal of Obstetrics and Gynecology, 140,* 165–172.

Pettay, O. (1979). Intrauterine and perinatal viral infections. *Annals of Clinical Research, 11,* 258–266.

Prechtl, H. F. R. (1968). Neurological findings in newborn infants after pre- and paranatal complications. In J. H. P. Jonxis, G. H. A. Visser, & J. A. Troelstra (Eds.), *Aspects of prematurity and dysmaturity* (pp. 303–321), Leiden: Stenfert Kroese.

Prechtl, H. F. R. (1977a). The neurological examination of the full term newborn infant. *Clinics in Developmental Medicine* (No. 63, 2nd ed.). London: Heinemann Medical Books.

Prechtl, H. F. R. (1977b). Assessment and significance of behavioral states. In S. R. Berenberg (Eds.), *Brain, fetal and infant* (pp. 79–90). Nijhoff: Hague.

Prechtl, H. F. R. Risk factors and the significance of early neurological assessment. In B. Brazelton & B. Lester (Eds.), *New approaches to developmental screening of infants. Proceedings of a Round Table Conference, Palm Beach. October* 1984.

Prechtl, H. F. R., & Stemmer, J. C. (1962). The choreiform syndrome in children. *Developmental Medicine and Child Neurology, 4,* 119–127.

Rothberg, A. D., Maisels, M. J., Bagnato, S., Murphy, J., Gifford, K., McKinley, K., Palmer, E. A., & Vannucci, R. C. (1981). Outcome for survivors of mechanical ventilation weighing less than 1,25O gm at birth. *Journal of Pediatrics, 98,* 106–111.

Sokoloff, L. (1977). Toxic effects of elevated oxygen tension on brain maturation. In S. R. Berenberg (ed.), *Brain, fetal and infant* (pp. 178–183). Nijhoff: Hague.

Stave, U., & Ruvalo, C. (1980). Neurological development in very-low-birthweight infants. Application of a standardized examination and Prechtl's optimality concept in routine evaluations. *Early Human Development, 4,* 229–241.

Steiner, E. S., Sanders, E. M., Phillips, E. C. K., & Maddock, C. R. (1980). Very low birth weight children at school age: Comparison of neonatal management methods. *British Medical Journal, 218,* 1237–1240.

Stewart, A. L., Reynolds, E. C. R., & Lipscomb, A. (1981). Outcome for infants of very low birthweight: Survey of world literature. *Lancet, i,* 1038–1041.

Teberg, A. J., Wu, P. Y. K., Hodgman, J. E., Mich, C., Garfinkle, J., Azen, S., & Wingert,

W. A. (1982). Infants with birthweight under 1500 g: Physical neurological and developmental outcome. *Critical Care in Medicine, 10,* 10–14.

Touwen, B. C. L. (1980). The preterm infant in the extrauterine environment. Implications for neurology. *Early Human Development, 4,* 287–300.

Touwen, B. C. L. (1981). Recovery of neurologically deviant infants. In M. W. van Hof, G. Mohn (Eds.), *Functional recovery from brain damage: Developments in neuroscience* (Vol. 13, pp. 77–94). Amsterdam: Elsevier North Holland.

Touwen, B. C. L., Bierman-van Eendenburg, M. E. D., & Jurgens-van der Zee, A. D. (1977). Neurological screening of full-term newborn infants. *Developmental Medicine and Child Neurology, 19,* 739–747.

Touwen, B. C. L., Huisjes, H. J., Jurgens-van der Zee, A. D., Bierman-van Eendenburg, M. E. D., Smrkovsky, M., & Olinga, A. A. (1980). Obstetrical condition and neonatal neurological morbidity. An analysis with the help of the optimality concept. *Early Human Development, 4*(3), 207–228.

Touwen, B. C. L., Huisjes, H. J., Lok-Meijer, T. Y., & Olinga, A. A. (1982). The recovery rate of neurologically deviant newborns. *Early Human Development, 7,* 131–148.

Treffers, P. E., De Leeuw, R., Huidekoper, B. L., Gubler, F., Leschot, N. J., & Verjaal, M. (1981). Congenital anomalies. A survey of 39,828 infants born during 21 years. In H. J. Huisjes (Ed.), *Aspects of perinatal morbidity.* Groningen: Universitaire Boekhandel Nederland.

Volpe, J. J. (1977). Neonatal intracranial hemorrhage. *Clinics of Perinatology, 4,* 77–102.

10

Behavioral Consequences of Cerebral Insult in Infancy

*Jack M. Fletcher, Harvey S. Levin**, *and Susan H. Landry*

Introduction

Many factors can influence the recovery of function and subsequent development of children who sustain early central nervous system insults, including the etiology and type of lesion, neurological complications, and treatment. Environmental variables such as the length of hospitalization, social class, quality of caretaking, and amount of stimulation also seem to influence recovery of function. Despite these multiple factors and the diversity of types of early brain injury, generalizations about the effects of early brain injury have been attempted. In fact, the traditional view of recovery maintains that the effects of brain injury are less deleterious for younger orga-

*Dr. Levin's research in this chapter was partially supported by grant #NS-07377, Center for the Study of Nervous System Injury.

Copyright © 1984 by Academic Press, Inc.
All rights of reproduction in any form reserved.
ISBN 0-12-052901-7

nisms than for older organisms. According to this view, the immature CNS (central nervous system) is less vulnerable to insult and recovers more completely than the adult CNS (Bastian, 1898; Lenneberg, 1967; Smith, 1981). Given the difficulties of generalizing across diverse and complicated etiologies, it is not surprising that the traditional view has been controversial. In the next section, this view and its limitations are examined. Then the implications of data on cerebral insult in human infants are reviewed in light of this viewpoint.

Neural Plasticity and Equipotentiality

There are several versions of the argument that recovery is better in younger organisms (Bastian, 1898; Lenneberg, 1967; Smith, 1981). However, better recovery is usually explained on the basis of one observable non-CNS variable (age) and two unobservable CNS variables (plasticity and equipotentiality). The traditional view of the effects of age is that neurobehavioral recovery is more extensive in children because of the greater plasticity of the immature CNS. This presumption of greater plasticity is sometimes extended to include the hypothesis that during the early stages of cerebral maturation, different brain areas are capable of subserving a variety of behaviors (i.e., equipotentiality) and that one hemisphere can support the functions of the other hemisphere in the event of early unilateral injury or operative removal of one hemisphere. Support for these presumptions is usually obtained by (1) comparing the development of younger and older brain-injured organisms with reported cases of superior neuropsychological recovery in children (Basser, 1962; Bastian, 1898; Byers & McLean, 1962; Lenneberg, 1967) or by (2) examining the development of cognitive skills in conjunction with presumed unilateral brain disease such as infantile hemiplegia or hemispherectomy for intractable seizures (Basser, 1962; Smith, 1981). In these latter studies, the development of language irrespective of the side of infantile hemiplegia (left or right) or early hemispherectomy is interpreted as evidence for both greater equipotentiality and plasticity of the immature CNS.

Age, of course, is an easily measured variable. Plasticity and equipotentiality, however, are inferences concerning presumed properties of the CNS. Plasticity is used to explain the hypothesized reduced vulnerability of the immature brain to injury (Kennard, 1936) and the greater potential for reorganization attributed to the younger

CNS (Lenneberg, 1967) in which focal regions of the brain are not fully committed to support specific functions. Equipotentiality has been used to describe one hypothesized mechanism of plasticity, namely the possibility that the CNS is organized in different regions that are equally adept at subserving different behaviors (Lashley, 1938). This concept has also referred more specifically to the notion that both cerebral hemispheres can subserve language during the early stages of brain maturation (Lenneberg, 1967). These concepts, along with the conclusion of better recovery in younger organisms, have not gone unchallenged (Isaacson, 1975; St. James-Roberts, 1979, 1981; Teuber, 1967).

LIMITATIONS OF AGE

While age is commonly invoked as a factor in recovery, it is not a variable with direct explanatory significance (Fletcher & Satz, 1983). Age can be used as an independent variable to demarcate periods of change and different developmental phases of the organism (Siegel, Bisanz, & Bisanz, 1983; Wohlwill, 1973). To suggest that age determines recovery inappropriately imputes age with explanatory significance. Age merely serves as an aid to marking the temporal course of development. It is neither a necessary nor a sufficient explanation of change over time or development (Siegel *et al.*, 1983; Wohlwill, 1973).

LIMITATIONS OF PLASTICITY

ANIMAL STUDIES

The concept of neural plasticity has been inferred from the results of animal experiments and human studies. Some animal ablation experiments showed sparing of function after early brain lesions that was not observed after similar injury to the mature brain. For example, Kennard (1936) reported in a widely cited article that ablations of the motor cortex in infant monkeys produced minor postoperative changes in motor function. Corresponding lesions in mature monkeys resulted in severe motor deficits. The author's observation of increased motor incoordination and spasticity as the operated infants matured is less widely appreciated than her description of the postsurgical motor behavior. Although ablation studies have demonstrated similar sparing of sensory function (see Finger, 1978, for a review), Goldman and her colleagues found that sparing of delayed-alternation task performance in young animals depended on the site of frontal lobe lesion and the postoperative interval before follow-up testing (Goldman, 1974; Goldman & Alexander, 1977). While more detailed reviews of lesion experiments in animals is provided in other chapters of this volume, one implication of this work for human neuropsychology is that the relative maturity of a given substrate influences the amount of recovery or sparing of neurobehavioral functions after brain injury. Furthermore, the developmental course of recovery can be appreciated only within a longitudinal design.

HUMAN STUDIES

Early human studies of the effects of brain damage sustained during infancy on language development have also been interpreted as support for neural plasticity (Lenneberg, 1967; Smith, 1981). These investigations have largely involved cases of infantile hemiplegia complicated by intractable seizures, hemispherectomy, and trauma. The most salient findings of the hemispherectomy studies include the absence of gross aphasia following removal of the left hemisphere during infancy (Basser, 1962). However, detailed analysis of language was not carried out as part of the follow-up examination in any of the studies. Two adults who underwent left hemispherectomy, both for excision of a malignant brain tumor, exhibited severe nonfluent expressive aphasia, but tumor regrowth precluded long-term follow up (Burkland & Smith, 1977; Smith, 1974). Consistent with this finding, Basser (1962) reported that removal of *either* hemisphere in children who had already acquired language greatly reduced or abolished expressive language. Again, the receptive lanaugage of these children and their long-term recovery was not described.

Relatively few cases of infantile left hemiplegia have been tested for visuospatial capacity after undergoing right hemispherectomy. The results indicate adequate development of visuospatial skills on simple tasks, but deficits are revealed on more complex tests (Kohn & Dennis, 1974). On standardized tests of global cognitive function, IQ scores were predominantly in the low normal to mildly impaired range for children who had received hemispherectomies prior to 1 year of age. However, verbal and nonverbal IQs were not consistent with the lateralization of hemispherectomy (Levin, Ewing-Cobbs, &

Benton, 1983). In contrast with the nonspecific cognitive deficit obtained after hemispherectomy during infancy, a more specific visuospatial impairment was apparent when the right hemisphere was removed after 1 year of age. (Woods, 1980). Removal of the left hemisphere after 1 year of age depressed verbal and nonverbal scores.

Reviewers of the literature concerning infantile hemiplegia and hemispherectomy have criticized Basser's (1962) unsystematic assessment of behavioral recovery (St. James-Roberts, 1979, 1981). Other authors have reanalyzed Basser's data and questioned the purported sparing of language after early left hemispherectomy (Satz & Bullard-Bates, 1981; Woods & Teuber, 1978). An intrinsic problem in research on infantile hemiplegia and hemispherectomy is the generalizability of the effects of this type of injury to infants with normal brains. Furthermore, St. James-Roberts (1979) suggested that plasticity might not be necessary for a parsimonious theory of recovery because other observable variables including type and extent of lesion, length of recovery, and environmental enrichment could be sufficient to explain the available data. Consequently, plasticity might not be needed to explain recovery from early brain injury.

Limitations of Equipotentiality

The concept of equipotentiality is incompatible with evidence suggesting that the left hemisphere is predisposed for language. Neuroanatomical studies of infants have confirmed that the planum temporale is larger in the left hemisphere than the homologous region of the right hemisphere (Wada, 1974). Clinical studies of children with early hemiplegia and hemispherectomy—the conditions that were interpreted by Lenneberg (1967) to support the equipotentiality hypothesis—have shown differences in the behavioral organization of language and nonlanguage skills between the isolated right and left hemisphere (Dennis, 1980; Dennis & Whitaker, 1976, 1977). As with the plasticity studies, detailed assessments of cognitive skills that extend beyond the conventional neurological examination and intelligence tests have been necessary to demonstrate these differences in cognitive organization. For example, Dennis and associates (Dennis, 1980; Dennis & Kohn, 1975; Dennis & Whitaker, 1976, 1977; Kohn & Dennis, 1974) applied a variety of linguistic and spatial tasks to left- and right-hemispherectomized children. Differences in linguistic skills were demonstrated primarily on tasks associated with language structure (i.e., syntax and grammar), and not on tasks associated with language content (e.g., vocabulary). The omission of tests of language structure may account for the failures of some researchers to show differences between left- and right-hemispherectomy cases (e.g., Smith, 1981). Although the concept of equipotentiality has also failed to receive support from other studies, no other mechanism has been proposed to explain the development of language after the left hemisphere is removed during infancy (Satz & Bullard-Bates, 1981).

Unresolved Issues

Despite the aforementioned problems, the traditional concepts of plasticity and equipotentiality remain popular. However, there are some factors that underlie the continued acceptance of these concepts. First, most clinical studies are based on children with infantile hemiplegia, hemispherectomy, or head trauma. The possibility of bilateral cerebral insult associated with these disorders cannot be eliminated until noninvasive techniques (e.g., nuclear magnetic resonance) that permit more definitive examination of structural and functional alterations of the brain are employed. For example, initial cranial computerized axial tomography (CAT) findings after head injury in children are in most cases compatible with diffuse brain insult (Levin, Benton, & Grossman, 1982). Consequently, while plasticity can be examined in relation to diffuse brain insult, it is difficult to test hypotheses concerning equipotentiality in children with these types of injuries. Despite these constraints, neurosurgical studies using global outcome measures and showing increased survival after severe head injury in children have been interpreted as support for greater resilience of the young brain (Bruce, Schut, Brown, Wood, & Sutton, 1978). In contrast, investigations of neuropsychological recovery have provided no evidence for preferential recovery from traumatic brain injury in young children (Brink, Garrett, Hale, Woo-Sam, & Nickel, 1970; Levin, Eisenberg, Wigg, & Kobayashi, 1982). Corresponding studies of cognitive development after brain trauma in infants have not been reported.

A second factor—seldom discussed in the literature—is that most clinical studies do not include a sufficiently broad age range to test hypotheses based on neural plasticity. Many studies of recovery from aphasia that fail to produce age-related findings acknowledge the possibility of a period early in development during which the equipotentiality hypothesis might hold. For example, Krashen's (1973) reanalysis of the Basser (1962) cases implied that equipotentiality might be operative before 5 years of age. Satz and Bullard-Bates (1981) conceded that equipotentiality might be present prior to 1 year of age, but Annett (1973) concluded that "after the age of 13 months, right and left [infantile] hemiplegic children show a difference in the incidence of speech problems which is as marked as that found in adults" (p. 11). However, there were relatively few cases in these studies with lesion onset prior to 1 year. Follow-up studies of head trauma, a prominent etiology for the infantile hemiplegic cases, were never systematically conducted for injuries sustained during infancy. Finally, many cases of hemiplegia had lesion onset after 1 year of age, and many hemispherectomy cases underwent surgery after age 1.

There are other etiologies of brain injury in children that occur prior to the age of 1 year. Although these etiologies (e.g., hydrocephalus) are diffuse in nature, they do bear on plasticity hypotheses. In the next section, representative data from these types of cases are reviewed.

Other Insults to the Infant Brain

Relevance to Equipotentiality and Plasticity

Apart from infantile hemiplegia and trauma, CNS insults that occur in infancy include (1) complications associated with prematurity and very low birthweight (VLBW), such as intraventricular hemorrhage (IVH) and hydrocephalus (2) hydrocephalus that is not associated with prematurity, such as aqueduct stenosis, Dandy-Walker syndrome, and dysgraphic conditions of the spine or skull (e.g., spina bifida), (3) cerebral palsy, and (4) early infectious diseases such as encephalitis and meningitis. The etiologies of these insults are diverse, diffuse, and often lead to significant handicaps. There are few neurological disorders in adults to which these conditions can be compared, but this problem arises for most comparative studies of children and adults (St. James-Roberts, 1979). Although the results of studies of children with these disorders may have relatively little bearing on equipotentiality, they are relevant to the plasticity issue and may elucidate mechanisms of recovery and behavioral sparing.

Hence, in the following sections we selectively review studies of the development of children with (1) prematurity and VLBW and (2) hydrocephalus not secondary to prematurity. We focus on studies that evaluate children with these conditions prior to 3 years of age. Cerebral palsy is not directly discussed, because it occurs frequently in conjunction with prematurity; but it is referred to when appropriate. Taylor reviews studies of recovery in children with infectious disease in Chapter 16 of this volume.

Prematurity and Early Medical Complications

A variety of early medical complications can occur during the pre- and postnatal development of infants. The most commonly studied complication is respiratory distress syndrome (RDS), which results in episodic anoxia at birth. Follow-up studies of infants who experience extended RDS have yielded mixed results. Early studies were largely retrospective (see Caputo & Mandell, 1970; Pasamanick & Knoblock, 1966) but were frequently interpreted to show a higher frequency of prematurity, anoxia, or other birth complications in the medical histories of older children with learning problems. Because of these findings, Pasamanick and Knobloch (1966) postulated a continuum of reproductive casualty in which pre- and postnatal medical complications were precursors to a variety of childhood learning and behavioral disorders. Because of (1) the large number of culturally disadvantaged children in these studies, (2) the null results of subsequent investigations (Minde, Webb, & Sykes, 1968; Rutter, Graham, & Yule, 1970), and (3) the limitations of diagnostic criteria and outcome measures, this continuum has been questioned (Sameroff & Chandler, 1975). Moreover, prospective studies have shown that the cognitive development of premature infants becomes increasingly similar to that of normal children over time (Graham, Ernhart, Thurston, & Craft, 1962) and that sociocultural factors may be major influences on outcome (Drillien, 1964; Sameroff & Chandler, 1975). In light of these data, Sameroff and Chandler (1975) argued for a continuum of caretaking casualty through which early medical problems such as anoxia have enduring effects on development because of the persistent, deleterious effects of the environment on the child. This continuum is assumed to pertain to all premature infants except those with severe biological problems.

The importance of social and cultural influences on the development of premature infants is supported by the literature (Sameroff & Chandler, 1975; St. James-Roberts, 1979). At the same time, prospective-outcome studies have frequently shown relationships between early risk signs and later developmental problems (Caputo & Mandell, 1970; Stewart & Reynolds, 1975). These findings are consistent with neuropathological studies that have shown morphological changes in the brains of infants and adults with histories of perinatal anoxia (Towbin, 1981). Deleterious effects on development are most consistently reported for premature infants with VLBW (less than 1501 g), possibly because of the high frequency of perinatal anoxia, IVH, and related disorders (Desmond, Wilson, Alt, & Fisher, 1980; St. James-Roberts, 1979). Moreover, CAT and ultrasound findings have disclosed that 40–50% of all VLBW infants sustain some degree of IVH (Papile, Burstein, Burstein, & Koffler, 1978). This finding, which exceeds earlier estimates of IVH in VLBW infants, reflects in part the increased survival rate for this high-risk group as well as the greater sensitivity of CAT scanning and ultrasonography.

Intraventricular Hemorrhage and Outcome

Given the reported incidence provided by noninvasive CAT -scan and ultrasound findings, it appears that many surviving VLBW infants in early studies had IVH that was largely undetected. IVH occurs primarily as a sequel to severe perinatal anoxia. Papile *et al.* (1978) classified four grades of IVH severity. Grade I hemmorrhage involves an isolated hemorrhage in one or both germinal matrices; Grade II is a rupture of the germinal matrix hemorrhage with bleeding into the lateral ventricles but with no swelling; Grade III refers to a rupture complicated by lateral ventricle swelling; Grade IV refers to dilated, blood-filled ventricles with extension of the hemorrhage of the germinal matrices into adjacent brain parenchyma. Intraventricular hemorrhage (particularly Grades III and IV) is the major cause of progressive hydrocephalus in neonates.

Studies investigating the effects of IVH on development prior to 3 years of age have yielded conflicting results. Some studies comparing infants with varying degrees of IVH have reported a strong relationship between severe IVH and subsequent developmental problems (Chaplin, Goldstein, Myerberg, Hunt, & Tooley, 1980; Desmond *et al.*, 1980; Dykes, Lazzara, Ahmann, Blumenstein, Schwartz, & Brann, 1980; Papile, Munsick, Weaver, & Pecha, 1979). Other studies have shown either a weak relationship between IVH and developmental outcomes or no differences between infants with and without IVH (Koons, Sun, & Koenigsberger, 1982; Krishnamoorthy, Todres, Kuehnle, Shannon, DeLong, Davis, 1980; Ment, Scott, Ehrenkranz, Rothman, Duncan, & Warshaw, 1982; Naulty, Binder, Murray, Markle, Barnet, & Wagman, 1982; Schub, Ahmann, Dykes, Lazzara, & Blumenstein, 1981). Attempts to compare the development of VLBW infants with IVH across studies have been hindered by differences in the type and range of IVH severity as well as by the inclusion of infants in IVH groups who have other severe medical complications (e.g., bronchopulmonary dysplasia). Furthermore, conflicting results could also reflect small samples, the absence of appropriate comparison groups, and the absence of longitudinal data to characterize later childhood.

The relationship of IVH with RDS and hydrocephalus is also unclear. Respiratory distress syndrome (RDS) has been frequently associated with poor developmental outcome (Field, Dempsey, & Shuman; 1981; Harrod, L'Heureaux, Wangensteen, & Hunt, 1974; Johnson, Malachowski, Grobstein, Welsh, Daily, & Sunshine, 1974). Since IVH rarely appears without RDS, it is unclear whether reported developmental delays for IVH infants are due to the hemorrhage or to other factors such as RDS (e.g., Koons *et al.*, 1982; Ross & Schechner, 1982; Shinnar, Molteni, Grammon, D'Souza, Altman, & Freeman, 1982; Williamson, Desmond, Wilson, Garcia-Pratt, & Andrews, 1982). It is unfortunate that many studies of IVH have not included RDS infants without IVH as a comparison group (e.g., Koons *et al.*, 1982; Ross & Schechner, 1982). Papile *et al.* (1979) compared groups of VLBW infants with RDS and no IVH and infants with both RDS and IVH. They found that severe developmental delay was found only in IVH infants with severe hemorrhage. However, Schub *et al.* (1981) compared similarly formed groups and were not able to show differential effects of IVH severity on subsequent development. Differences in sample size and the follow-up interval may help explain these contrasting results.

An additional dimension of the severity of IVH is the development of progressive hydrocephalus. Deleterious effects of IVH on later outcomes in association with hydrocephalus have been reported (Papile, Burstein, Burstein, Koffler, Koops, & Johnson, 1980). However, other studies suggest a more benign developmental outcome for IVH infants with hydrocephalus (Krishnamoorthy *et al.*, 1980; Naulty *et al.*, 1982). Again, it is difficult to compare results because in many studies IVH infants with and without hydrocephalus were grouped together (Koons *et al.*, 1982; Naulty *et al.*, 1982; Ross & Schechner, 1982; Williamson *et al.*, 1981).

In order to assess the differential effects of IVH on development, Landry, Fletcher, Chapieski, & Francis (1983) compiled scores from the Bayley Scales of Infant Development on a large cohort (N = 142) of VLBW infants. These infants were all under 1501 g with at least 4 weeks prematurity. For the purposes of this chapter, scores at four time intervals (6, 12, 24, and 36 months) are compared for three groups of infants in this cohort. These groups consisted of (1) an IVH–RDS group (n = 35) with IVH ranging from Grades I–IV but without progressive hydrocephalus, (2) an RDS–no IVH group representing infants who developed RDS but not IVH (n = 48), and (3) a hydrocephalus (HYD) group (n = 24) consisting of infants with both IVH and RDS who subsequently developed progressive hydrocephalus. Although all of the infants in each of the groups suffered at least briefly from RDS, there was a tendency for the more severe forms of RDS to be associated with IVH, particularly in those infants who developed hydrocephalus. None of these infants had severe respiratory complications such as bronchopulmonary dysplasia. It should be noted that these groups did not differ in birthweight, gestational age, socioeconomic status, or other demographic variables potentially related to outcome. Furthermore, the sample size decreased with longer study intervals, reflecting dropouts and infants who had not yet attained 36 months of age. However, analyses for attrition effects have shown that the samples were comparable with respect to their 6-month Bayley scores and initial demographic and medical variables (Landry *et al.*, 1983).

Figure 1 presents results for the three groups on Bayley Mental Development Index (MDI) scores at 6, 12, and 24 months and the IQ score from the Stanford-Binet at 36 months: Figure 2 presents the same results for the Bayley Physical Development Index (PDI) scores and the Perceptual–Performance scale from the McCarthy Scales of Children's Abilities. These figures permit a comparison of the degree of catching-up on scores that presumably reflect mental and motor–perceptual development. Although it is traditional to correct scores for gestational age as a control for degree of prematurity, uncorrected scores are presented to illustrate differential rates of development in the three groups. It is seen that at each age level the RDS–no IVH group and the IVH–RDS group perform better than the HYD group. Over time, the RDS–no IVH group and the IVH–RDS group show cognitive and motor development that exceeds that of the HYD group. In contrast, the HYD group shows little evidence for change

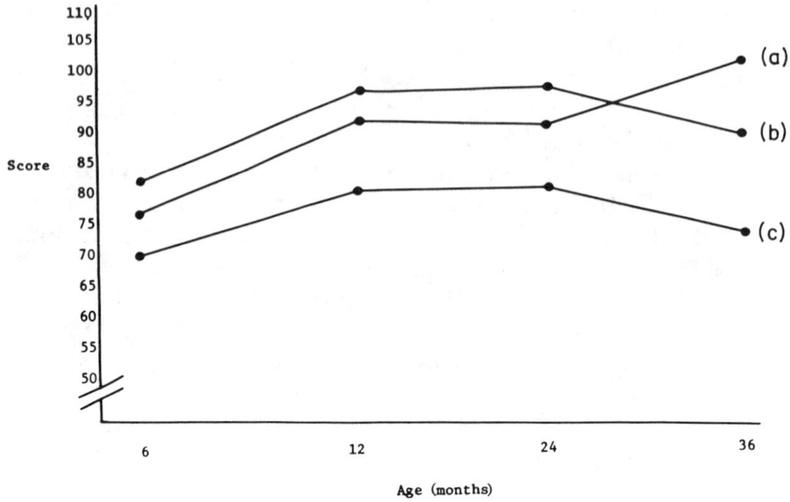

Figure 1. Uncorrected Bayley MDI scores (6, 12, and 24 months) and Stanford-Binet IQ score (36 months) in three prematurity groups: (a) IVH–RDS group; (b) RDS–no IVH group; (c) HYD group.

over time. Although there is substantial variability within these groups, the results imply that the outcome of the IVH–RDS infants is comparable to that of the RDS–no IVH infants for up to 3 years. When progressive hydrocephalus accompanies IVH, outcomes are much poorer.

Similar results are obtained if the IVH–RDS and the HYD groups are combined to examine relationships of IVH severity and outcome. For this analysis, infants were placed in three IVH-severity groups: Grades I–II, Grades III–IV, and hydrocephalus. Percentages of infants with scores below 70 were computed at each age level. There were no significant differences in the percentage of infants with scores below 70 between the performance of Grades III–IV IVH infants and the performances of Grades I–II IVH infants at each age. Although a small percentage of infants with Grades III–IV IVH showed significantly delayed MDI and PDI scores at 6 and 12 months (<70), all IVH infants without hydrocephalus had MDI and PDI scores above 70 by 24 months. In contrast, those infants with IVH who subsequently developed hydrocephalus showed a higher proportion of delayed scores. In summary, the studies indicate that the development of progressive hydrocephalus may be the most useful prognostic feature of IVH.

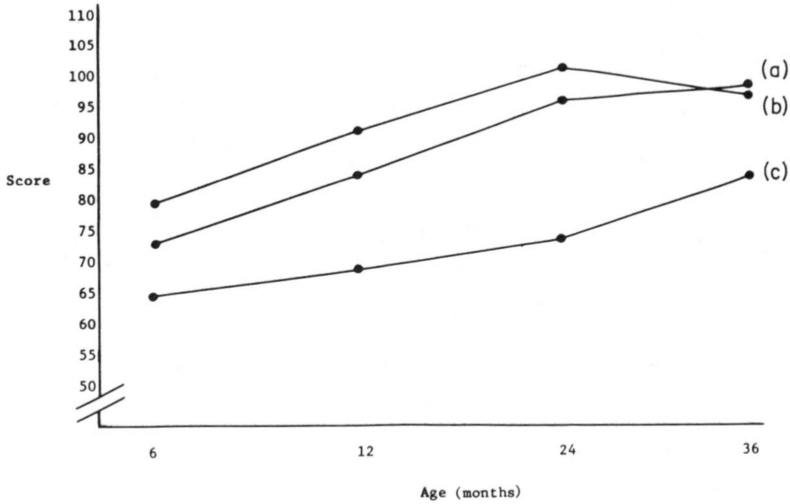

Figure 2. Uncorrected Bayley PDI scores (6, 12, and 24 months) and McCarthy Perceptual–Performance score (36 months) in three prematurity groups: (a) IVH–RDS group; (b) RDS–no IVH group; (c) HYD group.

OUTCOME IN CONGENITAL FORMS OF HYDROCEPHALUS

Hydrocephalus is not always associated with prematurity. The studies reviewed in this section are directed toward hydrocephalus that is usually associated with fullterm birth and complications other than IVH. The congenital ("uncomplicated") etiologies include aqueduct stenosis, conditions of the spine or skull (e.g., spina bifida), and the Dandy-Walker syndrome (agenesis of the cerebellar vermis). The major postnatal ("complicated") etiologies of hydrocephalus include meningitis and trauma. Hydrocephalus can be associated with complications such as seizures that can adversely effect cognitive functioning. Visual disturbances involving gaze, eye-movement disorders, and a variety of motor difficulties are also common. These symptoms vary substantially across individual children.

OUTCOME AFTER 3 YEARS OF AGE

There are many studies of the development of children with hydrocephalus. Although some studies have reported delays in language development (Hagberg, 1962; Tew, 1979), the most consistent deficits involve nonverbal cognitive abilities (e.g., visuomotor skill in copying designs) and motor skills (Dennis, Fitz, Netley, Sugar, Derek, Harwood-Nash, Hendrick, Hoffman, & Humphreys, 1981; Soare & Raimondi, 1977; Zeiner & Prigatano, 1982). For example, one of the more systematic studies (Dennis *et al.*, 1981) administered the Wechsler Intelligence Scale for Children—Revised (WISC-R) to 78 children of age 5–15 years who suffered hydrocephalus during the 1st year of life. In a series of elegant and sophisticated analyses, Dennis *et al.* (1981) showed that nonverbal skills (reflected by WISC-R Performance IQ) were less well developed than verbal skills on the WISC-R Verbal IQ scale. This dissociation was related to the presence of brain anomalies, but not to the etiology or treatment of the hydrocephalus. For example, discrepancies in verbal and nonverbal skills were related to a selectively thin vertex and occipital lobe in hydrocephalus with aqueduct stenosis. The discrepancies were also related to the cerebellar and oculomotor deficits characteristic of the sample as a whole.

Dennis *et al.* (1981) obtained WISC-R IQ scores that were generally within one standard deviation of the mean (100) for most of the etiological groups. Other studies, particularly those including children with encephalocele and spina bifida, show relative preservation of intellect in the face of discrepant verbal and nonverbal development (Brunt, 1981; Sand, Taylor, Hill, Kasky, & Rawlings, 1973; Soare & Raimondi, 1977; Spain, 1974). Dennis and her co-workers demonstrated that IQ discrepancies were related to indices of regional cortical thinning, oculomotor functioning, and motor impairment. Relatively few studies have demonstrated these types of relationships, with null results frequently occurring for comparisons of cognitive functioning and indices of hydrocephalus severity, etiology, and treatment (see Dennis *et al.*, 1981, for a review).

INFANT STUDIES

The tendency for congenitally hydrocephalic children—particularly those with spina bifida and encephalocele—to display relatively intact intellect is interesting in light of the IVH studies that show a higher proportion of severely delayed children when hydrocephalus is secondary to prematurity. The most obvious explanation for this apparent disparity is related to the complicated etiology of the hydrocephalus cases in the Landry *et al.* (1983) study, who were quite premature. However, this is only a partial explanation, because the other infants in the Landry *et al.* (1983) study were equally premature and were often less delayed in their development.

Another explanation concerns the age at which the infants were tested and the assessment instruments used. Infant cognitive tests may measure different abilities and do not predict scores on IQ tests appropriate to preschool and school-age children (McCall, 1979). Consequently, extension of the IVH results obtained with infants requires evaluation of a series of subjects that are studied as neonates with CAT or ultrasound and examined later in middle childhood. Similarly confounding, only a few studies have evaluated hydrocephalus subjects younger than 3 years of age who had not necessarily been VLBW infants.

Nelson (1980) evaluated 30 hydrocephalic children at 6, 18, 36, and 72 months of age. A progressive increase in IQ scores from 6 to 72 months was apparent; furthermore, mean IQ scores even at 6 months were much higher than those scores reported in the IVH literature. Given the different composition of the groups at each age point, selective sampling should be recognized as a possible source of bias in this study. In a second study, Spain (1974) reported on 145 children with encephalocele (n = 16) and spina bifida (n = 129) at 3 years of age. Although relatively few children were severely delayed, lower nonverbal than verbal scores were obtained, particularly for shunted patients.

Thompson, Eisenberg and Levin (1982) administered the Bayley scales to 29 infant hydrocephalics (age range 4.2–29.1 months) who had CAT scans performed within 24 hours of developmental testing. The infants had diverse etiologies for their hydrocephalus, including meningitis (n = 5), myelomeningocele or meningocele (n = 8), encephalocele (n = 2), and trauma or hemorrhage (n = 2). Only 4 infants were premature: the etiology of the hydrocephalus was unknown in the remaining cases. The infants were divided into two major groups: complicated hydrocephalus (n = 17), that is, those infants sustaining a primary brain injury (e.g., infection, hemorrhage), and uncomplicated hydrocephalus (n = 12), consisted of infants who did not sustain a primary brain injury (e.g., meningocele). All infants had shunt diversion of cerebrospinal fluid during their first few months of life.

As depicted in Table 1, comparison of Bayley MDI scores revealed a trend for lower corrected Bayley scores in the complicated group (median = 70) than in the uncomplicated group (median = 91). To compare Bayley scores with CAT scan results, ventricular brain ratios (VBR) representing the ratios of the size of the lateral ventri-

TABLE 1

Gestation-Corrected Bayley Mental Development Index Scores and Ventricular Brain Ratios in Hydrocephalic Infants

	Complicated[a]		Uncomplicated[b]	
	Median	Range	Median	Range
Bayley MDI	70	40–122	91	40–122
VBR[c]	14	1–54	12	1–52
Left VBR[d]	14	1–17	19	1–49
Right VBR[d]	18	1–62	8	1–54

[a]Complicated hydrocephalic subjects sustained primary brain injury.
[b]Uncomplicated hydrocephalic subjects did not sustain primary brain injury.
[c] $\frac{\text{Area of lateral ventricle}}{\text{Area of total intracranial contents}} \times 100$
[d] $\frac{\text{Area of lateral ventricle}}{\text{Area of total intracranial contents of hemisphere}} \times 100$

cles to the size of total intracranial contents were computed. Separate VBRs were also obtained for each hemisphere. Table 1 shows that there was no difference in median VBRs between complicated and uncomplicated cases. However, a modest inverse relation between the total VBR and the Bayley MDI score emerged that, according to the Spearman rank order correlation coefficient (r = .44), was significant in the total series. Although this relation was confirmed for the unilateral left and right hemispheres (r = .34 and .48 respectively), no correlation reached significance when the complicated and uncomplicated groups were considered separately. These inverse correlations suggest that larger VBRs are associated with lower Bayley MDI scores in both hydrocephalus groups.

Of potential relevance to the role of hemispheric functional asymmetry in development after early hydrocephalus was the finding by Thompson *et al.* (1982) of unilateral VBR that was more than two times greater than the contralateral VBR in 7 patients. Figure 3 presents a CAT scan from one of these cases to illustrate this asymmetry. In 6 of these cases of asymmetric VBRs, the shunt tip had been inserted into the lateral ventricle of the hemisphere with the smaller VBR. Although these infants apparently had adequate shunt function and their Bayley scores did not differ from those of other cases, the implications of their gross hemispheric structural asymmetry for subsequent neuropsychological functioning remains unclear.

A comparison of these three investigations of hydrocephalus with

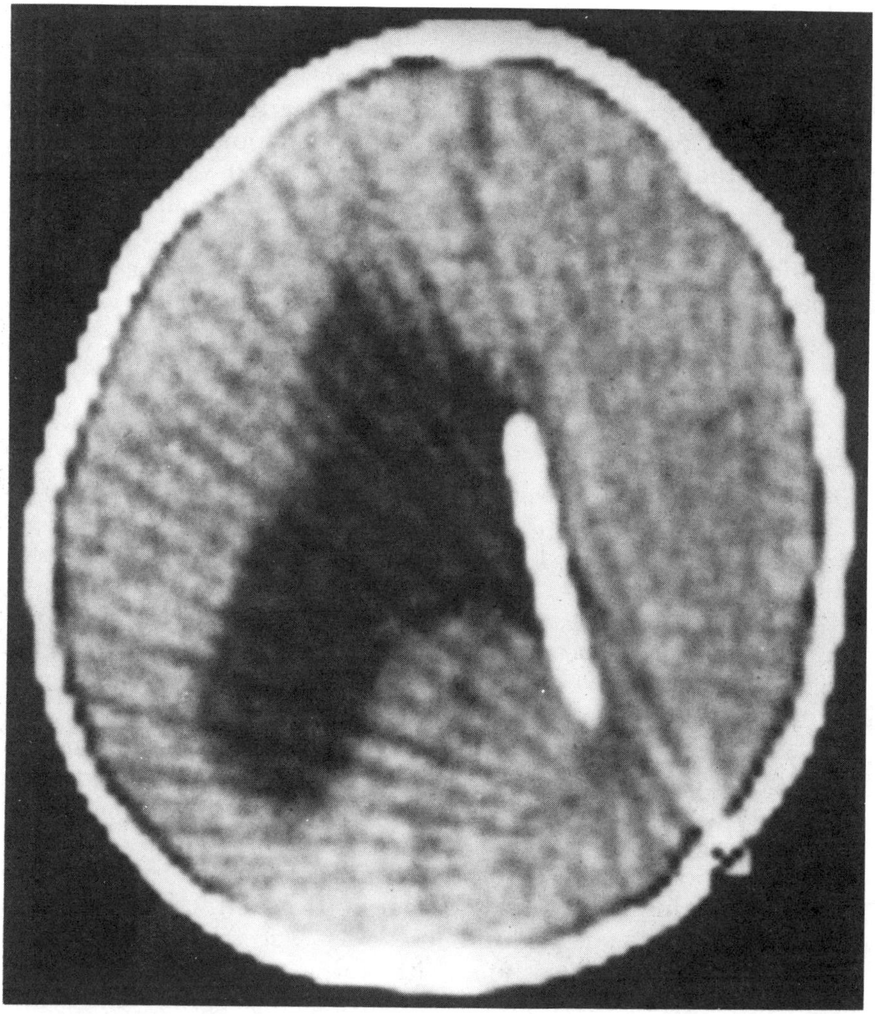

Figure 3. Asymmetry of ventricular size after shunting. The patient was a 14-month-old girl with myelomeningocele; her Bayley MDI was 122.

the IVH studies show that different etiologies yield contrasting results in developmental follow-up. Thompson *et al.* (1982), Spain (1974), and Nelson (1980) included large number of infants with congenital (uncomplicated) hydrocephalus etiologies. These infants did better on developmental follow-up than did premature infants with IVH-related hydrocephalus or in whom hydrocephalus was associated with primary brain injury. In order to explain these disparities, however, two types of data are necessary. First, longer-term follow-up of VLBW infants, especially those infants with IVH and hydrocephalus, would be informative. Second, relations between injury indices in IVH-related hydrocephalus and developmental functioning should be studied using procedures analogous to those employed by Thompson *et al.* (1982) and Dennis *et al.* (1981). Systematic follow-up of hydrocephalic infants that includes these data may provide important information concerning behavioral sparing after early diffuse cerebral insult.

Conclusions

What can we conclude from studies of infant cerebral insult involving prematurity, hydrocephalus, and other disorders regarding recovery of function and behavioral sparing? It is obvious that cognitive functioning is hardly unitary within these diagnostic groups; there is substantial variability across subjects. Furthermore, assessment procedures continue for the most part to be restricted to IQ tests. More specific analyses of cognitive skills may show subtle but important differences in the organization of abilities across these groups. The persistent documentation of better development of verbal than nonverbal skills in many cases of early cerebral insult is consistent with this possibility. This dissociation is especially apparent for hydrocephalic cases with congenital, uncomplicated etiologies. Whether this dissociation obtains with VLBW infants with hydrocephalus is unclear, reflecting the relative absence of sufficiently long follow-up studies. However, some preliminary evidence suggests that IVH and hydrocephlus may be associated with slower motor than mental development. Poorer development of nonverbal cognitive skills and motor skills has also been reported for nonretarded children evaluated for cerebral palsy (Abercrombie, 1968) and for early infectious and metabolic disorders (Chapter 16). However, somewhat different results have been reported for early cases involving hemiplegia and hemispherectomy, cases in which language skills have frequently been more impaired than nonlanguage skills, depending on the age of insult and the hemisphere damaged (Dennis, 1980; Woods & Carey, 1979). Further research is necessary to elucidate these disparities.

The possibility that diffuse cerebral insult in infancy leads to poorer nonverbal and motor skills in some types of cases may be important for models of recovery of function. Hydrocephalic infants frequently suffer generalized disturbances of motor and oculomotor functioning that severely limit environmental exploration. They are often delayed in walking, perhaps reflecting the greater influence of the motor handicaps in these infants than in infants with hemiplegia. Several developmental psychologists have emphasized the importance of sensorimotor experience and environmental exploration from 6 to 18 months as precursors for the development of nonverbal intelligence (Bruner, 1973; McCall, Hogarty & Hurlburt, 1972; Piaget, 1952). It is also plausible that the marked dilatation of the posterior portion of the lateral ventricles characteristic of hydrocephalus might partially disrupt connections to the primary and associative visual cortices, thereby constraining integration of visual input with other sensory modalities and stored engrams. Finally, it is possible that characteristics of the infant brain are predisposed to preferential development of verbal ability in cases of diffuse cerebral insult. However, the interaction of hydrocephalus-related motor and oculomotor deficits with the reduction in sensorimotor experience early in development could be related to the decrement in nonverbal skills observed in many cases of diffuse cerebral insult in infancy.

With respect to recovery of function, studies of diffuse cerebral injury provide opportunities to investigate the cumulative effects of experience in relation to early brain insult. Many longitudinal studies investigating the effects of biological and environmental variables on outcomes associated with prematurity have included only relatively low-risk infants with presumed early brain insult (e.g., RDS; Field, Dempsey, & Shuman, 1979, 1981; Hunt, 1981). Environmental effects on the development of infants with documented early brain damage such as IVH and hydrocephalus have not been systematically studied, even when the children are older. Investigations of these effects should include traditional social and cultural variables in addition to specific measures of parental caretaking abilities. For example, early infant characteristics were found to relate indirectly to later outcome by influencing maternal responsiveness (Sigman, Cohen, & Forsythe, 1981). Other studies have suggested that the degree and consistency of maternal responsiveness is related to several infant factors, including attentional differences within premature infants (Sigman & Beckwith, 1980), variability of infant response modes (Horowitz, 1981), and chronicity of illness over the first year (Beckwith & Cohen, 1983). At the same time, it is becoming apparent that cognitive differences between preterm and term infants can be observed early in development. For example, Rose (1981) found differences in the amount of time required to encode visual information between preterm and term infants at 4 months. Leslie (1982) showed that the inability to control focus of attention was related to the presence of IVH within a group of 6-month-old VLBW infants. As these studies suggest, a variety of infant behaviors and environmental factors could be examined in relation to degree and type of early brain insult. With the use of (1) improved documentation of neurological complications associated with prematurity and early brain injury, (2) additional indices of environmental influences, (3) more sensitive measures of early infant development, and (4) de-emphasis of standardized IQ tests as sole outcome measures, we may begin to better understand how biological and social factors influence development subsequent to early brain insult.

With regard to the plasticity hypotheses, studies of diffuse cerebral insult in infancy are consistent with research on neuropsychological recovery from severe head injury in children. These studies have provided little support for the view that the young brain is less vulnerable to diffuse insult or that it recovers more completely than the mature brain. The limitations inherent in studies confined to global measures of cognition, particularly in providing support for or against the concept of plasticity, should be carefully noted. For example, IQ test scores in hydrocephalic children are quite variable and do not support a strict interpretation of plasticity. Perhaps more important are the subtle dissociations among specific abilities in nonretarded children with congenital hydrocephalus. A more adequate model of recovery will include explorations of the nature and relationship of the multiple factors underlying the development of specific abilities in these children—not just global indices of functioning provided by IQ test scores. Whether plasticity will be a part of explanations of recovery awaits careful, systematic studies of the relationship of early cerebral insult and developmental outcome. One important aspect of the types of diffuse CNS insult emphasized in this chapter is that such cases occur more frequently than infantile hemiplegia cases. Advanced techniques for brain imaging can potentially make visible the degree of involvement of neuroanatomical regions of interest. Future studies of the consequences of diffuse cerebral insult in infancy with careful collection of injury data, environment variables, and detailed cognitive assessments beyond IQ tests may shed light on models of neurobehavioral development and recovery.

References

Abercrombie, M. L. J. (1968). Some notes on spatial disability: Movement, intelligence quotient, and alertness. *Developmental Medicine and Child Neurology, 10,* 206–213.

Annett, M. (1973). Laterality of childhood hemiplegia and the growth of speech and intelligence. *Cortex, 9,* 4–33.

Basser, L. S. (1962). Hemiplegia of early onset and the faculty of speech with special reference to the effects of hemipherectomy. *Brain, 85,* 427–460.

Bastian, H. C. (1898). *A treatise on aphasia and other speech defects.* New York: Appleton.

Beckwith, L., & Cohen, S. (1983). *Continuity of caregiving with preterm infants.* Paper presented at the Society for Research in Child Development, Detroit, MI.

Brink, J. D., Garrett, A. L., Hale, W. R., Woo-Sam, J., & Nickel, V. L. (1970). Recovery of motor and intellectual function in children sustaining severe head injuries. *Developmental Medicine and Child Neurology, 12,* 565–571.

Bruce, D. A., Schut, L., Brown, L. A., Wood, J. H., & Sutton, L. N. (1978). Outcome following severe head injury in children. *Journal of Neurosurgery, 97,* 721–727.

Bruner, J. S. (1973). The organization of early skilled action. *Child Development, 44,* 1–11.

Brunt, D. (1981). Predictive factors of perceptual motor ability in children with meningomyelocele. *American Corrective Therapy Journal, 35,* 42–46.

Burkland, C. W., & Smith, A. (1977). Language and the cerebral hemisphere. *Neurology,* 627–633.

Byers, R. K., & McLean, W. T. (1962). Etiology and course of certain hemiplegias with aphasia in children. *Pediatrics, 29,* 376–383.

Caputo, D. W., & Mandell, W. (1970). Consequences of low birthweight. *Developmental Psychology, 3,* 363–383.

Chaplin, E. R., Goldstein, G. W., Myerberg, D. Z., Hunt, J. V., & Tooley, W. H. (1980). Posthemorrhagic hydrocephalus in the preterm infant. *Pediatrics, 65,* 901–909.

Dennis, M. (1980). Language acquisition in a single hemisphere: Semantic organization. In D. Caplan (Ed.), *Biological studies of mental processes.* Cambridge: MIT Press.

Dennis, M., Fitz, C. R., Netley, C. T., Sugar, J., Derek, C. F., Harwood-Nash, M. B, Hendrick, H. B., Hoffman, H. J., & Humphreys, R. P. (1981). The intelligence of hydrocephalic children. *Archives of Neurology, 38,* 607–615.

Dennis, M., & Kohn, B., (1975). Comprehension of syntax in infantile hemiplegics after cerebral hemidecortication: Left hemisphere superiority. *Brain and Language, 2,* 472–482.

Dennis, M., & Whitaker, H. A. (1976). Language acquisition following hemidecortication: Linguistic superiority of the left over the right hemisphere. *Brain and Language, 3,* 404–433.

Dennis, M., & Whitaker, H. A. (1977). Hemispheric equipotentiality and language acquisition. In S. Segalowitz & F. Gruber (Eds.), *Language development and neurological theory.* New York: Academic Press.

Desmond, M. D., Wilson, G. S., Alt, E. J., & Fisher, E. S. (1980). The very low birth weight infant after discharge from intensive care: Anticipatory health care and developmental course. *Current Problems in Pediatrics, 10,* 1–50.

Drillien, C. M. (1964). *The growth and development of the prematurely born infant.* Baltimore: Williams & Wilkins.

Dykes, F. D., Lazzara, A., Ahmann, P., Blumenstein, B., Schwartz, J., & Brann, A. W. (1980). Intraventricular hemorrhage: A prospective evaluation of etiopathogenesis. *Pediatrics, 66,* 42.

Field, T. M., Dempsey, J. R., & Shuman, H. H. (1979). Developmental assessments of infants surviving the respiratory distress syndrome. In T. Field, A. Sostek, S. Goldberg, & H. H. Shuman (Eds.), *Infants born at risk.* New York: Spectrum.

Field, T. M., Dempsey, J. R., & Shuman, H. H. (1981). Developmental follow-up of pre and postterm infants. In S. L. Friedman & M. Sigman (Eds.), *Preterm birth and psychological development* (pp. 299–312) New York: Academic Press.

Finger, S. (1978). *Recovery from brain damage: Research and theory.* New York: Plenum.

Fletcher, J. M., & Satz, P. (1983). Age, plasticity, and equipotentiality: A reply to Smith. *Journal of Consulting and Clinical Psychology. 51,* 763–767.

Goldman, P. S. (1974). Plasticity of function in the CNS. In D. G. Stein, J. J. Rosen, & N. Butters (Eds.), *Plasticity and recovery of function in the central nervous system.* London: Academic Press.

Goldman, P. S., & Alexander, G. G. (1977). Maturation of prefrontal cortex in the monkey revealed by focal reversible cyrogenic depression. *Nature, 267,* 613–615.

Graham, F. K., Ernhart, C. B., Thurston, D. L., & Craft, M. (1962). Development three years after perinatal anoxia and other potentially damaging newborn experiences. *Psychological Monographs, 76,* 3(Whole no. 522).

Hagberg, B. (1962). The sequelae of spontaneously arrested hydrocephalus. *Developmental Medicine and Child Neurology, 4,* 583–587.

Harrod, J. R., L'Heureaux, P., Wangensteen, D. O., & Hunt, C. D. (1974). Long-term follow-up of severe respiratory distress syndrome treated with IPPV. *Journal of Pediatrics, 84,* 277.

Horowitz, F. D. (1981). Toward a model of early infant development. In C. C. Brown (Ed.), *Infants at risk: Assessment and intervention.* Skillman, NJ: Johnson & Johnson Baby Products.

Hunt, J. V. (1981). Predicting intellectual disorders in childhood for preterm infants with birthweight below 1501 gm. In S. L. Friedman & M. Sigman (Eds.), *Preterm birth and psychological development.* New York: Academic Press.

Isaacson, R. L. (1975). The myth of recovery from early brain damage. In N. E. Ellis, (Ed.), *Aberrant development in infancy.* London: Wiley.

Johnson, J. D., Malachowski, N. C., Grobstein, R., Welsh, D., Daily, W. J. F., & Sunshine, P. (1974). Prognosis of children surviving with the aid of mechanical ventilation in the newborn period. *Journal of Pediatrics, 84,* 272.

Kennard, M. A. (1936). Age and other factors in motor recovery from precentral lesions in monkeys. *American Journal of Physiology, 115,* 138–146.

Kohn B., & Dennis, M. (1974). Selective impairments of visuo-spatial abilities in infantile hemiplegics after right cerebral hemidecortication. *Neuropsychologia, 12,* 505–512.

Koons, A., Sun, S., & Koenigsberger, R. (1982). Intraventricular hemorrhage, ventricular dilation, and outcome. *Pediatric Research, 16,* 55A.

Krashen, S. (1973). Lateralization, language learning and the critical period: Some new evidence. *Language and Learning, 23,* 63–74.

Krishnamoorthy, K. S., Todres, D. D., Kuehnle, K. J., Shannon, D. C., DeLong, G. R., & Davis, K. R. (1980). Neurologic sequelae in the survivors of neonatal intraventricular hemorrhage. *Perinatal Intracranial Hemorrhage Conference Syllabus.* Columbus, OH: Ross Laboratories Publications.

Landry, S. H., Fletcher, J. M., Chapieski, L., & Francis, D. J. (1983, February) *Differen-*

tial outcomes associated with early medical complications in premature infants. Paper presented at the Annual Meeting of the International Neuropsychological Society, Mexico City, D. F.

Lashley, K. S. (1938). Factors limiting recovery after cerebral nervous lesions. *Journal of Nervous and Mental Disease, 88,* 733–755.

Lenneberg, E. (1967). *Biological foundations of language.* New York: Wiley.

Leslie N. (1982). *Visual attention in premature infants with intraventricular hemorrhage and respiratory distress syndrome.* Unpublished doctoral dissertation, University of Houston.

Levin, H. S., Benton, A. L., & Grossman, R. G. (1982). *Neurobehavioral consequences of closed head injury.* New York: Oxford University Press.

Levin, H. S., Eisenberg, H. M., Wigg, N. R., & Kobayashi, K. (1982). Memory and intellectual ability after head injury in children and adolescents. *Neurosurgery, 11,* 668–673.

Levin, H. S., Ewing-Cobbs, L., & Benton, A. L. (1983). Age and recovery from brain damage: A review of clinical studies. In S. Scheff (Ed.), *Aging and recovery of function.* New York: Plenum.

McCall, R. B. (1979). Development of intellectual functioning in infancy and the prediction of later IQ. In J. D. Osofsky (Ed.), *Handbook of infant development.* New York: Wiley.

McCall, R. B., Hogarty, P. S., & Hurlburt, N. (1972). Transitions in infant sensorimotor development and the prediction of childhood IQ. *American Psychologist, 27,* 728–748.

Ment, L. R., Scott, D. T., Ehrenkranz, R. A., Rothman, S. G., Duncan, C. C., & Warshaw, J. B. (1982). Neonates of 1,250 grams birthweight: Prospective neurodevelopmental evaluation during the first year post-term. *Pediatrics, 70,* 292–296.

Minde, K., Webb, G., & Sykes, D. (1968). Studies on the hyperactive child: II. Prenatal and perinatal factors associated with hyperactivity. *Developmental Medicine and Child Neurology, 10,* 355–363.

Naulty, C. M., Binder, H., Murray, S. L., Markle, B., Barnet, A., & Wagman, B. (1982). Neurodevelopmental outcome of birthweight infants at 18–36 months with and without intraventricular hemorrhage (IVH). *Perinatal intracranial hemorrhage conference syllabus.* Washington, D.C.: Ross Laboratories Publications.

Nelson, H. E. (1980). A longitudinal study of the psychological aspects of myelomeningocele. *Scandinavian Journal of Psychology, 21,* 45–54.

Papile, L. A., Burstein, J., Burstein, R., & Koffler, H. (1978). Incidence and evaluation of subependymal and intraventricular hemorrhage: A study of infants with birth weight less than 1500 grams. *Journal of Pediatrics, 92,* 529.

Papile, L. A., Burstein, J., Burstein, R., Koffler, H., Koops, B. L., & Johnson, J. D. (1980). Posthemorrhagic hydrocephalus in low birthweight infants: Treatment by serial lumbar punctures. *Journal of Pediatrics, 97,* 273–277.

Papile, L., Munsick, G., Weaver, N., & Pecha, S. (1979). Cerebral intraventricular hemorrhage in infants (CVHY) 1500 grams: Developmental follow-up at one year. *Pediatric Research, 13,* 528.

Pasamanick, B., & Knoblock, H. (1966). Retrospective studies on the epidemiology of reproductive casualty: Old and new. *Merrill Palmer Quarterly of Behavioral Development, 12,* 7–26.

Piaget, J. (1952). *The origins of intelligence in children.* New York: International Universities.

Rose S. A. (1981). Lags in the cognitive competence of prematurely born infants. In S.

L. Friedman & M. Sigman (Eds.), *Preterm birth and psychological development.* New York: Academic Press.

Ross, G., & Schechner, S. (1982). *Peri/intraventricular hemorrhage as a risk factor in the development of premature infants.* Paper presented at the International Conference on Infancy, Austin, TX.

Rutter, M., Graham, P., & Yule, W. (1970). A neuropsychiatric study in childhood. *Clinics in developmental medicine* (Nos. 35/36). Philadephia: Lippincott.

St. James-Roberts, I. (1979). Neurological plasticity and recovery from brain insult. In H. W. Reese & L. P. Lipsitt (Eds.), *Advances in child development and behavior.* (Vol. 5, pp. 253–319). New York: Academic Press.

St. James-Roberts, I. (1981). A reinterpretation of the hemispherectomy data without functional plasticity of the brain. *Brain and Language, 13,* 31–53.

Sameroff, A. L., & Chandler, M. J. (1975). Reproductive risk and the continuum of caretaking casualty. In F. D. Horowitz (Ed.), *Handbook of child development research* (Vol. V). Chicago: University of Chicago Press.

Sand, P. L., Taylor, N., Rawlings, M., & Chitnis, S. (1973). Performance of children with spina bifida manifesta on the Frostig Developmental Test of visual perceptual skills. *Perceptual and Motor Skills, 37,* 539–546.

Satz, P., & Bullard-Bates, C. (1981). Acquired aphasia in children. In M. T. Sarno (Ed.), *Acquired aphasia.* New York: Academic Press.

Schub, H. S., Ahmann, P. A., Dykes, F. D., Lazzara, A., & Blumenstein, B. (1981). Prospective long-term follow-up of prematures with subependymal/intraventricular hemmorrhage (SEH/IVH). *Pediatric Research, 15,* 711.

Siegel A. W., Bisanz, J., & Bisanz, G. L. (1983). Developmental analysis: A strategy for the study of psychological change. *Controbutions to human development, 8,* 53–80.

Shinnar, S., Molteni, R. A., Gammon, K., D'Souza, B. J., Altman, J., & Freeman, J. M. (1982). Intraventricular hemorrhage in the premature infant: A changing outlook. *The New England Journal of Medicine, 306,* 1464–1468.

Sigman, M., & Beckwith, L. (198O). Infant visual attentiveness in relation to caregiver–infant interaction and developmental outcome. *Infant Behavior and Development, 3,* 141–154.

Sigman, M., Cohen, S., & Forsythe, A. (1981). The relation of early infant measures to later development. In S. L. Friedman & M. Sigman (Eds.), *Preterm birth and psychological development.* New York: Academic Press.

Soare, P. L., & Raimondi, A. J. (1977). Intellectual and perceptual–motor characteristics of treated myelomeningocele children. *American Journal of Disabled Children, 131,* 199–204.

Smith, A. (1974). Dominant and nondominant hemispherectomy. In M. Kinsbourne & W. L. Smith (Eds.), *Hemisphere disconnection and cerebral function.* Springfield, IL: Thomas.

Smith, A. (1981) On the organization, disorganization and reorganization of language and other brain functions. In Y. Lebrun & O. L. Zangwill (Eds.), *Lateralization of language in the child.* Lisse: Swets.

Spain, B. (1974). Verbal and performance ability in pre-school children with spina bifida. *Developmental Medicine and Child Neurology, 16,* 773–780.

Stewart, D. L., & Reynolds, E. O. R. (1975). Improved prognosis for infants of very low birthweight. *Pediatrics, 54,* 724–735.

Teuber, H. L. (1967). Lacunae and research approaches to them. In C. H. Millikan & F. L. Darley (Eds.), *Brain mechanisms underlying speech and language.* New York: Grune & Stratton.

Tew, B. (1979). The "Cocktail Party Syndrome" in children with hydrocephalus and spina bifida. *British Journal of Disorders of Communications, 14,* 89–101.

Thompson, M. G., Eisenberg, H. M., & Levin, H. S. (1982). Hydrocephalic infants: Developmental assessment and computed tomography. *Child's Brain, 9,* 400–410.

Towbin, A. (1981). Neuropathological aspects: II. Perinatal brain damage and its sequels. In P. Black (Ed.), *Brain dysfunction in children: Etiology, diagnosis, and management.* New York: Raven.

Wada, J. A. (1974). Morphologic asymmetry of human cerebral hemispheres: Temporal and frontal speech zones in 100 adult and 10 infant brains. *Neurology, 24,* 349.

Williamson, W. D., Desmond, M., Wilson, G. S., Andrew, M. S., & Garcia-Prats, J. A. (1982). Early neurodevelopmental outcomes of low birth weight infants surviving neonatal intraventricular hemorrhage. *Journal of Perinatal Medicine, 304,* 886–891.

Wohlwill, J. (1973). *The study of behavioral change.* New York: Academic Press.

Woods, B. T. (1980). The restricted effects of right-hemisphere lesions after age one: Wechsler test data. *Neuropsychologia, 18,* 65–70.

Woods, B. T., & Carey, S. (1979). Language deficits after apparent clinical recovery from childhood aphasia. *Annals of Neurology, 6,* 405–409.

Woods, B. T., & Teuber, H. L. (1978). Changing patterns of childhood aphasia. *Annals of Neurology, 3,* 273–280.

Zeiner, H. K., & Prigatano, G. P. (1982). Information processing deficits in hydrocephalic and letter reversal children. *Neuropsychologia, 20,* 483–492.

11

Neuropsychological Correlates of Early Generalized Brain Dysfunction in Children

Daniel S. O'Leary
and Thomas J. Boll

Introduction

As with most brain–behavior issues, knowledge concerning effects of early brain damage has been gained through two major stategies: (1) laboratory study of the behavioral effects of purposively placed lesions in animals and (2) clinical study of behavior following naturally occurring disease or trauma in humans. Although both strategies have weaknesses, they also have complementary strengths (Benton, 1978; Glassman, 1978). Through interaction, perspectives can be achieved that are not accessible to either approach in isolation. A continuing dialogue between those who do animal research and those who work with human clinical populations is therefore extremely important. Volumes such as the present provide a valuable forum for such dialogue.

Copyright © 1984 by Academic Press, Inc.
All rights of reproduction in any form reserved.
ISBN 0-12-052901-7

This chapter discusses knowledge gained from human clinical studies of early generalized brain damage. This type of damage has not received much attention from animal researchers interested in brain–behavior relationships, perhaps because traditional laboratory methodologies emphasize the study of lesions that are as discrete and as well localized as possible (Woosley, 1978). However, laboratory studies as well as clinical studies of the effects of early generalized brain damage are important for a number of reasons. Of the naturally occurring forms of early brain damage, generalized damage is much more common than is focal damage. The brain appears to be more vulnerable to damage during its early period of rapid growth than it is later (Brazier, 1975), and a variety of agents (anoxia, hypoxia, infection, nutritional deficiencies, chemical pollutants, etc.) can cause early generalized damage (Renis & Goldman, 1980). Furthermore, there is evidence that even focal damage may have generalized effects if it occurs very early in development. Small focal lesions produced at or near the time of birth have been shown to reduce overall brain size in animals (Isaacson & Nonneman, 1973), and Isaacson (1975) has argued that many of the effects of early focal damage are due to more generalized and permanent changes in brain structure that are secondary to the damage.

Given that early generalized brain damage occurs relatively frequently, knowledge of its effects on the neuronal and the behavioral level has both practical and theoretical importance. From a practical and humanitarian perspective, such knowledge is necessary to allow the development of adequate techniques for the assessment and treatment of children with early generalized brain damage. For example, it would be important to know if techniques such as environmental enrichment might help to alleviate the behavioral deficits caused by early damage. From a more theoretical perspective, knowledge of the relationship between neuronal changes caused by early generalized damage and resulting behavioral changes in animals may allow new insights into brain–behavior relationships. As is noted in the following, there is evidence that early generalized damage may differentially effect higher cognitive functions but allow relative sparing of more elementary sensory and motor functions. Thus, despite the complexities involved, study of the behavioral effects of early generalized brain damage should yield information not available from the study of the effects of discrete lesions.

Several findings have emerged from both laboratory and clinical studies of the behavioral effects of localized brain lesions that have relevance to studies of the effects of early generalized damage. The first is that the effects of brain damage are frequently task specific, with some behaviors showing deficits while others are unaffected (Isaacson, 1975; Teuber & Rudel, 1962). The relevance of this fact for clinical studies of humans with early generalized damage is that a wide variety of behaviors need to be sampled in order to ensure an accurate assessment of the pattern of behavioral deficits and strengths that result from the damage. A second finding is that different types of deficits may be seen at different ages following early brain damage (Johnson & Almli, 1978). This has particular relevance for clinical studies because human behavior shows dramatic developmental changes across the life-span. Knowledge of the effects of early brain damage on behavior in the childhood years is particularly important because this is the period during which knowledge and skills must be acquired that will be used throughout adult life. Thus, the following review will concentrate on the effects of early generalized brain damage in children.

Effects of Early Generalized Damage

Sensory and Motor Effects

Vygotsky (1962) suggested that early brain damage may differentially affect complex abilities, leaving elementary functions relatively intact. Support for this position can be found in the effects of early generalized damage on simple sensory functions. Rudel, Teuber, and Twitchell (1974) found that children with cerebral palsy due to pre- or perinatal brain injury had normal or better than normal sensitivity for light touch. Two-point discrimination, discrimination of passive movement of the fingers and toes, and response to double simultaneous stimulation were also normal in a majority of these children. In contrast, more complex sensory tasks requiring recognition of objects by touch or cross-modal sensory transfer showed significant impairment, as did all tasks with a motor component.

Klonoff and Low (1974) found similar motor impairment in two groups of children with early brain damage due to either meningitis, maternal rubella, kernicterus, or encephalitis. Studies that have grouped children with early generalized brain damage with children with other types of early damage have also found that the brain-damaged groups performed more poorly than normal children on tasks measuring motor speed and coordination (Boll, 1972, 1974; Reitan, 1974; Reitan & Boll, 1973). However, Boll (1972) found that abilities requiring higher-level conceptual abilities were significantly more impaired by the presence of brain damage than were abilities of motor speed or auditory, visual, or tactile perception.

Despite the frequent suggestion that hyperactive children have a form of minimal brain dysfunction resulting from early brain damage (Pasamanick & Knoblock, 1966; Strauss & Lehtinen, 1947), there is no evidence that early brain damage results in increased motor output. Graham, Ernhart, Thurston, and Craft (1962), in a study of children who suffered from fetal anoxia, and Seidel, Chadwick, and Rutter (1975), in a study of children with cerebral palsy, found no evidence of hyperactivity in any of the children studied. Similarly, Rutter (1982a), in a review of studies in which subclinical brain injury may be presumed to have occurred (perinatal complications and lead intoxication), found no evidence of a consistent behavioral syndrome that included hyperactivity as a symptom.

INTELLIGENCE

The effects of brain damage on intelligence as measured by standardized IQ tests differ strikingly in adults and children. Many studies of adults have found that even serious brain damage may have little effect on psychometric IQ, with vocabulary showing particular sparing (see Boll, 1978 for a review). In contrast, IQ deficits are extremely common following brain damage in children, with vocabulary being particularly likely to show deficits (Boll & Barth, 1981). Rutter (1981), in a review of the effects of brain damage in children, noted that bilateral widespread damage is usually associated with substantial cognitive retardation. He suggested that brain damage in children, unlike that in adults, tends to have its main effect on general intelligence (Rutter, 1982b). Reitan (1974) stated that the Weschler Intelligence Scale for Children (WISC) is one of the most sensitive measures of brain dmage in children. He suggested that early brain damage limits the potential for normal development and therefore has more serious consequences with respect to higher cognitive functions than does damage to the adult brain.

The IQ data might seem to indicate that brain damage affects qualitatively different cognitive abilities in children and adults. However, the data may instead indicate that the seemingly similar child and adult IQ tests actually measure very different sorts of abilities (Boll, 1978). Halstead (1947), Hebb (1949), and Goldstein (1952) have all argued that brain damage at any age primarily impairs the ability to learn, to solve unfamiliar problems, and to abstract. Hebb labeled these abilities type A *intelligence* and postulated that this form of intelligence is heavily relied upon by children for daily living. These abilities are also heavily tapped by children's IQ tests, which explains the sensitivity of the WISC to brain damage. Type *A* intelligence is also impaired by brain damage in adults, but performance on adult IQ tests depends more upon the retrieval and proper use of previously learned material. Hebb labeled these functions type B *intelligence* and suggested that this ability is less disrupted by brain damage. Thus, brain damage may have relatively little effect on IQ test performance in adults, who rely predominantly on type *B* intelligence.

One other major difference between IQ test performances in brain damaged children and in adults concerns the significance of discrepancies between verbal and performance IQ scores. In adults, lesions localized to the left and right cerebral hemispheres may differentially affect verbal and nonverbal abilities, causing verbal–performance splits on the Weschler Adult Intelligence Scale. Rutter (1981) concluded that localized cerebral lesions in children are much less likely to cause specific deficits in verbal or nonverbal processes and are therefore less likely to result in verbal–performance splits. On the other hand, Boll and Barth (1981) reviewed studies that indicate that in children with *generalized* brain damage there was a much higher incidence than in adults of relatively large discrepancies between verbal and performance IQ scores. In the majority of these cases, verbal IQ scores surpassed the performance scores. Although the significance of these findings is unknown, it would appear that in children there is much less of a relationship between verbal and performance IQ score discrepancies and localization of damage than there is in adults.

Other Cognitive Measures

Several authors have criticized the use of intelligence tests as the sole behavioral measure of central nervous system (CNS) damage (St. James-Roberts, 1979; Spreen, 1976; Yule, 1978). Although experienced clinical researchers have consistently reported intelligence tests to be among the most sensitive measures of brain damage in children (Benton, 1974; Boll, 1972; 1974; Boll & Barth, 1981; Reitan, 1974; Rutter, 1981), they have also consistently reported that there is no homogenous pattern of deficit associated with such damage. That is, there are large individual differences in the patterns of behavioral deficit that are exhibited by brain-injured children.

Modern intelligence tests are designed to measure a broad range of cognitive abilities, and IQ scores have for this reason been found to have moderately high correlations with a number of other commonly administered neuropsychological measures (Klonoff & Low, 1974; Knights & Tymchuck, 1968). Nevertheless, it is possible for a child with early brain injury to have a subtle and highly specific cognitive deficit that is not detectable by an IQ test (Benton, 1974; Boll, 1982; Rutter, 1982b). If relationships between brain systems and specific cognitive abilities are to be uncovered, then neuropsychological measures that tap narrow and well-defined cognitive abilities need to be administered along with wider-band measures such as intelligence tests.

A number of types of early generalized brain damage impair communicative functions in children (Dreifuss, 1975; Pirozzolo, Campanella, Christensen, & Lawson-Kerr, 1981). In contrast to the acquired aphasias of childhood that can result from later brain injury, early generalized damage can disrupt the normal development of language. Benton (1978) has differentiated several subgroups of children who have problems in the development of speech and language. He cautions about the problems of interpretation that arise when studies of developmental language disorders fail to adequately control for such subgroups.

Thoman (1978) has argued that early CNS damage may disrupt the early nonverbal communication that takes place between a child and its mother. This early communication is primarily emotional and is carried out with the whole body rather than with speech. It establishes the communicative ties between mother and infant that are essential for the later acquisition of language and other cognitive and social skills. Thus, disruption of early nonverbal communication by CNS damage can seriously disrupt the normal process of both cognitive and social development.

Personality and Emotional Disturbance

The effects of early brain damage on personality and emotional disturbance has been assessed in a series of careful studies by Rutter and his associates (see Rutter, 1977, 1981, 1982a, 1982b for review).

In brief, Rutter found that children with early brain injury are twice as likely as children with nonneural physical handicaps such as diabetes or heart disease to show behavioral disorders. Even when matched for degree of physical handicap with children with neural damage below the brainstem (e.g., polio and muscular dystrophy), children with early brain damage (mostly cerebral palsy) had twice the incidence of behavioral disturbance of the matched controls. Behavioral disorders were significantly more common when the brain damage was bilateral than when it was unilateral, and there was a tendency for behavioral disorder to be more frequent when brain injury was accompanied by seizures or abnormal EEG discharges.

Despite the high incidence of psychological disturbance, there was no stereotyped pattern of behavior that was characteristic of brain-damaged children in the Rutter studies. In the Isle of Wight study (Rutter, Graham, & Yule, 1970), children with brain damage showed an excess of symptoms of all types but had no characteristic symptom cluster. Brain-damaged children showed patterns of emotional disturbance that were similar to those exhibited by children without brain damage. The brain-damaged children simply had a higher incidence of such disturbance. Rutter (1981) concluded that behavioral abnormalities such as impulsivity or hyperactivity, which have been associated with brain injury, are in fact characteristic of psychiatric disorder regardless of the presence or absence of brain damage.

Areas in Need of Further Research

Anatomical Basis of Damage

Benton (1974) has noted that clinical researchers who study humans must frequently rely on much less precise knowledge of the nature, extent, and locus of brain injury than do researchers who use laboratory animals. In no area is this truer than in the study of the behavioral effects of early generalized brain damage in children. Early brain damage of a generalized nature may be caused by a variety of agents, all of which differ significantly in the specific brain systems that they affect. Renis and Goldman (1980), for example, note that anoxia, a brief but total absence of oxygen available to a fetus, causes damage that is typically concentrated in the brainstem. Hypoxia, or a reduction in partial pressure of oxygen, is more likely to damage the cerebral hemispheres. Other agents such as chemical and viral teratogens, radiation damage, and nutritional deficiencies may also affect different brain systems, and their specific effects undoubtedly depend upon the maturational state of the pre- or postnatal brain at the time of the insult.

Chelune and Edwards (1981) reviewed the effects of a number of different types of early brain damage. They found evidence that, for generalized damage caused by infectious diseases and diffuse anoxic conditions, early injury typically has a worse prognosis than does later injury. For closed head-injury, however, the earlier the injury the better the prognosis. The developmental neural mechanisms that underlie this interaction between age and causal agent are unknown.

Seizures are a manifestation of an underlying neurophysiological dysfunction that frequently has an unknown etiology and anatomical basis. Children with both generalized tonic–clonic and partial seizures that begin early in life exhibit, as a group, poorer neuropsychological performance than do children whose seizures begin later (O'Leary, Lovel, Sackellares, Giordani, Seidenberg, Berent & Boll, 1983; O'Leary, Seidenberg, Berent & Boll, 1981). However, children with seizures of early onset typically begin antiepilepsy medication early, so the effects of seizure variables are difficult to disentangle from the effects of drugs on the developing brain.

In general, there is a great deal to be learned about the specific anatomical effects of early generalized brain damage in humans and about the relationship between anatomical changes and resulting behavioral deficit. It is clear that abnormal brain functioning caused by early diffuse injury can have much more deleterious effects on behavior than does complete loss of neural tissue (Dreifuss, 1975; Rutter, 1981). The continuous presence of abnormal neural tissue throughout development would not allow recovery from long-distance effects, as might occur with a discrete lesion (i.e., von Monakow's, 1914/1969 diaschisis concept, [1914/1969]). Neither could there be replacement of destroyed neuronal connections through sprouting or other structural neural changes. Thus, most anatomical models of recovery of function following discrete damage to the brain are not appropriate for early generalized damage.

Subclinical or Minimal Brain Damage

The lack of knowledge concerning the effects of early brain damage has resulted in a great deal of controversy as to the effects of subclinical or minimal brain damage. The lack of hard anatomical or neurological criteria has frequently led to the diagnosis of brain damage by purely behavioral criteria. The underlying assumption of

Logistic regression

① Mortality ?

② WH

③ Outcome

SIMILAC® Infant Formulas
Providing growth . . .
plus metabolic response
closest to the breastfed infant

Switch first to
ISOMIL® Soy Protein Formulas
When the baby
can't take milk

Z312/6860

ROSS

LITHO IN USA

Haith has described certain Rules that babies look by

Healthy

compelled to seek an edge in a homogeneous field and then scan briefly.

this approach is that early brain damage results in a characteristic behavioral pattern with hyperactivity and distractability as major symptoms.

Problems with the minimal brain-dysfunction concept have been discussed in detail elsewhere (Boll, 1982, Reitan & Boll, 1973; Rutter, 1981, 1982a, 1982b). It is worth stressing, however, that review of the effects of demonstrable early brain damage lends no support to the hypothesis that there is a consistent behavioral syndrome that results from early damage. Rather, one of the primary effects of early brain damage would seem to be an increase in the variability of behavior, and there are large individual differences in the behavioral patterns exhibited by children with seemingly similar damage. Although generalized brain damage in early childhood is likely to lead to later cognitive impairment, there is no evidence that it leads to a specific pattern of either cognitive or behavioral deficit.

Environmental Interactions

As Johnson and Almli (1978) have noted, brain damage sustained early in life automatically precludes normal ontogeny. Thus, even if the brain were susceptible to similar forms of damage in infancy and adulthood (which is clearly not the case), the effects of early and late damage would not be comparable. Human cogitive development is highly dependent on the interaction of a child with both the social and the physical environment. If, as Thoman (1978) suggests, early CNS damage seriously disrupts this interaction, then the result on the developing brain could be similar to that caused by environmental deprivation. That is, disruption of normal environmental interactions would result in functionally lower levels of stimulation to the brain, which could interact with and compound the effects of the initial damage. Thus, a full understanding of the effects of early generalized brain damage will depend on an understanding of the manner in which interactions with the environment normally influence neural and cognitive development.

Normal Developmental Process

We understand relatively little about the normal developmental course of brain–behavior relationships. For example, although a great deal is known about the differential functions of the two hemispheres in adults, there is controversy concerning the development of the adult pattern. The prevailing view has been that the two hemispheres are equipotential at birth and became asymmetrically specialized only as language and other cognitive abilities are acquired (Lenneberg, 1967). But this view has been challenged, and there is a variety of evidence that indicates that the two hemispheres possess innate specializations (see Kinsbourne, 1981 for a review of this data).

Questions concerning the development of cerebral asymmetries are related to questions concerning possible developmental changes in the use of cognitive strategies that rely on left and/or right hemisphere mechanisms. For example, it is possible that very young children rely predominantly upon perceptually based, right hemisphere mechanisms whereas older children rely more on verbal, left hemisphere mechanisms (O'Leary, 1982).

The manner in which the two hemispheres interact during the normal use of language and other cognitive functions is also currently unknown. There is anatomical evidence that the corpus callosum is not completely myelinated until at least the age of 10 years (Yakovlev & Lecours, 1967), and there is behavioral evidence that transfer of information between the two hemispheres becomes increasingly efficient throughout childhood (Galin, Johnstone, Nakell, & Herron, 1979; O'Leary, 1980). Goldman (1971, 1972, 1974) demonstrated (with monkeys) that there are developmental changes in the neural structures that are used to perform particular behaviors. It is likely that such changes occur in humans also. In children, these may involve developmental changes in the neural mechanisms that are unique to the left and right hemispheres, as well as developmental changes in the nature, quality, and extent of interaction between the left and right hemispheres. Damage to the brain that occurs very early in development may not only disrupt the neural systems that are functional at that time, but may also be the cause of deficits that are not seen until much later in development—at the time at which the damaged structures or connections would normally become functional.

Summary and Conclusions

Early generalized brain damage is not a unitary phenomenon. Diffuse damage to the CNS may be caused by a variety of agents. These agents may effect different brain systems, and the specific effect of a particular agent may differ depending upon the maturational level of the brain at the time of insult. In general, earlier damage has a worse prognosis than does later damage, but closed head-injury may be an exception to this generalization. Early generalized damage may spare simple sensory functions, but more complex sensory tasks are likely to show impairment, as are most tasks with a motor component. The greatest impairment, however, is typically seen in cognitive performance. The WISC, which measures a variety of cognitive functions but tests learning, abstraction, and problem-solving abilities particularly heavily, is very likely to show impairment. There is some evidence that verbal IQ may be less impaired than performance IQ, but there is no consistent pattern of cognitive impairment that is exhibited by a majority of children with early diffuse damage. Children with early damage have a much higher than normal incidence of psychological disturbance, but again, there is no specific pattern of disturbance that is characteristic of such children. In particular, hyperactivity and distractability are not characteristic behavioral features of children with early damage.

The human brain undergoes considerable postnatal development, and a child's interactions with both the social and the physical environment appear to be extremely important for the normal development of brain structure and function. When damage occurs early and is diffusely distributed throughout the brain, not only are the damaged neural structures themselves impaired, but the normal ontogenetic process, which requires interaction with the environment, is also disrupted. The preceding human clinical data reviewed earlier indicate that this can have a profound effect on a child's cognitive development. The ultimate effect of early generalized damage depends on a complex interaction of a variety of variables, including the individual differences in genetic endowment, the nature and locus of the damage, the possible continuous presence of impaired neural tissue throughout development, and the extent to which interaction with the environment is impaired. Given this complexity, it is not surprising that there is a great deal of individual variability in the effects of early generalized brain damage.

Data concerning the effects of early generalized damage do not address the traditionally important issues of developmental change in neuronal plasticity and recovery of function. Unlike laboratory lesions that damage or remove specific cortical or subcortical structures, naturally occurring early brain damage may be more likely to affect functional brain systems. Also unlike laboratory lesions, the affected tissue, while damaged, may remain in place and continue to function, albeit in an abnormal fashion. There may be no opportunity for undamaged tissue to assume the functions of the affected neural systems, and issues relating to neuronal plasticity cannot, therefore, be addressed. Similarly, when damage occurs very early in development, issues concerning recovery of function are largely irrelevent because behavioral function, for the most part, has not been established. Questions that can be addressed by data concerning the effects of early generalized damage are more closely related to the developmental process through which the brain establishes function and the manner in which early impairment of neural systems effects this process. In answering such questions, a great deal of attention must be paid to the possibly cumulative effects of early damage on an organism's interaction with environment.

References

Benton, A. (1974). Clinical neuropsychology of childhood: An overview. In R. M. Reitan & L. A. Davison (Eds.), *Clinical neuropsychology: Current status and applications.* New York: Wiley.

Benton, A. (1978). The cognitive functioning of children with developmental dysphasia. In M. A. Wyke (Ed.), *Developmental dysphasia.* London: Academic Press.

Benton, A. (1978). The interplay of experimental and clinical approaches in brain lesion research. In S. Finger (Ed.), *Recovery from brain damage.* New York: Plenum.

Boll, T. J. (1972). Conceptual versus perceptual versus motor deficits in brain-damaged children. *Journal of Clinical Psychology, 28,* 157–159.

Boll, T. J. (1974). Behavioral correlates of cerebral damage in children aged 9–14. In R. M. Reitan & L. A. Davison (Eds.), *Clinical neuropsychology, current status and applications.* New York: Wiley.

Boll, T. J. (1978). Diagnosing brain impairment. In B. Wolman (Ed.), *Diagnosis of mental disorders: A handbook.* New York: Plenum.

Boll, T. J. (1982). Neuropsychological assessment of the child: Myths, current status and future prospects. In L. E. Walker & M. C. Roberts (Eds.), *Handbook of clinical child psychology.* New York: Wiley.

Boll, T. J., & Barth, J. T. (1981). Neuropsychology of brain damage in children. In S. B. Filskov & T. J. Boll (Eds.), *Handbook of clinical neuropsychology.* New York: Wiley.

Brazier, M. A. B. (Ed.) (1975). *Growth and development of the brain. Nutritional, genetic and environmental factors* (Vol. 1). International Brain Research Organization Monograph Series. New York: Raven Press.

Chelune, G. J., & Edwards, P. (1981). Early brain lesions: Ontogenetic–environmental considerations. *Journal of Consulting and Clinical Psychology, 49*(6), 777–790.

Dreifuss, F. E. (1975). The pathology of central communicative disorders in children. In D. B. Tower (Ed.), *The nervous system: Human communication and its disorders* (Vol. 3). New York: Raven.

Galin, D., Johnstone, J., Nakell, L., & Herron, J. (1979). Development of the capacity for tactile information transfer between hemispheres in normal children. *Science, 204,* 1330–1332.

Glassman, R. B. (1978). The logic of the lesion experiment and its role in the neural sciences. In S. Finger (Ed.), *Recovery from brain damage, research and theory.* New York: Plenum.

Goldman, P. S. (1971). Functional development of the prefrontal cortex in early life and the problem of neuronal plasticity. *Experimental Neurology, 32,* 366–387.

Goldman, P. S. (1972). Developmental determinants of cortical plasticity. *Acto Neurobiologica, 32,* 495–511.

Goldman, P. S. (1974). An alternative to developmental plasticity: Heterology of CNS structures in infants and adults. In D. G. Stein, J. R. Rosen, & N. Batters (Eds.), *Plasticity and recovery of function in the central nervous system.* New York: Academic Press.

Goldstein, K. (1952). The effects of brain damage on personality. *Psychiatry, 15,* 245–260.

Graham, F. K., Ernhart, C. B., Thurston, D., & Craft, M. (1962). Development three years after perinatal anoxia and other potentially damaging new born experiences. *Psychological Monographs, 76,*(Whole No. 522).

Halstead, W. C. (1947). *Brain and intelligence: A quantitive study of the frontal lobes.* Chicago: University of Chicago Press.

Hebb, D. O. (1949). *The organization of behavior.* New York: Wiley.

Isaacson, R. L. (1975). The myth of recovery from early brain damage. In N. E. Ellis (Eds.), *Aberrant development in infancy.* London: Wiley.

Isaacson, R. L., & Nonneman, A. J. (1973). Early brain damage and later development. In P. Satz & J. Ross (Eds.), *The disabled learner, early detection, and intervention.* Rotterdam, The Netherlands: Rotterdam University Press.

Johnson, D., & Almli, C. R. (1978). Age, brain damage and performance. In S. Finger (Ed.), *Recovery from brain damage: Research and theory.* New York: Plenum.

Kinsbourne, M. (1981) The development of cerebral dominance. In S. B. Filskov & T. J. Boll, Handbook of Clinical Neuropsychology New York: Wiley.

Klonoff, H., & Low, M. (1974). Disordered brain function in young children and early adolescents: Neuropsychological and electroencephalographic correlates. In R. M. Reitan & L. A. Davison (Eds.), *Clinical neuropsychology: Current status and applications.* New York: Wiley.

Knights, R. M., & Tymchuck, A. J. (1968). An evaluation of the Halstead–Reitan category tests for children *Cortex, 4,* 403–414.

Lenneberg, H. (1967). *Biological foundations of language.* New York: Wiley.

O'Leary, D. S. (1980). A developmental study of interhemispheric transfer in children aged five to ten. *Child Development, 51,* 743–750.

O'Leary, D. S. (1982). Cerebral specialization and cognitive mode—a developmental perspective. In R. N. St. Clair & N. Von Raffler-Engel (Eds.), *Language and cognitive styles.* Lisse: Swets & Zeitlinger.

O'Leary, D. S., Lovell, M. R., Sackellares, C., Berent, S., Giordani, B., Seidenberg, M., & Boll, T. J. (in press). The effects of age of onset of partial and generalized seizures on neuropsychological performance in children. *Journal of Nervous and Mental Disease.* 1983, *171*(10), 624–629.

O'Leary, D. S. Seidenberg, M., Berent, S., & Boll, T. J. (1981). Effects of age of onset of tonic–clonic seizures on neuropsychological performance in children. *Epilepsia, 22,* 197–204.

Pasamanick, B., & Knoblock, H. (1966). Retrospective studies on the epidemiology of reproductive casuality; old and new. *Merrill-Palmer Quarterly of Behavioral Development, 12,* 7–26.

Pirozzolo, F. J., Campanella, D. J., Christensen, K., & Lawson-Kerr, K. (1981). Effects of cerebral dysfunction on neurolinguistic performance in children *Journal of Consulting and Clinical Psychology, 49*(6), 791–806.

Reitan, R. M. (1974). Psychological effects of cerebral lesions in children of early school age. In R. M. Reitan & L. A. Davison (Eds.), *Clinical neuropsychology current status and applications.* New York: Wiley.

Reitan, R. M., & Boll, T. J. (1973). Neuropsychological correlates of minimal brain dysfunction. *Annals of the New York Academy of Sciences, 205,* 65–88.

Renis, S., & Goldman, J. M. (1980). *The development of the brain.* Springfield, IL: Thomas.

Rudel, R. G., Teuber, H. L., & Twitchell, T. E. (1974). Levels of impairment of sensory–motor functions in children with early brain damage. *Neuropsychologia, 12,* 95–108.

Rutter, M. (1977). Brain-damage syndromes in childhood: Concepts and findings. *Journal of Child Psychology and Psychiatry, 18,* 1–21.

Rutter, M. (1981). Psychological sequelae of brain damage in childhood. *American Journal of Psychiatry, 138,* 1533–1544.

Rutter, M. (1982a). Syndromes attributed to "minimal brain dysfunction" in childhood. *American Journal of Psychiatry, 139,* 21–33.

Rutter, M. (1982b). Developmental neuropsychiatry: Concepts, issues and prospects, *Journal of Clinical Neuropsychology, 4,* 91–115.

Rutter, M., Graham, P., & Yule, W. (1970). *A neuropsychiatric study in childhood: Clinics in developmental medicine 35/36.* London: Heinemann/Simp.

St. James-Roberts, I. (1979). Neuronal plasticity, recovery from brain insult, and child development. In H. W. Reese & L. P. Lipsitt (Eds.), *Advances in child development and behavior* (Vol. 14). New York: Academic Press.

Seidel, U. P., Chadwick, O. F. D., & Rutter, M. (1975). Psychological disorders in crippled children. A comparative study of children with and without brain damage. *Developmental Medicine and Child Neurology, 17,* 563–573.

Spreen, O. (1976). Neuropsychology of learning disorders: Post-conference review. In R. Knicht & D. Bakker (Eds.), *The neuropsychology of learning disorders.* Baltimore, MD: University Park Press.

Strauss, A. A., & Lehtinen, V. (1947). *Psychopathology and education of the brain-injured child* (Vol. 1). New York: Grune & Stratton.

Teuber, H. L., & Rudel, R. G. (1962). Behavior after cerebral lesions in children and adults. *Developmental Medicine and Child Neurology, 4,* 3–20.

Thoman, E. B. (1978). CNS dysfunction and nonverbal communication between mother and infant. In C. L. & M. E. Doran-Quine (Eds.), *NINCDS Monograph No. 22; The neurological bases of language disorders in children: Methods and directions for research.* Bethesda, MD: U. S. Department of Health, Education & Welfare.

van Hof, M. W., & Mohn, G. (1981). Introductory overview. In M. W. van Hof & G. Mohn (Eds.), *Functional recovery from brain damage.* Elsevier/North-Holland, Amsterdam: Biomedical Press.

von Monakow, C. (1969). Diaschisis. Excerpted in K. H. Pribram (Ed.), *Mood, states and mind* (pp. 27–37). London: Penguin Books. (Original work published 1914).

Vygotsky, L. S. (1962). *Thought and language.* Cambridge, MA: MIT Press.

Woolsey, T. A. (1978). Lesion experiments: Some anatomical considerations. In S. Finger (Ed.), *Recovery from brain damage; research and theory*. New York: Plenum.

Yakovlev, P. I., & Lecours, A. R. (1967). The myelogenetic cycles of regional maturation of the brain. In A. Mikowski (Ed.), *Regional development of the brain in early life*. Philadelphia: Davis.

Yule, W. (1978). Diagnosis: Developmental psychology assessment. In A. F. Kalverboer, H. M. Van Proag, & J. Mendlewicz (Eds.), *Advances in biological psychiatry* (Vol. 1). Basel, Switzerland: Karger.

IV

Cerebral Lateralization and Higher-Order Functions

12

Functional and Neuronal Plasticity: The Evidence from Callosal Agenesis

Malcolm A. Jeeves

Introduction

The apparent absence of changes in behavior and cognition, accompanied by the presence of a major structural abnormality in the primate brain raises the question, What sort of compensation has taken place? Such is the situation of those few people born without the corpus callosum and, in some cases, also without the anterior commissure. In order to explore possible compensatory mechanisms, we need to know how the corpus callosum develops normally, what additional structural changes may be present when it is absent, and whether acallosal people are indeed as free from behavioral or cognitive deficits as has been assumed. With those three lines of evidence at hand, we may then try to relate the overall behavioral picture with the structural information, to indicate the most likely compensatory mechanisms.

Copyright © 1984 by Academic Press, Inc.
All rights of reproduction in any form reserved.
ISBN 0-12-052901-7

The plan of this chapter is, first, to summarize what is known of the normal development of the neocortical commissures together with the available evidence of structural reorganization in acallosal brains. This is followed by a summary of deficits seen in "split-brain" patients but absent in acallosal patients, as well as deficits reported in acallosal patients. That sets the scene for a discussion of compensatory mechanisms that may account for the overall pattern of abilities and deficits in acallosals. Finally, I briefly summarize the limited evidence of the effects of postnatal–prematurity callosal lesions and compare it with the well-documented effects of commissurotomy in adulthood.

Background

Changing Views

Several bundles of nerve fibers directly connect the two cerebral hemispheres. They include the anterior commissure and the hippocampal commissure (and for some purposes, the massa intermedia), but the largest by far is the corpus callosum, which contains approximately 200 million fibers. In the late 1930s a surgical procedure was introduced that involved the total or partial sectioning of the neocortical commissures, usually the corpus callosum and the anterior commissure. It was aimed at reducing the effects of epilepsy focused in one or the other of the cerebral hemispheres. (Van Wagenen & Herren, 1940). Psychological studies of patients who had undergone this operation (Akelaitis, 1943, 1944) reported few, if any, behavioral or cognitive consequences. In the 1950s, however, Sperry and his colleagues in California (e.g., Sperry, 1968a) undertook careful studies of animals in which the neocortical commissures had been totally sectioned, and they discovered that the two cerebral hemispheres learned independently and did not communicate with one another. Around the same time, the commissurotomy procedure for humans was reintroduced by Bogen and Vogel (e.g., 1962). Adapting the testing techniques used in the animal studies, it was now discovered that in response to lateralized sensory input, whether tactile, visual, or auditory, the patients also showed marked effects of the commissurotomy procedures. As a result, the *disconnection syndrome* became well known and emphasized beyond any doubt the important role of the callosum in the interhemispheric transfer and integration of information.

Around the time that Bogen and Vogel were beginning their new series of commissurotomies, we became interested in the very small group of people who are born without the corpus callosum (Jeeves & Rajalakshmi, 1964). As the results of the California human-commissurotomy studies became widely publicized, the apparent absence of deficits, whether behavioral or cognitive, in those born without the corpus callosum became an embarrassment, to say the least. It was also a challenge, for here was a naturally occurring lesion whose cause was still unknown and whose consequences had not been subjected to careful experimental study. The question arose—and still remains—if the corpus callosum is of such vital importance for the normal interhemispheric transfer and integration of information, how is it that those born without the major neocortical commissural pathway may appear to lead normal lives without consequences of its absence?

Commissural Development: Normal and Abnormal

Since the early 1960s the normal development of the neocortical commissures and the detailed structure of acallosal brains have been studied, the former primarily by Yakovlev and Lecours (1967) and Rakic and Yakovlev (1968) and the latter by Bossy (1970), Stefanko and Schenck (1979), and others. The reports of Rakic and Yakovlev (1968) showed that the corpus callosum is not fully myelinated until about 10 years of age, thus confirming an earlier report by Tomasch (1954). If incomplete myelination reflects a continuing functional plasticity, then we can raise the question of how prematurity lesions of the callosum compare in their effects with the well-documented postmaturity lesions. Likewise, knowledge of the structural changes in acallosal brains could be combined with the findings of psychological and behavioral abilities and deficits in acallosal patients. We could thus begin to ask how the psychological and behavioral results might be understood in the light of the known structural changes in acallosal brains.

Development of the Neocortical Commissures

The first interhemispheric fibers to appear are those of the anterior and hippocampal commissures. The process of further commissuralization involving the corpus callosum is then a rapid one. The first callosal fibers are seen in embryos of about 11 and 12 weeks, and the growth of the fibers toward and across the midline is generally complete after 18–20 weeks. The anterior part of what is to become the body of the corpus callosum develops first and extends caudally with the parallel development of the cortices. The genu and the splenium are the last parts to develop. The onset of myelinization of the fibers of the corpus callosum is later than that of most other cortical fiber tracts, beginning during the period from the second week to the second month of extrauterine life (Yakovlev & Lecours, 1967). Myelinization of the callosum is complete by the 10th year of life, but as Tomasch (1954) points out, not all of the fibers of the corpus callosum become myelinated. The distribution of callosal fibers is principally to homologous areas in the two cerebral hemispheres, although heterotopic connections also occur. The distribution to the various layers of the cerebral cortex is orderly.

Although there is as yet no full understanding of the nature of the developmental insult that prevents the normal development of the corpus callosum, it is clear that the time at which the insult occurs affects the extent of absence of the callosum. So, for example, if the insult occurs before the 10th embryonic week of life, this will prevent the development of all forebrain commissures. An insult in the 10th to 11th weeks will spare only the anterior commissure. At a slightly later stage a defect will not affect the anterior and nascent hippocampal commissures, but it will result in callosal agenesis. In acallosal brains the posterior commissure is normal because its development is independent of the forebrain commissures. There is some evidence to show that when the corpus callosum has failed to develop, certain functioning "callosal" fibers can still cross via the anterior commissure (Geschwind, 1974).

STRUCTURAL CHANGES IN CALLOSAL AGENESIS

Rakic and Yakovlev (1968) believe that callosal agenesis is not a failure of the fibers to grow, but is rather a misdirection of their growth. Three cerebral anomalies are frequently found in conjunction with callosal agenesis. First and perhaps the most important is the occurrence of the so-called Probst bundle. This is a massive longitudinal bundle lying above the fornix and running frontooccipitally in the medial wall of each hemisphere (Figures 1 and 2). The second abnormality is a radial patterning of the sulci found in the medial aspect of the hemispheres. The radial patterning is interpreted as a mechanical result of callosal absence, because most sulci develop

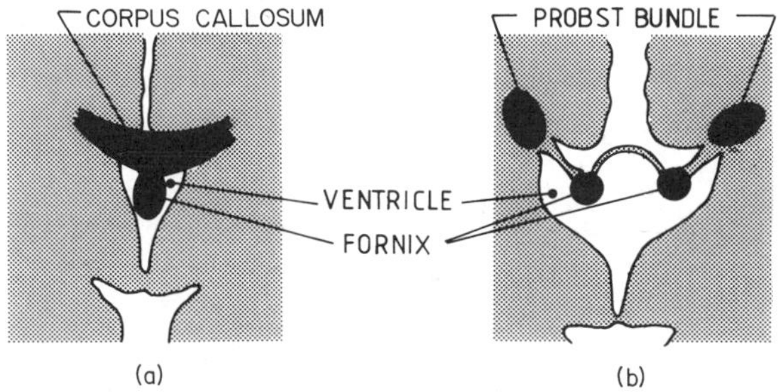

Figure 1. Coronal sections of normal (a) and acallosal (b) brains at the level of the foramen of Monro (Taken from Stefanko and Schenk, 1979.)

after the corpus callosum has been established. Third, the lateral ventricles are often abnormally shaped, with dilation of the posterior horns due to the absence of the forceps major. This feature is especially important in the diagnosis of corpus callosum agenesis. In recent years a series of reports have indicated the existence of normal cytoarchitecture in some acallosal brains (Bossy, 1970; Stefanko & Schenk, 1979).

Bossy (1970) reported a case of what he regarded as pure agenesis: a man who died of natural causes at age 66 and who, during life, gave no evidence of any cerebral abnormality. The brain fell well within the normal range of weight and volume. Microscopic studies of the cortex showed no abnormalities. The anterior commissure, however, was slightly increased in size and included a group of "callosal" fibers. Shoumura, Ando, and Kato (1975) studied two acallosal brains and found that the microstructure of a narrow zone of cortex of Brodmann's area 18 at the boundary area 17 (OBg) differed from normal. Layer III of OBg contained a reduced number of smaller pyramidal cells, whereas the large pyramidal cells were scarcely detectable. These cells in the normal brain send axons through the callosal splenium.

Evidence for the plasticity of callosal connections comes from animal studies by Innocenti and others. Innocenti, Fiore, and Caminiti (1977) have shown that those callosal neurons that interconnect the first and second visual areas in cats (VI and V2) acquire their distribution postnatally by disappearing (dying or eliminating their callosal connections) from most of areas 17 and 18 and decreasing in number in Layer VI. They have also shown that visual experience is one factor that can effect which juvenile callosal neurons (or axons) are stabilized or eliminated. They believe that the reduction of the cortical efferent zone is probably one aspect of a more general on-

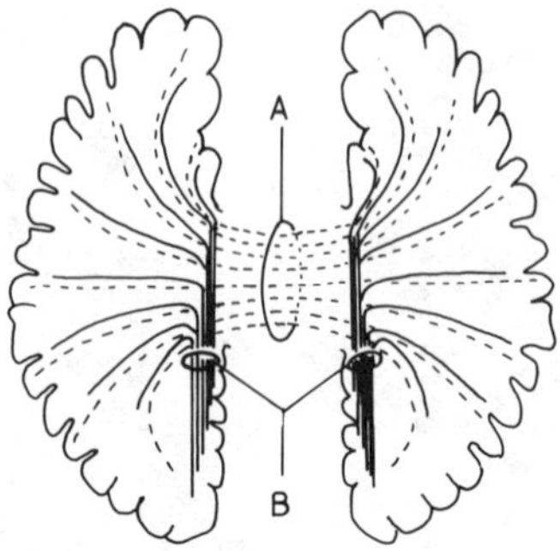

Figure 2. Failure of commissuration without agenesis of callosal fibers. The commissural fibers of corpus callosum (a) in a normal brain are shown by dashed lines. The abnormal longitudinal bundles (Balkenlängsbündels of Probst) (b) consist of normal callosal fibers that failed to cross in agenesis of corpus callosum (solid lines). (Taken from Stefanko and Schenk, 1979, in *Structure and Function of Cerebral Commissures*, Macmillan Press Ltd.).

togenetic diminution of neurons and neuronal connections. They also believe that their results on cats, taken together with others on monkeys, suggest that the transitory neonatal connections can provide a substrate for the plasticity of neuronal connectivity.

Ptito and Lepore (1983), studying interocular transfer in cats with early callosal transections, have emphasized the functional plasticity of the commissural system and have shown that in cats the period of susceptibility to plastic changes is very brief, seeming to end once the corpus callosum becomes anatomically and physiologically mature. Their work on the visual system confirms and extends our own earlier work using tactile tasks (Jeeves & Wilson, 1969). They speculate that the two most likely candidates through which their observed recovery was possible were the intercollicular commissure and the anterior commissure, and that such pathways may help to explain the lack of the disconnection syndrome in human callosal agenesis and in callosotomized children.

DIAGNOSIS OF CALLOSAL AGENESIS

Since 1934, ventriculograms and pneumoencephalograms have been used to detect callosal agenesis. In some cases, carotid angiograms have helped to confirm a diagnosis. Computerized tomography has provided a noninvasive diagnostic technique. Acallosal patients who can thus be identified during life only by the use of nonroutine neurological procedures present a wide variety of signs suggestive of brain dysfunction. Although truly asymptomatic cases have been identified at autopsy (e.g., Bossy 1970), it is always possible that in such cases subliminal deficits were present. The most frequently reported associated brain disorder in acallosals is epilepsy. This is so in the sample reviewed by Chiarello (1980) and referred to in this chapter, as well as in several of the additional cases reported here. Other recurring themes in case notes of acallosal patients include macrocephaly, clumsiness, poor motor control, and low intelligence.

Behavioral and Cognitive Consequences of Callosal Agenesis

The Absence of Expected Deficits

When the corpus callosum and anterior commissure are sectioned in adulthood, the well-documented disconnection syndrome becomes evident under suitable testing conditions (Gazzaniga, 1970). In people born without the corpus callosum (and in some cases, additionally, without the anterior commissure) there is an apparent absence of the disconnection syndrome even when testing is carried out using the same techniques and under the same stringent conditions as in the California split-brain studies. Chiarello (1980) has presented a detailed and comprehensive account of cognitive functioning in callosal agenesis and has tabulated the findings from studies of the 29 cases she reviews. Combining her summary conclusions with the results of our own ongoing investigations, we can produce a consolidated list of the abilities of acallosals as they contrast with the deficits in commissurotomized patients.

In contrast to the split-brain patients, acallosal patients can do the following:

1. read words and name drawn objects when presented in the left visual field (there is one exception to this in the report by Solursh, Margulies, Ashem, and Stasiak (1965);
2. cross-match verbal or nonverbal stimuli presented in opposite visual fields and judge the alignment or misalignment of horizontal lines presented to the two half-fields;
3. name out-of-sight objects by palpation with either hand;

4. carry out cross-tactile localization, although not at the 100% level shown by normal adults;
5. perform dichotic listening tasks without left-ear extinction.

Because split-brain deficits are not evident even with careful testing that involves the lateralized presentation of visual, auditory, and tactile stimuli—it is hardly surprising that it became widely accepted that callosal agenesis did not result in behavioral and cognitive deficits. However, in recent years a number of studies have shown that there are deficits associated with callosal agenesis. The next section describes the extent to which these occur in all acallosal patients and are attributable solely or primarily to the absence of the callosum.

Deficits in Callosal Agenesis

The following are the most frequently reported and clearly demonstrated deficits of callosal agenesis:

1. lengthened interhemispheric transmission times (ITT) with manual responses to lateralized light stimuli; whereas normal subjects show ITTs of approximately 2 msecs, acallosal subjects show ITTs of 10–20 msecs (Jeeves, 1965, 1969; Reynolds & Jeeves, 1977);
2. significant slowing on tasks which require bimanual visual–motor coordination performed as quickly as possible; for example, threading wooden beads, winding a string onto a stick, placing pegs in holes, buttoning up (Jeeves, 1969; Jeeves & Rajalakshmi, 1964; Reynolds & Jeeves, 1977; Sperry, Gazzaniga, & Bogen, 1969);
3. dimished transfer of the learning of a tactual form board or a finger or stylus maze; what is learned with one hand transfers less readily to the other hand (Jeeves, 1965, 1969, 1981; Jeeves & Rajalakshmi, 1964; Reynolds & Jeeves, 1977; Russell & Reitan, 1955; Solursh *et al.*, 1965);
4. the presence of the unintentional synkinetic movements of the fingers of one hand when the fingers of the other hand are required to make specific movements (Dennis, 1976);
5. subnormal levels of cross-localization (between hands) of touch, together with marked deficits in tactile discrimination when required to determine the number of fingers between two that are lightly touched (Jeeves, 1979).

The following deficits were reported in only one study or in only one patient:

1. lengthened ITTs to lateralized light stimuli when the stimulus intensity is decreased—a lengthening that is not found in normals (Milner, 1982);
2. lengthened ITTs with vocal responses to left visual-field light-stimuli as compared with right visual-field stimuli (Milner, 1982);
3. failure to detect (or reduced accuracy in detecting) difference between the constituent half-faces that form a chimeric face (the joint falling along the vertical meridian of the visual field) (Jeeves, 1979, 1981; Mackay, 1976; Milner & Jeeves, 1979);
4. difficulty in detecting variation between the densities of patterns of dots in the two halves of the visual field (dot size as well as density was varied to compensate for brightness differences) (Ettlinger, Blakemore, Milner & Wilson, 1972);
5. difficulty in judging stereoscopic depth in the midline (Jeeves, 1979, 1981; Mackay, 1976);
6. difficulty in using or understanding the syntactic–pragmatic component of language. This was shown by a variety of tasks that required either
   a. the matching of active or passive, affirmative or negative sentences to simple line drawings, for example, "the boy is pushed by the girl"; or
   b. the accuracy of repetition of such sentences of varying complexity, or the production of words that rhymed with given words and that defined animals or objects, for example, "rhymes with 'aion,' lives in a jungle, and has a mane." A further task called for the identification of words against a background of what was called "cafeteria" noise. (Dennis, 1981; Jeeves, 1981).

Compensatory Mechanisms: Neurological, Functional, and Behavioral

A number of suggestions have been made about compensatory mechanisms present in acallosal patients that permit them, to all intents and purposes, to overcome the disconnection syndrome of the split-brain patients whose commissures have been sectioned at maturity. We examine these and at the same time consider how such compensatory mechanisms may in turn be responsible for some of the deficits that have been demonstrated in some acallosal patients. We stress at this point the need for further detailed studies of acallosal subjects, because our own ongoing studies make it clear that some of the most interesting and convincing demonstrations of cognitive deficits in some acallosal cases do not occur in them all. For example, Dennis's (1981) detailed account of the linguistic deficits in an acallosal girl of above-normal intelligence not only demonstrated how sophisticated testing can bring to light hitherto hidden deficits, but also how a compensation model proposed to handle previously reported deficits (Dennis, 1976) can also explain the new ones. However, our own recent testing of four more subjects, using Dennis's techniques, has shown that not all acallosal patients show the deficits evident in Dennis's patient. Indeed, in some cases they are not evident at all, which again raises the question of whether the deficits reported by her may be due to other undetected brain abnormalities. With those cautionary comments in mind, we now turn to a consideration of possible compensatory mechanisms.

Bilateral Representation of Functions that Are Normally Lateralized

In order to explain how acallosal subjects could make appropriate responses to lateralized visual or tactual inputs on either side, Gazzaniga, Bogen, and Sperry (1962) proposed that speech and language mechanisms were represented in both cerebral hemispheres (Sperry, 1968b). Their hypothesis was supported by the results of Gott and Saul (1978), who used unilateral intracarotid barbiturate injection "to put to sleep" each hemisphere in turn (the Wada test) and reported that their patient performed as if speech and language were represented in both hemispheres. B. Milner (cited in Gazzaniga, 1970), using the same technique, had reported normal left hemisphere lateralization for language in a right-handed patient.

Another technique that has been claimed to indicate language lateralization is dichotic listening (Geffen & Caudrey, 1981). Superior dichotic monitoring performance for stimuli presented to the right ear was taken as evidence of speech lateralization to the left cerebral hemisphere, and superior left ear monitoring was taken as evidence of right hemisphere speech lateralization. Their method required subjects to make a manual response on detecting a target word that was presented to either ear when words were presented simultaneously to the two ears. Geffen has reported that an acallosal subject performs better on this task than a normal subject, and this she believes is further evidence for bilateral representation of speech and language. However, it is possible that Geffen might have used a level of task difficulty that gave rise to a ceiling effect, and so with increased difficulty, the usual asymmetry might be reported. Certainly, other researchers using the dichotic listening task and using Geffen's own tapes have found asymmetries of performance within the normal range (Jeeves & Silver, 1983; Milner & Jeeves, 1979).

The Elaboration of Ipsilateral Pathways

The possibility of elaborated ipsilateral pathways has been cogently presented by Dennis (1976, 1981). It assumes that sensory input has access to both hemispheres via the simultaneous use of crossed and uncrossed projections because callosal suppression of such effects is absent. If motor pathways are likewise elaborated, then either hemisphere alone could direct responses by both hands.

This proposal helps to explain the *absence*, in acallosal subjects, of deficits found in the patients whose commissures had been split in adulthood. But it also may account for the *presence* of some of the deficits reported in acallosal patients. As regards the absence of deficits, it suggests that by relying on ipsilateral as well as contralateral projections, sensory information is transmitted in parallel to each hemisphere even when the input is lateralized (the exception to this would be the visual input). As regards the residual deficits, Dennis (1976) argues that the dissociation shown by acallosal patients between discrimination and localization on a number of tactile tests supports her view that the sensory information is available through (unsuppressed) uncrossed and extralemniscal pathways that are known to give poor coding of stimulus topography.

With regard to motor deficits, the acallosal subjects show a deficiency in discriminatory selective movements that is characteristic of motor output mediated by uncrossed projections. She gives evidence of unintended associated movements accompanying voluntary finger movements in acallosal subjects and argues that they may be attributed to the elaborated ipsilateral motor pathways that are now not being suppressed in the normal way via the callosum. Evidence in support of the elaboration of sensory ipsilateral pathways is available (Bach-y-rita, 1972). There is evidence from Dennis (1976), Preilowski (1972), and Brinkman and Kuypers (1973) for how the use of ipsilateral together with contralateral motor pathways might give rise to interference effects on a bimanual motor task. An account along this line could help to explain the ability to recall words from the left ear in a dichotic listening task. Although the ipsilateral auditory pathway appears to operate effectively in monaural presentation conditions (Milner, Taylor & Sperry, 1968) and perhaps even in dichotic conditions after practice (Sparks & Geschwind, 1968) following commissure section, it could be argued that it can also provide the necessary compensatory pathway in callosal agenesis (Ettlinger, Blakemore, Milner, & Wilson, 1974). Such an absence of the suppressive function of the corpus callosum in auditory input is used by Dennis (1981) to explain one of the difficulties encountered by her acallosal subjects in acoustic tasks: She notes that when the auditory features of two stimuli interact, as, for example, in a dichotic situation, the input from one ear is typically suppressed according to the degree of interaction involved; the difference between the two ears concerns not dominance as such, but how ipsilateral information is transmitted or suppressed.

What all this means is that the compensatory benefits that accrue through the bilateral reception of sensory input have to be balanced against the loss of efficiency on motor tasks and the difficulties encountered on some acoustic tasks (Dennis, 1981). Once again, however, caution is needed. The same deficits are not evident in all patients. For example, in our 1981 report (Jeeves, 1981) we showed that an acallosal patient performed as well as normal subjects in a task that required simply reaching to a target, but significantly worse than normal subjects in a task that required the fine distal manipulation of the fingers and the grasping of a target. We argued that this was possibly due to competition between the crossed information and the unsuppressed, uncrossed information. However, more recently another acallosal subject has performed as well as normal subjects on the same task (Jeeves & Silver, 1983). As mentioned earlier, Dennis has argued (1981) that the basis of certain linguistic deficits that she observed in an acallosal subject could be due to now unsuppressed, elaborated ipsilateral pathways. However, in using her same tasks with four more acallosal subjects, we have not found any consistent picture of linguistic deficits.

Subcortical and Anterior Commissural Pathways

The evidence for intact cross-visual integration in acallosal patients, based such things as tachistoscopic matching, the phiphenomenon, and crossed visual reaction times require one to postulate some form of compensatory specialization in terms of extracallosal commissures. Two mechanisms have been proposed for such crossed communications. The first is the commissures of the midbrain visual system (Jeeves, 1965; Ettlinger *et al.*, 1972; Sperry, 1968b); the second is an increased usage of the anterior commissure (Doty & Negrao, 1973). The results of the study by Ptito and Lepore (1983) are interpreted by them as lending support to these possibilities. Some have suggested that the information required to permit cross-judgments of onset and place, such as would be required in apparent movement and judgments of temporal order, could be handled by the former system even without supernormal development (Ettlinger & Blakemore, 1969). Trevarthen and Sperry (1973) found that even in patients with presumed complete callosal section there was some evidence of crossed integration of simple visual patterns when the stimuli were moving or changing and were in the periphery of vision. It is now conceivable that this midbrain system could, in callosal agenesis, develop sufficiently to account for the observed tachistoscopic findings. Alternatively, there is good evidence for visual function in the anterior commissure of primates (e.g., Hamilton, 1982). There is the further evidence, cited earlier, of some callosal fibers crossing along with the fibers of the anterior commissure, and since we know from other studies that very few fibers are necessary for maintenance of apparently normal functioning, it is possible that these fibers could play a major part in acallosal vision.

The evidence concerning the perception of asymmetry about the vertical meridian remains controversial. Some studies have suggested that acallosal patients are unaware, for example, of chimeric figures. Risse, LeDoux, Springer, Wilson, and Gazzaniga (1978) argued for the role of an intact anterior commissure, which is known to be present in some acallosal subjects, as a multisensory system. However, a further report questioned their results (McKeever, Sullivan, Ferguson & Rayport, 1981). It must also be remembered that in some acallosal patients the anterior commissure is not present and therefore does not provide an adequate explanation for the absence of deficits in all acallosal subjects.

Behavioral Strategies

Sperry (1968a) and Gazzaniga (1970) described their commissurotomized patients' subtle behavioral strategies for overcoming the limits imposed by the experimental conditions to which they were subjected—strategies that were aimed at enabling the cerebral hemispheres to react in independent fashion. Certainly we have evidence of acallosal subjects developing behavioral strategies *within* a long session: On the task of touch localization we have observed patients making *gross* movements of the finger touched on one hand before indicating on the other hand which finger corresponded to the one touched. Such gross movements involving more proximal musculature gave cues to the correct response. It could be argued that acallosal patients have had a lifetime in which to develop such cross-cuing methods and might therefore have them deeply ingrained into their everyday behavior. Contrarily, one might argue that they have also had a lifetime to develop appropriate neurological compensation and therefore would have less need for such behavioral compensation. One possible strategy that Sperry (1968b) argued for is continuous ocular-motor scanning of the visual world so that both hemispheres are kept fully informed. This kind of activity could become ingrained and therefore difficult to suppress. In an unpublished study by Lassonde, Laurencelle, and Geoffrey (personal communication, 1983), evidence is given, showing that acallosal patients produce significantly more rapid-eye movements (REMs) from side to side across the vertical meridian than do normals. Again, however, caution is necessary: This study is based on only two acallosal patients, and in one of those the above-average eye movements did not occur in one of the experimental conditions.

Summary: Compensatory Mechanisms in Acallosals

There can be no doubt that the study of acallosal patients produces strong evidence for the remarkable ability of the human brain to compensate, whether neurally or behaviorally, for the absence from birth of the major commissure linking the left and right cerebral hemispheres. It would seem that superficially intact behavior is ensured in these patients by virtue of the immature brain's ability to reprogram its development in response to an early developmental error by making use of alternative neural structures or developing behavioral skills. The evidence available, however, both structural and behavioral, also suggests that there are limits to the amounts of compensation, of whatever kind, that can occur. Moreover, just those mechanisms that help to compensate for the absence of the commissures can also arguably be responsible for some of the deficits observed in these patients. Compensation, whether neural or behavioral, has a cognitive and behavioral price attached to it.

Effects of Postnatal–Prematurity Callosal Lesions

The results of the studies by Rakic and Yakovlev (1968) referred to earlier indicate that the neocortical commissures continue the process of myelination until the 10th year. Whether this lack of neural maturity until the 10th year confers the commissural system a corresponding degree of plasticity until the 10th year remains an unanswered empirical question. The evidence from human and animal studies is meager. As mentioned earlier, studies by Ptito and Lepore (1983) on cats indicate a period, albeit brief, of functional plasticity before the corpus callosum becomes anatomically and physiologically mature.

When there are prematurity partial lesions of the callosum, any absence of expected deficits could exist either because not all the fibers that normally carry specialized information have been destroyed or because, although these fibers have all been destroyed, other fiber pathways have taken over the relevant role. We can compare the evidence, both animal and human, for the effects of partial callosal lesions in adults (Gordon, Bogen, & Sperry, 1971; Preilowski, 1972) with the effects of similar prematurity lesions.

Winston, Cavazzuti, and Arkins (1979) reported a study of four children whose ages ranged from 18 months to 10 years and who had undergone 2-cm longitudinal incisions in the anterior body of the corpus callosum. Only one child, age 6 years, had both pre- and postoperative testing. Their tests examined memory, visual perception, motor integration and dexterity, tactile recognition, intermanual localization, and graphesthesia. They reported that none of the symptoms or signs found in more extensive disruption of the neocortical commissures in adults were to be found in these patients. Moreover, although adults with lesions in the anterior commissure and the anterior two thirds of the corpus callosum did not show the full disconnection syndrome, they did perform poorly on memory and bimanual motor tasks. (Preilowski, 1972).

I have published preliminary results (Jeeves, (1981) of an ongoing study of a 6-year-old girl, with a cyst in the third ventricle for whom the neurosurgeon's preferred approach was a longitudinal section through the body of the corpus callosum. It was possible to administer preoperative testing, and to follow the operation after 3 hours and then at intervals over a period now amounting to 4 years, with further tests. I compared the results of these tests with those of adult patients, both my own and from other published studies. The tasks given tested tactile localization, both ipsilateral and contralateral; tactile shape discrimination using Milner and Taylor's nonsense wire shapes (1972); and aspects (three tasks) of bimanual visual–motor coordination of movement. I was also able to measure this girl's ITTs using thousands of manual responses to lateralized visual stimuli. There was no evidence of any difference in the ITT from that which would normally be expected for children of her age. It is evident that the patient, who was 6 years old at the time of the operation, showed no evidence of any deficit on any of the tasks. I have also used Preilowski's technique (1972) to study this girl's learning of a bimanual motor task, and I found none of the deficits reported by him on his adult patients with partial commissurotomy.

In contrast, patients who, as adults, have undergone partial commissurotomy of the same parts of the callosum (Geffen, Walsh, Simpson, & Jeeves, 1980; Jeeves, Simpson, and Geffen, 1978) showed deficits in postoperative performance of the finger localization task, as did an adult female patient who was tested both pre- and postoperatively. These same patients also showed deficits on tasks involving bimanual coordination and tactile shape discrimination. Thus, our results, together with those of Winston *et al.*, suggest that deficits that are evident with small longitudinal lesions (1–3 cm) of the body of the callosum in adults are not found with similar lesions in young children. Clearly, caution must be exercised in generalizing from these studies, because the precise extent of the lesions is not known with certainty. However, they do provide some support for the view that prematurity partial callosal lesions do not have the same sequelae as do late-occurring lesions. Like Winston *et al.*, (1979), I presume that the function of the interrupted fibers is taken over by other interhemispheric pathways, although restitution could also be due to synaptic reorganization within the affected cortex.

General Conclusions

Taken together, evidence from studies of patients who were born without a corpus callosum or who have suffered surgical lesions of the callosum before the age of 10 years suggests that a considerable degree of reorganization and compensation is possible. Results suggest that those who have postnatal–prematurity lesions show considerable plasticity of function, which is not evident when similarly placed and sized lesions occur after the age of 10. However, as has been stressed several times, this could indicate either functional plasticity or the survival of a very few of the normally specialized interhemispheric fibers. Studies examining the effects of splenial lesions have indicated that if any splenial fibres are intact, deficits may not appear.

The evidence from the cases of agenesis is more compelling. Here we consider the effects of very early prenatal lesions, and the evidence suggests a number of possible forms of reorganization and compensation. These include the elaboration of ipsilateral sensory and motor pathways, the routing of a small number of callosal fibers through the anterior commissure, and the use of midbrain pathways. The suggestion of bilateral representation of function seems, on balance, to remain unproven. Finally, there is evidence for behavioral compensation in terms of such things as cross-cuing and increased amounts of ocular scanning in order to supply information from the two visual half-fields.

References

Akelaitis, A. J. (1943). Studies on corpus callosum; study of language functions (tactile and visual, lexia and graphia) unilaterally following section of corpus callosum. *Journal of Neuropathology and Experimental Neurology, 2,* 226.

Akelaitis, A. J. (1944). Study of gnosis, praxis and language following section of corpus callosum and anterior commissure. *Journal of Neurosurgery, 1,* 94.

Bach-y-rita, P. (1972). *Brain mechanisms in sensory substitution.* New York: Academic Press.

Bogen, J. E., & Vogel, P. J. (1962). Cerebral commissurotomy in man. Preliminary case report. *Bulletin of the Los Angeles Neurological Society, 27,* 169.

Bossy, J. G. (1970). Morphological study of a case of complete, isolated and asymptomatic agenesis of the corpus callosum. *Archives d'anatomie, d'histologie et d'embryologie, 53,* 289–340.

Brinkman, J., & Kuypers, H. G. J. M. (1973). Cerebral control of contralateral and ipsilateral arm, hand, and finger movements in the split-brain rhesus monkey. *Brain, 96,* 653–674.

Chiarello, C. (1980). A house divided? Cognitive functioning with callosal agenesis. *Brain and Language, 11,* 128–158.

Dennis, M. (1976). Impaired sensory and motor differentiation with corpus callosum agenesis: A lack of callosal inhibition during ontogeny? *Neuropsychologia, 14,* 455–469.

Dennis, M. (1981). Language in a congenitally acallosal brain. *Brain and Language, 12,* 33–53.

Doty, R. W., & Negrao, N. (1973). Forebrain commissures and vision. In R. Jung (Ed.), *Handbook of sensory physiology* (pp. 543–582. Berlin: Springer.

Ettlinger, G., & Blakemore, C. B. (1969). The behavioral effects of commissure section. In A. L. Benton (Ed.), *Contributions to clinical neuropsychology* (chap. 2). Chicago: Aldine.

Ettlinger, G., Blakemore, C. B., Milner, A. D., & Wilson, J. (1972). Agenesis of the corpus callosum: A behavioural investigation. *Brain, 95,* 327–346.

Ettlinger, G., Blakemore, C. B., Milner, A. D., & Wilson, J. (1974). Agenesis of the corpus callosum: A further behavioural investigation. *Brain, 97,* 225–234.

Gazzaniga, M. S. (1970). *The bisected brain.* New York: Appleton-Century-Crofts.

Gazzaniga, M. S., Bogen, J. E., & Sperry, R. W. (1962). Some functional effects of sectioning the cerebral commissures in man. *Proceedings of the National Academy of Sciences, 48,* 1765–1769.

Geffen, G., & Caudrey, D. (1981). Reliability and validity of the dichotic monitoring test for language laterality. *Neuropsychologia, 19,* 413–424.

Geffen, G., Walsh, A., Simpson, D., & Jeeves, M. A. (1980). Comparison of the effects of transcortical removal of intraventricular tumours. *Brain, 103,* 773–788.

Geschwind, N. (1974) Late changes in the nervous system: An overview. In D. G. Stein, J. J. Rosen, & N. Batters (Eds.), *Plasticity and recovery of function in the central nervous system.* New York: Academic Press.

Gordon, J. W., Bogen, J. E., & Sperry, R. W. (1971). Absence of deconnexion syndrome in two patients with partial section of the neocommissures. *Brain, 94,* 327–336.

Gott, P. S., & Saul, R. E. (1978). Agenesis of the corpus callosum: Limits of functional compensation. *Neurology, 28,* 1272–1279.

Hamilton, C. R. (1982). Mechanisms of interocular equivalence. In D. Ingle, M. A. Goodale, & R. J. W. Mansfield (Eds.), *Analysis of visual behaviour* (pp. 693–717). Cambridge, MA: M.I.T. Press.

Innocenti, G. M., Fiore, L., & Caminiti, R. (1977). Exuberant projection into the corpus callosum from the visual cortex of newborn cats. *Neuroscience Letters, 4,* 237–242.

Jeeves, M. A. (1965). Psychological studies of three cases of congenital agenesis of the corpus callosum. In E. G. Ettlinger (Ed.), *Functions of the Corpus Callosum* (pp. 77–94). London: Churchill.

Jeeves, M. A. (1969). A comparison of hemispheric transmission time in acallosals and normals. *Psychonomic Science, 16,* 245–246.

Jeeves, M. A. (1979). Some limits to interhemispheric integration in cases of callosal agenesis and partial commissurotomy. In I. Steele Russell, M. S. van Hof, and G. Berlucchi (Eds.), *Structure and function of the cerebral commissures* (pp. 449–474). London: Macmillan.

Jeeves, M. A. (1981). Age related effects of agenesis and partial sectioning of the neocortical commissures. In M. W. van Hof & G. Mohn (Eds.), *Developments in neuroscience: Functional Recovery from Brain Damage* (Vol. 13). Elsevier: North Holland.

Jeeves, M. A., & Rajalakshmi, R. (1964). Psychological studies of a case of congenital agenesis of the corpus callosum. *Neuropsychologia, 2,* 237–252.

Jeeves, M. A., & Silver, P. H. (1983). Dichotic listening performance in acallosals. Unpublished manuscript.

Jeeves, M. A., Simpson, D., & Geffen, G. (1978). Functional consequences of the transcallosal removal of intraventricular tumours. *Journal of Neurology, Neurosurgery and Psychiatry, 42,* 134–142.

Jeeves, M. A., & Wilson, A. F. (1969). Tactile transfer and neonatal callosal section in the cat. *Psychonomic Science, 16,* 235–237.

Mackay, B. (1976). M. A. thesis, University of St. Andrews. An investigation into two perceptual impairments with agenesis of the corpus callosum: depth perception and the completion of one visual half-field for a chimeric stimulus.

McKeever, W. F., Sullivan, K. F., Ferguson, S. M., & Rayport, M. (1981). Typical cerebral hemisphere disconnection deficits following corpus callosum section despite sparing of the anterior commissure. *Neuropsychologia, 19,* 745–755.

Milner, A. D. (1982). Simple reaction times to lateralized visual stimuli in a case of callosal agenesis. *Neuropsychologia, 20,* 411–419.

Milner, A. D., & Jeeves, M. A. (1979). A review of behavioural studies of agenesis of the corpus callosum. In I. Steele Russell, M. W. van Hof, & G. Berlucchi (Eds.), *Structure and function of the cerebral commissures* (pp. 428–448). London: Macmillan.

Milner, B., & Taylor, L. (1972). Right-hemisphere superiority in tactile pattern-recognition after cerebral commissurotomy: Evidence for nonverbal memory. *Neuropsychologia, 10,* 1–15.

Milner, B., Taylor, L., & Sperry, R. W. (1968). Lateral suppression of dichotically presented digits after commissural section in man. *Science, 161,* 184–186.

Preilowski, B. F. B. (1972). Possible contribution of the anterior forebrain commissures to bilateral motor coordination. *Neuropsychologia, 10,* 267–277.

Ptito, M., & Lepore, F. (1983). Interocular transfer in cats with early callosal transection. *Nature, 301,* 513–515.

Rakic, P., & Yakovlev, I. (1968). Development of the corpus callosum and carum septum in man. *Journal of Comparative Neurology, 132,* 45–72.

Reynolds, D. M., & Jeeves, M. A. (1977). Further studies of tactile perception and motor coordination in agenesis of the corpus callosum. *Cortex, 8,* 257.

Risse, G. L., LeDoux, J., Springer, S. P., Wilson, D. H., & Gazzaniga, M. S. (1978). The anterior commissure in man: Functional variation in a multisensory system. *Neuropsychologia, 16,* 23–31.

Russell, J. R., & Reitan, R. M. (1955). Psychological abnormalities in agenesis of the corpus callosum. *Journal of Nervous and Mental Diseases,* 1955, *121,* 205–214.

Shoumura, K., Ando, T., & Kato, K. (1975). Structural organization of 'callosal' OBg in human corpus callosum agenesis. *Brain Research, 93,* 241–252.

Solursh, L. P., Margulies, A. I., Ashem, B., & Stasiak, E. A. (1965). The relationship of agenesis of the corpus callosum to perception and learning. *Journal of Nervous and Mental Diseases, 141,* 180–189.

Sparks, R., & Geschwind, N. (1968) Dichotic listening in man after section of neocortical commissures. *Cortex, 4,* 3–16.

Sperry, R. W. (1968a). Mental unity following surgical disconnection of the cerebral hemispheres. *The Harvey Lecture Series, 62,* 293–323.

Sperry, R. W. (1968b). Plasticity of neural maturation. *Developmental Biology Supplement, 2,* 306, 327.

Sperry, R. W., Gazzaniga, M. S., & Bogen, J. E. (1969). Interhemispheric relationships: The neocortical commissures: Syndromes of hemisphere disconnection. In P. J. Vinken & G. W. Bruyn (Eds.), *Handbook of clinical neurology* (Vol. 4, chap. 14). Amsterdam: North Holland.

Stefanko, S. Z., & Schenk, V. W. D. (1979). Anatomical aspects of the agenesis of the corpus callosum in man. In I. Steele Russell, M. W. van Hof, & G. Berlucchi (Eds.), *Structure and function of the cerebral commissures* (pp. 479–483). London: Macmillan.

Tomasch, J. (1954). Size, distribution and number of fibres in the human corpus callosum. *Anatomical Record, 119,* 119–135.

Trevarthen, C., & Sperry, R. W. (1973). Perceptual unity of the ambient visual field in human commissurotomy patients. *Brain, 96,* 547–570.

Van Wagenen, W. P., & Herren, R. Y. (1940). Surgical division of commissural pathways in corpus callosum: Relation to spread of epileptic attack. *Archives of Neurology and Psychiatry Chicago, 44,* 740–759.

Winston, K. R. Cavazzuti, V., & Arkins, T. (1979). Absence of neurological and behavioural abnormalities after anterior transcallosal operation for third ventricular lesions. *Neurosurgery, 4,* (5), 386–393.

Yakovlev, P. I., & Lecours, A. R. (1967). Myelogenetic cycles in regional maturation of the nervous system in man. In A. Minkowski (Ed.), *Regional development of the brain in early life* (pp. 3–65). London: Blackwell.

13

Early Brain Damage and the Ontogenesis of Functional Asymmetry*

Rolando R. Henry, Paul Satz, and Eric Saslow

Introduction

This chapter reviews findings suggesting that early injury to the left hemisphere may produce alterations in lateral development that affect manual dominance, the hemispheric control of higher cognitive functions, and trophic changes in the extremities. It is also suggested that these alterations in lateral development may be seen in a number of different neurological disorders as well as in individuals who are clinically asymptomatic. We attempt to show that identification of these individuals could provide new insights into the ontogeny

*Supported in part by a National Institute of Mental Health Grant MHO8865-01 to the senior author and a National Institute of Health Grant 5 ROI N518462-02 to the second author.

Copyright © 1984 by Academic Press, Inc.
All rights of reproduction in any form reserved.
ISBN 0-12-052901-7

of cerebral and manual dominance and could help to increase our understanding of the brain's reorganization of its functional systems subsequent to early insult.

Brain Damage and Manual Dominance

Evidence suggests that the determinant of hand dominance in some individuals is early injury to the left hemisphere. In this section, data from a number of different clinical populations in which there is unequivocal unilateral brain damage are used to provide new insights into environmental and genetic theories of handedness. An adequate explanation of the development of hand dominance has been elusive.

It is well established that an elevated incidence of non right-handedness exists within a variety of neurologically atypical populations. Clinical populations in which this elevated incidence has been observed include individuals with epilepsy (Bolin, 1953), mental retardation (Hicks & Barton, 1975), and autism (Colby & Parkinson, 1977). Prevalence estimates have consistently revealed an incidence of approximately 17% in these groups, which represents at least a twofold increase over that reported for normal populations (Hardyck & Petrinovich, 1977).

Several hypotheses have been advanced to account for this increase in manifest left-handedness (MLH). At the extremes are explanations based largely on genetic factors (e.g., Annett, 1978) and those that argue that all occurrences of MLH are consequences of early brain insult (Baken, Dibb, & Reed, 1973). Neither of these hypotheses, however, has received strong empirical support. A more parsimonious explanation for this increase in MLH is that early damage to the left hemisphere, in a small proportion of natural right-handers, causes a mild hypofunction of the contralateral hand, which causes the individual to switch to the opposite hand for manual activities, thus becoming a pathological left-hander (PLH) (Bingley, 1958).

Satz (1972, 1973) has developed a statistical model of the concept of PLH. Satz's model elaborates and extends Bingley's notion of PLH to include (1) the concept of pathological right-handedness: natural left-handers who experience right hemisphere damage and subsequently switch to the right hand for manual activities and (2) probability statements about the likelihood of manual transfer (switch) in natural left- and right-handers that would account for the twofold increase of MLH in various clinical populations. Satz's model is built on two basic assumptions. First, the lateralization of brain lesions is a random process. Thus, unilateral brain damage in statistical terms is a binomial function. Second, lesions lateralized to the left hemisphere lead to the greatest incidence of switched handedness. Since a significantly larger proportion of the general population are naturally right-handed than are naturally left-handed, it follows that the switching of hand dominance as a function of early brain injury will exist to a greater degree as PLH than as pathological right-handedness. Based on these assumptions, the model predicts that the frequency of MLH increases largely as a function of injury to the left cerebral hemisphere. We next examine empirical evidence garnered from several studies that tested this prediction.

Studies attempting to elucidate the relationship between MLH and early brain insult can be divided into two groups: (1) retrospective birth-stress studies and (2) clinical studies involving cases of known or suspected brain damage (e.g., mental retardation, epilepsy). For convenience these reports could be conceptualized along a continuum of CNS severity, ranging from mild (birth stress) to moderate (epilepsy) to severe (mental retardation, autism).

Birth-Stress Studies

Several studies have examined the relationship between handedness and birth stress. In general these reports have operationalized birth stress in terms of estimates of birth complications (e.g., prematurity, prolonged labor), maternal age, and/or parity. The impetus for these investigations was the contention of Bakan (1971, 1977) that MLH results from stressful perinatal experiences. Results from investigations that tested this hypothesis have been equivocal.

A few studies have provided some support for the prediction that there is a raised incidence of MLH in populations purported to have experienced early insult to the brain (Bakan, 1971, 1977; Bakan, *et al.*, 1973; Leviton & Kilty, 1979; Coren & Porac, 1980). These results, however, are not compelling. A major methodological flaw in almost all of these investigations is the reliance on subjective and retrospective indices of birth stress. This type of flaw seriously constrains the kinds of assumptions and conclusions one can make regarding the incidence of brain damage in the index cases used in these studies. One is therefore limited in making conclusive statements about the relationship, if any, between MLH and early brain injury when the basis of such statements rests on subjective and retrospective indices.

Most studies have been unable to demonstrate a relationship between MLH and perinatal central nervous system (CNS) trauma, that is, birth stress. For example, studies conducted by Hicks and his colleagues (Hicks & Barton, 1975; Hicks, Dusek, Larsen, Williams, & Pellegrini, 1980; Hicks, Elliott, Garbesi, & Martin, 1979; Hicks, Evans, & Pellegrini, 1978; Hicks, Pellegrini, & Evans, 1978) consistently report a near zero correlation between handedness and birth stress and thus find Bakan's hypothesis untenable. However, the Hicks *et al.* data do suggest that mild trauma (birth stress) sustained by the developing CNS may result in a modification in the degree of handedness instead of a change in the direction of handedness. If this were true, early left hemisphere damage in some individuals would manifest itself as a diminution in the absolute strength of manual dominance rather than as a reversal in the direction of manual dominance.

Birth-stress studies can, however, provide useful additions to the data pool on the origin of handedness. This is particularly true when the study takes a prospective rather than a retrospective approach. For example, Liederman and Coryell (1982) examined functional asymmetry in two groups of infants with (e.g., toxemia, prematurity) and without (e.g., normal gestation, vaginal delivery) a history of perinatal complications. The groups were matched for age, gender, and parental handedness. Between 4 and 10 weeks of age all subjects were observed for spontaneous rightward-turning bias in a repeated measures design. The results of the study were that children in the perinatal-complication (PC) group did not show the right-turning bias observed in the nonperinatal-complication (NPC) group. This difference was statistically significant. Additionally, it was shown that PC children who were homozygous for right-handedness lacked the lateralization of the asymmetric tonic neck reflex (ATNR) observed in NPC children who were also homozygous for right-handedness. It has been shown that children without a history of perinatal complications are more likely to exhibit the ATNR when turning to the nonpreferred side than when turning to the preferred side (Liederman & Coryell, 1981). In the Liederman and Coryell (1982) study, PC children did not discriminate between preferred and nonpreferred side when exhibiting the ATNR. The authors interpreted their findings to be supportive of the Satz rather than the Bakan *et al.* model of PLH.

Despite the methodological advantages in this prospective study, one could question whether head-turning bias and the lateralization of the ATNR in a 4–10-week-old infant are reliable and valid indices of future hand preference. We do not know whether either of these are predictive of handedness. If such a relationship is to be confirmed, it will require a longitudinal prospective design. The approach seems promising because it has the potential to provide useful data that can be brought to bear on the question: Does early brain damage alter manifest handedness?

An equally valuable approach to dealing with this issue of early brain insult and handedness is to look at MLH in populations with known or suspected brain damage. It would be of particular interest to study samples in which lesion loci and time of lesion onset could be specified. We next consider evidence garnered from such samples.

Clinical Studies

The following sections present results from several studies in which three clinical probands were used to examine the issue of the origin of pathological handedness. Specifically, tests of the prediction generated from Satz's model were conducted on three epilepsy subject populations and one mental retardation subject population. In addition to an examination of the incidence of MLH in these probands, the relationships among MLH, absence or presence of brain abnormality (lesion or abnormal EEG), locus of brain abnormality (unilateral versus bilateral), and age at time of brain insult were assessed. Locus of brain abnormality was examined to determine whether the high incidence of MLH predicted by Satz's model for cases of unilateral left-side abnormality is altered under conditions of bilateral brain abnormality.

EPILEPSY STUDIES

Examinations of epileptic populations have consistently revealed the incidence of MLH to be approximately 17–20% (e.g., Satz, Baymur, & Van der Vlugt, 1979; Satz, Yanowitz, & Willmore, 1983; Silva & Satz, 1979). We briefly present the findings of several exemplary studies which support Satz's model.

Penfield and Roberts (1959) examined 522 adult patients with intractable epilepsy. All patients underwent unilateral cortical lobectomy. The incidence of MLH was approximately two times the expected level for the normal population. It is interesting to note that the incidence of MLH was 8% after excluding those individuals whose seizures began before the age of 2 years. This finding suggests that age at the time of brain insult is a critical variable for the expression of PLH. Within this sample of patients, the raised incidence of MLH was due, to a large extent, to those PLHs who had sustained early brain damage.

Baymur (1977) studied 192 epileptic children (mean age = 10.16 years). The incidence of MLH in this sample was 17%. Readings from routine EEGs were taken and classified, independent of handedness, as normal or abnormal (left, right, bilateral). Of those with abnormal EEGs, 19% (31/166) were MLH. In contrast, 4% (1/26) of those having normal EEGs were MLH. The incidence of MLH in the normal-EEG group was similar to that observed in a control group without brain injury (17/242 = 7%). The prevalence of MLH in both the normal-EEG and the control groups was lower than that observed in most normative studies. A plausible explanation of this discrepancy is that handedness within these two groups was significantly influenced by cultural pressures against left-handedness. That the abnormal-EEG group's handedness was not influenced by environmental factors is explained by the fact that the damaged nervous system may not be readily responsive to certain environmental constraints.

Satz *et al.* (1983) examined the incidence of MLH in a large sample of epileptic patients ($N = 230$). All patients were classified on the basis of seizure onset into one of the following three groups: early (birth–age 2 years), middle (ages 2–17 years), and late onset (ages 17–55 years). Each of these three groups was further divided into two groups on the basis of type of brain abnormality (focal or nonfocal abnormal EEG). In addition to these six groups, a group of patients with no history of clinical seizure and with normal EEGs served as controls ($n = 50$). The following results were reported: (1) consistent with the model's predictions, a raised incidence of MLH, but only in the early-onset focal-EEG group (22%) and (2) a robust relationship between EEG focus and manifest hand preference, but only in the early- and middle-onset groups. These results strongly suggest that MLH is directly related to lesion locus (left hemisphere), lesion severity (unilateral or bilateral–asymmetric), and lesion onset (birth–age 6 years). The expression of PLH seems to depend on the presence of each of these factors. It appears that none of these factors in isolation is sufficient to cause a shift in handedness.

MENTAL RETARDATION

As occurred with the epileptic population, studies of the mentally retarded have revealed an elevated incidence (approximately 20%) of MLH (e.g., Bingley, 1958; DeMyer, Hingtgen, & Jackson, 1981; Hicks & Barton, 1975; Silva & Satz, 1979). Hand-preference and brain-damage (EEG abnormality) data obtained from mentally retarded clients have been used to test Satz's model of PLH. Silva and Satz (1979) sampled 1230 mentally retarded patients. MLH was determined to be 17.8%. EEGs of 572 of these subjects were classified, independent of handedness, as abnormal (left, right, or bilateral–asymmetric) or normal. Of those with abnormal EEGs, 17% (82/476) were MLH. In contrast, only 9% (9/96) of those with normal EEGs were MLH. An incidence of 9% closely approximates the incidence of MLH reported for normal samples (Hardyck & Petrinovich, 1977).

Of significant note is the EEG data reported by these investigators. Contrary to the expected low frequency of unilateral or bilateral–asymmetric EEG abnormalities in the mentally retarded, a marked increase in the frequency of these abnormalities was found (136/572 = 24%). Furthermore, when these subjects were divided into lateralized EEG groups, it was found that the incidence of MLH was primarily associated with lesions to the left hemisphere.

INFANTILE-AUTISM STUDIES

Although evidence in support of an association between MLH and early brain injury is suggested from studies of mentally retarded clients, the status of this association within the autistic population is less clear. One reason for this discrepancy is that there is less known about the nature of the brain damage involved in autism. What is known is highly speculative (see review by DeMyer *et al.*, 1981). Although multiple CNS etiologies have been suggested for autism, the effects on brain function are most probably diffuse and bilateral. An early bilateral asymmetric lesion (left > right) is frequently invoked to account for the pronounced retardation observed in this population's speech and language functions. If the lesion is predominantly unilateral it might cause these functions to be transferred to the compromised right hemisphere. It seems reasonable to postulate that the same early, predominantly left hemisphere damage that causes speech and language to shift to the right hemisphere also causes hand dominance to shift to that hemisphere.

Tsai and Stewart (1982) investigated the relation between handedness and EEG status in autistics ($N = 40$). Of these subjects, 43% were classified as right-handed and 57% as non-right-handed. Within the right-handed group 35% had abnormal EEGs, as did 43% of the non-right-handers. The proportion of abnormal EEGs between the two groups was not statistically different. These investigators also reported no relationship between manifest handedness and abnormal EEG pattern. These negative findings can be attributed to methodological flaws. Tsai and Stewart classified subjects as non-right-handers if they were unable to use the right hand alone on any of five tasks. This procedure presents two problems: First, such classification assumes that in the normal population non-right-handers are only those individuals who exclusively use their left hands for unimanual tasks. The issue of degree of hand preference is not considered. Furthermore, this procedure assumes that neurologically compromised populations are dichotomous with respect to handedness. Both of these assumptions are probably untenable. The second problem is one that is ubiquitous to the handedness literature in general. Handedness, as determined by these and other investigators, was based on preference rather than dexterity. Preference is a particularly unreliable measure when writing hand is not used as one of the indexes of preference, which was the case in Tsai and Stewart's study. Since autistic individuals are severely compromised functionally, their skill of writing is generally not measurable. Use of some other dexterity measure, however, would yield a more parsimonious index of hand dominance in these individuals.

An examination of handedness from a performance (i.e., dexterity–skill) perspective was undertaken by Colby and Parkison (1977). These investigators compared the distribution of handedness in samples of autistic and age-matched normal subjects. A behavioral inventory was used to define handedness. Weights were assigned to each of the inventory items on the basis of the amount of dexterity required to successfully perform the activity. Colby and Parkison reported that the incidence of non-right-handedness (65%) in the autistic sample was elevated relative to the normal sample (12%). They concluded, "Since only 35% of our tested autistic children are definitely right-handed compared to 88% of our tested normals, this great difference suggests that the process of normal lateralization of cerebral functions fails in many autistic children . . . Failure to lateralize in the normal way is a clinical indicator of brain damage" (pp. 8,9).

Although Colby and Parkison's study represents a methodological improvement over previous studies, some caution should be raised concerning their conclusions. Several features of their study demand attention:

1. the subjective weighting applied to their behavioral inventory items;
2. the absence of any explanation of the decision rules used to create the criteria for assigning dexterity weights;
3. failure to indicate whether or not interobserver reliability was examined;
4. failure to include an appropriately matched, retarded control group. This is a severe limitation because there is evidence that shows a raised incidence of non-right-handedness in mental retardates (Hicks & Barton, 1975);
5. the use of young children (mean age = 4.3 years), which led the authors to invoke a "failure to lateralize" explanation of their autistic subjects' handedness responses.

Barry and James (1978) replicated Colby and Parkison's study but included older subjects (mean age = 10.11 years) as well as an appropriate control group of mental retardates. On the basis of their finding of no difference between groups, Barry and James invoked a "developmental lag" explanation. They concluded, "it is necessary to postulate that young autistics are severly retarded in the normal lateralization of cerebral functioning, and that this lateralization gradually develops throughout childhood. This is equivalent to postulating a developmental lag in the cerebral lateralization of autistics rather than the failure of lateralization proposed by Colby and Parkison" (p. 322).

Altogether, the studies of handedness in autistics present discordant findings. This discordance may be attributed to differences in methodological strategies. Studies that use appropriate control groups and more objective measures of handedness (preference plus performance measures) will no doubt strengthen and clarify this area of research.

Two of the present authors (Henry and Satz) and their colleagues initiated a large-scale examination of cerebral lateralization in a group of autistic clients. This study incorporated several improvements over previous studies:

1. In addition to the standard preference measures, objective and quantifiable performance measures were employed.
2. Handedness was examined several times within two temporally disparate assessment sessions.

3. Multivariate statistical procedures were used to determine whether handedness subgroups could be clustered along a preference and performance continuum.
4. Appropriately matched retarded controls were used.

Some preliminary data analyses from this study have been performed. Although the results are prefatory and cannot be viewed as definitive, the initial trend in the data indicates an elevated incidence of non-right-handedness. An interesting preliminary finding is that the non-right-handed group clusters into two subgroups: a strongly left-handed group and an ambiguous handed group. Data obtained from this examination should serve to more clearly elucidate the incidence of manifest handedness and its relationship to early brain damage in autistic probands.[1]

In general, handedness studies suggest an association between early brain trauma and the development of manual dominance. The exact nature of this association is, of course, unknown. However, several hypotheses can be drawn: (1) the expression of PLH is due, in large part, to a subset of natural right-handers who, because of insult to the left hemisphere, transfer hand dominance to the left hand (PLH); (2) brain insult must be sustained early in life (birth–age 6 years) in order for PLH to manifest itself; (3) the increased prevalence of MLH observed in some brain-injured populations is largely the result of early insult that is unilateral (primarily left-side) as opposed to bilateral in nature.

An interesting question raised by these data is what are the effects, if any, of bilateral brain damage (i.e., bilateral EEG abnormality) on MLH? In the clinical studies cited, the frequency of MLH was significantly lower in the abnormal bilateral-EEG groups. This observed diminution of MLH in the bilateral groups is intuitively reasonable if we assume that in these cases early injury is moderate or severe in intensity. With moderate or severe bilateral brain damage one would expect a concomitant increase in the likelihood of bimanual hypo-

[1]The original model of PLH, as presented in this chapter, uses only two handedness phenotypes (right, left) to predict lesion foci and pathological handedness in posited cases of mild brain injury (e.g., epilepsy). The existence of an ambiguous handed phenotype, if valid, helps to explain the presence of nonlateralized individuals in populations posited to have experienced more severe early bilateral brain trauma (e.g., mental retardation, autism). This third phenotypic handedness group has been incorporated into the original model of PLH and testable predictive statements have been generated. (Soper, H. V. & Satz, P. Pathological left-handedness and ambiguous handedness: A new explanatory model. *Neuropsychologia*, in press.)

function. Such an outcome would, of course, favor maintenance (rather than transfer) of the natural hand—most often the right.

Two important questions that emerge from the preceding review are examined in the remainder of this chapter. To a large extent, manual dominance accurately reflects cerebral dominance. This fact raises the first question: What happens to the functional organization of the brain following early trauma that produces a shift in handedness? More specifically, one wonders whether speech–language functions shift along with handedness in the PLH. An associated concern is the status of other cognitive functions normally subserved by the nondamaged hemisphere (e.g., visuospatial functions). Can we assume that the nondamaged hemisphere will share its physiological and anatomical resources equally with the damaged hemisphere? This issue is discussed in the final section of this chapter.

A second question concerns the identification of a true PLH. There are several reasons why it is important to differentiate between natural left-handers and the PLH. First, the identification of a true PLH would permit a more rigorous evaluation of the various genetic and environmental theories of handedness and cerebral dominance. There is a great deal of controversy and debate concerning the genetic and environmental determinants of handedness. The resolution of this controversy could come, in part, from the identification and systematic study of those natural right-handers who, because of early left hemisphere damage, masquerade as left-handers. Before genetic models can reasonably be constructed it is important to know how environmental influences, such as early brain injury, influence the observed phenotype.

A second reason for attempting to identify PLH is that it would afford a unique opportunity to examine higher cortical information-processing functions. If a shift in handedness is also associated with a shift in the hemispheric control of speech or an alteration in the integrity of spatial–perceptual processes, then brain–behavior researchers would be in an ideal position to study the phenomenon of intrahemispheric competition.

A third reason for seeking to identify PLH is that this phenotype may exist in subgroups of the population who are clinically asymptomatic. No reliable means of identifying the PLH exists. A biological marker is needed. There is evidence, some of it long known, that lateralized brain injury may alter growth of the limbs. What is known about the nature and timing of brain injury that limits somatic growth? Might these asymmetries be a useful marker of brain injury that might otherwise not be recognized?

Brain Damage and Trophic Changes

It has long been known that lateralized brain injury is a correlate of aberrant contralateral somatic development (e.g., Gowers, 1878). Indeed, a plethora of medical evidence exists that demonstrates that an appropriately localized and timed lesion will produce hypoplasia of the contralateral hand or foot. The present section reviews some of this evidence, specifically focusing on studies that demonstrate the potential for early left hemisphere lesions to produce trophic changes. An attempt is made to relate the notion of trophic changes to the concepts of handedness and cerebral lateralization to develop the contention that such changes can be used to help identify cases of PLH.

CNS injury that is sustained during development is an important mechanism of lateral underdevelopment. The extent of underdevelopment depends on the individual's age at the time of injury. Injuries sustained after completion of growth and development are likely to alter cell size (hypertrophy) rather than cell number (hyperplasia). In general, skeletal asymmetries suggest early nervous system injury; soft-tissue asymmetries alone suggest an insult occurring after the early developmental period.

Several researchers have reported an association between brain lesions localized to the area of the postcentral gyrus and underdevelopment of the contralateral limbs (Bastian & Horsley, 1881; Guthrie, 1918; Winkelman & Silverstein, 1935). Perhaps the most convincing evidence in support of this relationship is the 1943 report of Penfield and Robertson. Epileptic patients with localized cerebral pathology, somatic asymmetries, and evidence that lesion onset occurred in childhood were studied ($n = 13$). Asymmetries included lateralized differences in the length and thickness of the bones of the upper and lower arms, hands, feet, face, and chest. A control group ($n = 14$) of patients with early onset brain lesions but with no measurable somatic asymmetries was also examined. The critical determinants of the presence or absence of somatic asymmetry in these patients were age at onset of brain lesion and involvement of the postcentral gyrus. In every instance of somatic asymmetry, age at lesion onset was reported to be 2 years or younger. If the postcentral gyrus was spared, regardless of the timing of the insult, asymmetry did not develop.

These findings strongly suggest that lateralized brain injury involving the postcentral gyrus can produce unilateral underdevelopment of the limbs. However, several intriguing questions remain.

1. What, if any, is the extent of somatic asymmetry in neurologically intact individuals?
2. Does the degree of somatic asymmetry observed in unilaterally brain-damaged individuals always exceed that found in individuals without brain injury?
3. Do somatic asymmetries vary as a function of sex, handedness, or other factors?
4. Under what circumstances can somatic asymmetries allow reliable inferences about aspects of cerebral lateralization and organization?

We now consider data that address these questions.

Somatic asymmetry has long been of interest to scientists. Some of the earliest studies of asymmetry were conducted in the late nineteenth and the first half of the twentieth century. The consensus of these studies was that somatic asymmetries occur quite frequently in the normal population (e.g., Hasse & Dehner, 1893). In one early study of somatic asymmetries, Landauer (1939) reviewed a series of 22 literature cases of congenital hemiatrophy involving the arm or leg. These cases of unilateral underdevelopment were not associated with motor deficits. Of the 22 cases reported, 16 involved the left body side and 6 the right body side. Of particular interest, 5 of the 6 subjects with right-side underdevelopment were left-handed, whereas only 2 of the 16 subjects with left-side underdevelopment were left-handed. These findings strongly suggest a relationship between right-side underdevelopment and MLH. Interestingly, Landauer was puzzled by this association and failed to entertain early left hemisphere injury as a possible explanation.

The majority of the early studies of somatic asymmetry emphasized the length of a limb or of the long bones of the body. We now know that there is a poor correlation between the size of a body part and the amount of brain tissue devoted to its function. Although the mechanism by which the cortex mediates skeletal growth is unclear, the evidence supports a somatotopic correspondence for development that is similar to somatosensory development. Because the feet, hands, and face dominate the homunculus of the postcentral gyrus, these parts of the body might reasonably best reflect trophic changes due to early brain injury.

Means and Walters (1982) studied asymmetries of the hands and feet in children without known brain damage. A significant association among asymmetry of the hands, handedness, and sex was found. Right-handed males had longer right than left hands, whereas non-right-handed males had longer left than right hands. Asymmetries of the hands in female subjects were also found. No significant associations were found among asymmetry of the feet, handedness, and sex.

Levy and Levy (1978) measured the feet of neurologically intact females and males (n = 98 and 52, respectively). Eighteen of the 98 females and 17 of the 52 males were under the age of 6 years. Levy and Levy reported a difference in pedal length that varied as a function of gender and handedness. This finding suggests that, at the very least, pedal asymmetries, when present, may be indirectly related to handedness. If true, Levy and Levy's finding may have indirectly provided a clue to the identification of PLHs. Unfortunately, Levy and Levy's study contained a number of methodological problems (rating scale, statistical tests, sample composition, and measurement procedures). Four other studies (Mascie-Taylor, MacLaron, Lanigan, & McManus, 1981; Orsini & Satz, 1983; Peters, Perie & Oddie, 1981; Yanowitz, Satz, & Heilman, 1981) failed to replicate Levy and Levy's (1978) findings with these methodological problems corrected.

Although no significant differences in foot length were observed in the Yanowitz *et al.* (1981) replication of Levy and Levy (1978), an interesting incidental finding emerged. Yanowitz *et al.* found a larger variability in foot-length asymmetry in left-handed males than in females or right-handed males. This variability was due largely to 4 subjects whose differences in foot length were greater than two standard deviations compared to the study sample as a whole. This finding suggested that something other than normal variance was operative. Closer inspection of the data revealed that these 4 subjects were left-handed. Furthermore, in 3 of the 4 cases there was no positive family history for left-handedness, and the right foot length was significantly smaller than the left. Yanowitz *et al.* (1981) concluded that the magnitude of pedal asymmetry that they observed (>1.3 cm) was consistent with trophic changes in the extremities that have been reported in clinical cases with early birth trauma. They further concluded that the presence of a markedly shorter right foot in left-handers, especially in males, who are known to be at greater risk for birth injury and disease (Taylor & Ounsted, 1972), indirectly suggests the presence of PLH.

The findings of Yanowitz *et al.* (1981), although suggestive of a relationship between handedness and early brain injury, must be viewed with caution. The subjects in the Yanowitz *et al.* study were neurologically intact. However, it is tempting and reasonable to speculate that these subjects were asymptomatic individuals who had experienced early trauma to the left hemisphere that resulted in manual transfer (PLH) and underdevelopment of the bones of the right foot due to involvement of the left postcentral gyrus. But the relationship between handedness and trophic changes in subjects with known brain injury must be examined before this contention can be accepted.

In addition to testing Satz's (1972, 1973) model of PLH, the Satz *et al.* (1983) study cited earlier (see "Clinical Studies") also investigated the relationship among foot length, handedness, and early brain injury in a large group of epileptics. Results of this examination revealed a significant relationship between pedal asymmetry and lateralization of EEG abnormality only in those patients with early onset seizures. Individuals with early onset lesions and left-side EEG foci were found to have a significantly shorter right foot, whereas individuals with early onset lesion and right-side EEG foci had a shorter left foot. No differences in foot length were observed in the control group, which confirms earlier reports (Mascie-Taylor *et al.*, 1981; Yanowitz *et al.*, 1981).

Using these findings, Satz *et al.* (1983) hypothesized that cases of PLH would exist to a significantly greater extent in clusters of subjects with focal left hemisphere lesions and in whom brain damage had occurred before the age of 2 years. To test this hypothesis, all of the MLHs ($N = 33$) were assigned to one of four PLH suspect groups and an analysis of their foot-length differences was performed. The four groups were not suspect (non-left focal lesion regardless of onset, or no seizure history; control); low suspect (left-focal lesion, late onset, ages 17–55 years); moderate suspect (left focal lesion, middle onset, ages 2–17 years); high suspect (left focal lesion, early onset, birth–age 2 years). The analysis revealed a significant group difference. There was a significant relationship between pedal asymmetry and the different suspect groups ($r = -.67$). Negative pedal-asymmetry scores (shorter right foot) were generally associated with the moderate and high suspect groups, and null or slightly positive asymmetry scores tended to be associated with the low and not suspect groups. In fact, Satz *et al.* (1983) reported that all of the patients in the high PLH suspect group had a shorter right foot.

Multivariate analyses were also used to determine a foot-length difference (pedal asymmetry) cutoff score that would minimize the misclassification of a subject as either highly suspect or not suspect for PLH. The results showed that if a left-hander had a pedal-asymmetry score greater than or equal to -0.50 cm (smaller right foot), he or she would be highly suspect for PLH. Using this cutoff score, 4 of the 6 left-handers from the high suspect group were identified. In other words, patients with left-side brain lesions of early onset who have a right foot shorter than the left foot by 0.5 cm or more were likely to be left-handed. These data support the view that left hemisphere injury sustained before the age of 2 years retards skeletal growth in the right foot, producing a pedal asymmetry. Furthermore, under certain circumstances significant underdevelopment of the right foot and PLH may be causally related. Presumably, injury before 2 years of age to the left hemisphere, which includes the anterior parietal region, produces a partial failure of unilateral somatic development along with a change in hand preference.

If early brain injury leads to a reallocation of the hemispheric control of manual functions and a hypofunctioning of the cortical systems involved in the mediation of somatic growth, it seems reasonable to postulate that such damage may also adversely affect the organization of controls for other functional systems: Does early left hemisphere damage cause the right hemisphere to become dominant for language? What effect does early left hemisphere damage have on functions normally ascribed to the right hemisphere? The next section addresses such questions.

Brain Damage and Higher Cognitive Functions

Speech–Language Processes

Satz's (1972) model of PLH predicts that injury-induced shifts in manual dominance are concurrent with shifts in speech–language functions. It is intuitively reasonable to postulate this dual transfer of functions because presumably both handedness and speech–language functions are subserved by the same general brain areas, the perisylvian and perirolandic areas and the supplemental motor area. The following section examines data germane to this postulation.

There is, unfortunately, a paucity of studies that have examined the issue of trauma-induced shifts in the hemispheric control of higher cognitive functions. The contention that speech–language processes can be lateralized to either hemisphere subsequent to early unilateral brain damage was first advanced by Basser (1962) and later refined by Lenneberg (1967). Two clinical observations served as the impetus for this idea. First, children who sustained early unilateral brain damage (ages 2–6 years) were likely to become aphasic regardless of the hemisphere damaged. The implication of this observation was

TABLE 1

Speech Lateralization as Related to Handedness in Noninjured Patients[a,b]

Handedness	n	Speech representation		
		Left	Bilateral	Right
Right	140	134 (96%)	0 (0%)	6 (4%)
Left or mixed	122	86 (70%)	18 (15%)	18 (15%)

[a]Data from Rasmussen and Milner (1977).
[b]Patients have no clinical evidence of early left hemisphere damage.

that both hemispheres in young children are equally involved in facilitating language. The second observation was that the aphasia observed in children who sustained early left hemisphere damage was qualitatively different from the aphasia observed in adults who sustained left brain damage. Childhood aphasia appeared to be neither as severe nor as protracted as adult aphasia. Again, the implication was that in young children both hemispheres have the capacity to subserve speech–language functions. It was presumed that language functions in aphasic children were spared severe compromise because the right hemisphere, if undamaged, had the capacity to compensate for the damaged left hemisphere. It should be noted that these observations do not necessarily lead to the conclusion that both hemispheres are equipotent for language. Rather, these observations merely suggest tht the nondominant hemisphere has the capacity to subserve some, but not all, of the language functions normally ascribed to the dominant hemisphere.

Perhaps the strongest support for Satz's prediction of a concurrent shift in manual dominance and speech–language functions following early unilateral brain injury rests on the report by Rasmussen and Milner (1977), who reviewed the effects of unilateral injections of amobarbital on speech functions in epileptic patients. This report addressed the role of early left brain injury in determining lateralization of cerebral speech functions in a large sample of left- and right-handed patients. Tables 1 and 2 present the results. Table 1 presents estimates of speech lateralization as a function of handedness in patients without clinical evidence of early left-side injury. Inspection of this table reveals the well-established unilateral, left-side mode of speech in the right-handed (96%) and the more variable unilateral or bilateral mode of speech in the left-handed (left = 70%, right = 15%, bilateral = 15%) (Satz, 1979).

TABLE 2

Speech Lateralization as Related to Handedness in Patients with Definite Clinical Evidence of Early Left Hemisphere Lesions[a]

		Speech representation		
Handedness	n	Left	Bilateral	Right
Right	42	34 (81%)	3 (7%)	5 (12%)
Left or mixed	92	26 (28%)	17 (19%)	49 (53%)

[a]Data from Rasmussen and Milner (1977).

Table 2 presents similar data in patients with clinical evidence of an early left-side injury (before age 6 years). Inspection of this table reveals a dramatic increase in the incidence of right-side speech representation in the left-handed patients, whereas the majority of the right-handers still show the unilateral, left-side mode of speech. In fact, there was more than a threefold increase in the percentage of right-side speech representation in left-handers who had sustained early injury to the left cerebral hemisphere. Most of these MLHs were probably PLHs who had experienced alterations in both manual and cerebral dominance. Conversely, most of the right-handers with bilateral or right-side speech were probably natural right-handers who had experienced lateral transfer in speech functions only. This latter group, although much smaller, provides support for Rasmussen and Milner's (1977) suggestion that "an early lesion that does not modify hand preference is on the whole unlikely to change the side of speech representation" (p. 359).

Spatial–Perceptual Processes

Rasmussen and Milner's data strongly suggest that speech–language functions may be subsumed by an intact right hemisphere if the injury is sustained early. If one accepts this notion of cerebral reorganization one is faced with the problem of explaining what effect such reorganization would have on the functions normally mediated by the undamaged hemisphere. Specifically, one is confronted with the fact that additional cognitive functions must now be subserved by the undamaged hemisphere. Does the undamaged hemisphere reallocate its resources equally or does it favor one function over another? In general, visuospatial–perceptual functions are subserved by the right hemisphere. However, early injury to the left hemisphere that results in a shift in hand dominance and speech–language functions may compromise the right hemisphere's ability to carry out these functions.

Data germane to this issue are at best scant and indirect. Results from hemidecortication studies (Dennis & Whitaker, 1976, 1977) suggest that visuospatial–perceptual functions in the isolated right hemisphere are not diminished relative to the verbal functions taken on by this hemisphere. In fact, Dennis and Whitaker (1977) conclude that spatial functions develop more readily in the isolated brain region. These results conflict with the proposition of Satz (1972) and others (e.g., Lansdell, 1969) that language processing supersedes visuospatial processing in right hemisphere takeover. However, Dennis and Whitaker's small sample size precludes definitive conclusions.

One case report presents some support, albeit indirect, for the notion of diminished visuospatial–perceptual processing subsequent to right hemisphere takeover of speech–language functions. Bullard-Bates and Satz (1983) report the case of a 37-year-old nonfamilial left-handed woman. Neuropsychological evaluation of this patient revealed superior performance in language skills but rather dramatic impairment in visuospatial–constructive skills and on sensory–motor tasks with the nonpreferred, right hand. Further testing revealed a dramatically shorter right hand and foot, a slight right-side facial asymmetry, and a robust left-ear advantage on a dichotic word-pair task. A static lesion in the left hemisphere, presumed to be present from birth, was confirmed by computerized axial tomography (CAT). This case lends support to the claim that early injury to the left hemisphere (before age 6 years) spares normal language development at the expense of visuospatial functions. Most probably this sparing occurred because of early transfer of speech functions to the right hemisphere, which altered the functional space for visuospatial functions normally subserved by this hemisphere (Lansdell, 1969).

More direct support for the contention that normal visuospatial–perceptual functions of the right hemisphere are diminished due to right hemisphere takeover of speech–language functions is obtained from Tizard, Paine, and Crothers (1954). Of 4 cases of right hemiplegia described in detail by Tizard *et al.,* there was evidence of cortical sensory loss in 3. These 3 patients had documented visuospatial handicaps. The possible link between cortical sensory deficits and cognitive deficits was not discussed by the authors, though their limited data would support this association.

The issue of intrahemispheric competition between higher cognitive processes following early unilateral brain injury has not received ample attention. The resultant dearth of information precludes strong conclusive statements. However, several tentative conclusions can be made on the basis of the available data.

1. Although the two hemispheres are not necessarily equipotent for subserving higher cognitive functions, each can to a reasonable degree subserve those functions not normally ascribed to it if predominantly unilateral damage is sustained early.
2. Early unilateral brain damage leads to a transfer in manual dominance and a concomitant shift in speech–language functions in some indifivuals.
3. It is presently unclear what the effect of early left hemisphere damage is on the perceptual processes of the right hemisphere subsequent to right hemisphere takeover of speech–language functions. Indirect evidence suggests a detrimental effect.

Summary and General Conclusions

This chapter examined the effects of early CNS insult on three aspects of lateral development: (1) manual dominance, (2) hemispheric control of higher cognitive processes, and (3) somatic asymmetries. The studies reviewed strongly suggest that precisely timed and localized insults to the developing brain have deleterious effects on the ontogeny of functional asymmetry. Brain injury sustained prior to the age of 2 years and predominantly lateralized to the left hemisphere may cause a shift in manual dominance, a transfer in the hemispheric control of speech–language functions with concomitant hypofunctioning of visuospatial–perceptual processes, and a hypodevelopment of the limbs contralateral to the injury focus. Of course all of these consequences may or may not be present within one individual. In addition, the degree to which a given outcome is manifested varies from person to person. While early brain injury in some individuals leads to a right–left reversal in the normal pattern of lateralization, such injury in others results in an absence of lateralization or in a reduction in the degree of lateralization. The factors that determine the type and quality of injury-induced alterations in functional asymmetry are unknown. However, data reviewed in this chapter allow us to posit some reasonable speculations.

The determinants of injury-induced changes in functional asymmetry can best be characterized along two dimensions: a severity of injury dimension and an injury-focus dimension. The severity dimension ranges from mild to moderate to severe trauma, whereas the injury-focus dimension ranges from unilateral left hemisphere to bilateral asymmetric (left > right) to bilateral symmetric. The severity as well as the locus of the early injury dictates whether functional asymmetry will be disrupted and, if it is, what its direction (left versus right) and strength will be. In general, severe bilateral trauma is likely to result in an absence of functional asymmetry. That is, both hemispheres will be either equally competent or incompetent. In comparison, severe unilateral trauma is likely to result in a contralateral shift in lateral dominance. It is assumed that in cases of early unilateral damage the remaining hemisphere is reasonably intact and able to subserve those functional systems displaced by the insult. Thus, hemispheric control of a given functional system is transferred to the intact contralateral hemisphere. The result of this transfer is a right–left reversal of cerebral dominance. It is assumed that in cases of early bilateral trauma the amount of intact tissue is markedly reduced. Consequently, normal patterns of functional lateralization fail to develop.

In contrast to severe brain injuries, mild injuries, regardless of focus, may produce several aberrant patterns of lateralization. Mild trauma may lead to (1) maintenance of the innate pattern of functional asymmetry, (2) complete reversal in the innate pattern of functional asymmetry, or (3) maintenance of the innate pattern of functional asymmetry with significant reductions in the strength of lateralization (i.e., the function is not as strongly lateralized as would be expected).

Two intriguing conclusions emerge from this chapter. First, there exists within the normal population of MLHs a small subset of genotypic right-handers who, because of early unilateral brain injury, masquerade as left-handers (PLH). Differentiation of these "asymptomatic" individuals may help to advance research in and increase our knowledge of the ontogeny of cerebral and manual dominance and the course of transient changes in functional systems following mild brain injury. Second, insights obtained from the study of MLHs with a history of early unilateral CNS injury, trophic asymmetries, and right hemisphere speech–language functions with concomitant visuospatial–perceptual deficits may have etiological significance for a variety of neurological disorders. Systematic studies of these individuals may yield neuropsychological and neurological knowledge that can be applied to a variety of clinical subgroups (e.g., autism and schizophrenia) for whom putative alterations in hemispheric organization have already been suggested (DeMyer *et al.*, 1981).

References

Annett, M. (1978). Genetic and nongenetic influence on handedness. *Behavioral Genetics, 8,* 227–249.

Bakan, P. (1971). Handedness and birth order. *Nature, 229,* 195.

Bakan, P. (1977). Left handedness and birth order revisited. *Neuropsychologia, 15,* 837–839.

Bakan, P., Dibb, G., & Reed, P. (1973). Handedness and birth stress. *Neuropsychologia, 11,* 363–366.

Barry, R. J., & James, A. L. (1978). Handedness in autistics, retardates, and normals of a wide age range. *Journal of Autism and Childhood Schizophrenia, 8*(3), 315–323.

Basser, L. S. (1962). Hemiplegia of early onset and the faculty of speech with special reference to the effects of hemispherectomy. *Brain, 85,* 427–460.

Bastian, H. C., & Horsley, V. (1881). Arrest of development in the left upper limb in association with an extremely small right ascending parietal convolution. *Brain, 3,* 113–116.

Baymur, L. (1977). *The relationship between manifest handedness and EEG abnormalities in epileptic children.* Unpublished manuscript.

Bingley, T. (1958). Mental symptoms in temporal lobe epilepsy and temporal lobe gliomas with reference to laterality of lesion and the relationship between handedness and brainedness. *Acta Psychiatrica et Neurologica, 33,* (Suppl. 120).

Bolin, B. J. (1953). Left handedness and stuttering as signs diagnostic of epileptics. *Journal of Mental Science, 99,* 484–488.

Bullard-Bates, C., & Satz, P. (1983). A case of pathological left-hander. *Clinical Neuropsychology. 5,* 128–129.

Colby, K. M., & Parkison, C. (1977). Handedness in autistic children. *Journal of Autism and Childhood Schizophrenia, 7*(1), 3–9.

Coren, S., & Porac, C. (1980). Birth factors and laterality: Effects of birth order, parental age and birth stress on four indicies of lateral preference. *Behavior Genetics, 10,* 123–138.

DeMyer, M. K., Hingtgen, J. N., & Jackson, R. K. (1981). Infantile autism reviewed: A decade of research. *Schizophrenia Bulletin, 7*(3), 388–451.

Dennis, M., & Whitaker, H. A. (1976). Language acquisition following hemidecortication: Linguistic superiority of the left over the right hemisphere. *Brain and Language, 3,* 404–433.

Dennis, M., & Whitaker, H. (1977). Hemispheric equipotentiality and language acquisition. In S. J. Segalowitz & F. A. Gruber (Eds.), *Language development and neurological theory* (pp. 93–106). New York: Academic Press.

Gowers, W. R. (1878). The brain in congenital absence of one hand. *Brain, 1,* 386–390.

Guthrie, L. (1918). Muscular atrophy and other changes in nutrition associated with lesions of the sensory cortex of the brain, with especial reference to the possible existence of trophic representation in the postcentral areas. *Proceedings of the Royal Society of Medicine, 11*(1, 2), 21–26.

Hardyck, C., & Petrinovich, L. F. (1977). Left-handedness. *Psychological Bulletin, 84*(3), 385–404.

Hasse, C., & Dehner. (1893). Unsere Truppen in Korperlicher Beziehung. *Archiv fuer Anatomie und Physiologie, Anatomische Abteilung,* 249–256.

Hicks, R. A., & Barton, A. K. (1975). A note on left-handedness and severity of mental retardation. *Journal of Genetic Psychology, 127,* 323–324.

Hicks, R. A., Dusek, C., Larsen, F., Williams, S., & Pellegrini, R. J. (1980). Birth complications and the distribution of handedness. *Cortex, 15,* 135–137.

Hicks, R. A., Elliott, D., Garbesi, L., & Martin, S. (1979). Multiple birth risk factors and the distribution of handedness. *Cortex, 15,* 135–137.

Hicks, R. A., Evans, E. A., & Pellegrini, R. J. (1978). Correlation between handedness and birth order: Compilation of five studies. *Perceptual and Motor Skills, 46,* 53–54.

Hicks, R. A., Pellegrini, R. J., & Evans, E. A. (1978). Handedness and birth risk. *Neuropsychologia, 16,* 243–245.

Landauer, W. (1939). Supernumerary nipples, congenital hemihypertrophy and congenital hemiatrophy. *Human Biology, 11,*(4), 447–472.

Lansdell, H. (1969). Verbal and nonverbal factors in right-hemisphere speech: Relation to early neurological theory. *Journal of Comparative and Physiological Psychology, 69,* 734–738.

Lenneberg, E. (1967). *Biological foundations of language.* New York: Wiley.

Leviton, A., & Kilty, T. (1979). Birth risk and left-handedness reconsidered. *Archives of Neurology, 36,* 119–120.

Levy, J., & Levy, J. M. (1978). Human lateralization from head to foot: Sex-related factors. *Science, 20,* 1291–1292.

Liederman, J., & Coryell, J. (1982). The origin of left hand preference: Pathological and non-pathological influences. *Neuropsychologia, 20*(6), 721–725.

Mascie-Taylor, C., MacLarnon, A., Lanigan, P., & McManus, I. (1981). Foot-length asymmetry, sex and handedness. *Science, 212,* 1416–1417.

Means, L. W., & Walters, R. E. (1982). Sex, handedness and asymmetry of hand and foot length. *Neuropsychologia, 20*(6), 715–719.

Orsini, D., & Satz, P. (in Press). Pedal Asymmetries and Handedness *Journal of Clinical and Experimental Neuropsychology.*

Penfield, W., & Roberts, L. (1959). *Speech and brain mechanisms.* Princeton: Princeton University Press.

Penfield, W., & Robertson, J. S. M. (1943). Growth asymmetry due to lesions of the postcentral cerebral cortex. *Archives of Neurology and Psychiatry, 50*(4), 405–430.

Peters, M., Perie, B., & Oddie, D. (1981). Foot-length asymmetry, sex and handedness. *Science, 212,* 1417–1418.

Rasmussen, T., & Milner, B. (1977). The role of early left-brain injury in determining lateralization of cerebral speech functions. *Annals of the New York Academy of Sciences, 299,* 355–369.

Satz, P. (1972). Pathological left-handedness: An explanatory mode. *Cortex, 8,* 121–135.

Satz, P. (1973). Left-handedness and early brain insult: An explanation. *Neuropsychologia, 11,* 115–117.

Satz, P. (1979). A test of some models of hemispheric speech organization in left- and right-handers. *Science, 203,* 1131–1133.

Satz, P., Baymur, L., & Van der Vlugt, H. (1979). Pathological left-handedness: Cross-cultural tests of a model. *Neuropsychologia, 17,* 77–81.

Satz, P., Yanowitz, J., & Willmore, J. (1983). Early brain damage and lateral development. In R. Bell, J. Elias, R. Green, & J. Harvey (Eds.), *Interfaces in psychology*. Texas: Texas University Press.

Silva, D. A. & Satz, P. (1979) Pathological left-handedness: Evaluation of a model. *Brain and Language, 7*, 8–16.

Taylor, D. C., & Ounsted, C. (1972). The nature of gender differences explored through ontogenetic analysis of sex ratios in disease. In C. Ounsted & D. C. Taylor (Eds.), *Gender differences: Their ontogeny and significance*. Edinborough: Livingstone.

Tizard, J. P. M., Paine, R. S., & Crothers, B. (1954). Disturbances of sensation in children with hemiplegia. *Journal of the American Medical Association, 155*, 628–632.

Tsai, L. Y., & Stewart, M. A. (1982). Handedness and EEG correlation in autistic children. *Biological Psychiatry, 17*, 595–598.

Winkelman, N. W., & Silverstein, A. (1935). Unilateral amytrophy: Its diagnostic importance for cerebral localization. *American Journal of Syphilis and Neurology, 19*, 58–76.

Yanowitz, J., Satz, P., & Heilman, K. (1981). Hemispheric laterality and body asymmetries. *Science, 212*, 1418.

14

The Effects of Cortical Lesions in Children: Language and Visual Functions

Henri Hécaen, M. T. Perenin, and Marc Jeannerod

Introduction

Experimental data are now accumulating that progressively disclose the behavioral, physiological, and anatomical processes underlying functional recovery after early brain lesions. In this context, clinical material reveals itself to be an interesting source of information regarding the multiple factors (beneficial or detrimental) that may influence the course of recovery.

The role of the age at which a brain lesion occurs has been investigated both in animals and in humans. It is a common claim since the work of Margaret Kennard that brain lesions made in newborn animals produce less deficit than comparable lesions in adults. For instance, the motor deficit following destruction of the cortical motor

EARLY BRAIN DAMAGE, Volume 1
Research Orientations and Clinical Observations

Copyright © 1984 by Academic Press, Inc.
All rights of reproduction in any form reserved.
ISBN 0-12-052901-7

and premotor areas in newborn monkeys will be much less severe than that after destruction of the same areas in adult animals (Kennard, 1936, 1938). A similar functional sparing after early lesions has been observed in many brain areas and in many different animal species (see review in Jeannerod & Hécaen, 1979). There are important limitations to this so-called Kennard effect, however. A number of functional impairments may be permanent after early brain lesions. In addition, some aspects of the function may never even appear if the lesion is made before the function has fully matured. For example, monkeys in which area 4 is ablated (Passingham, Perry, & Wilkinson, 1978) or the bulbar pyramids are sectioned (Lawrence & Hopkins, 1972) during the first few days of life never develop the ability to make fine finger-movements.

Many of the concepts relating to the effects of age at which a lesion is made on subsequent functional sparing have been established with prefrontal lesions in newborn monkeys. Harlow *et al.* have shown in 1964 that an animal undergoing operation during the first weeks of life will not later present the typical loss of delayed responses observed after prefrontal lesions in adults. This functional sparing has been confirmed by Goldman, Rosvold, and Mishkin in 1970. Prolonged observation of the same animals, however, has shown that they become impaired at the age at which the destroyed areas should normally mature (Goldman, 1971). These observations have led to the conclusion that functional recovery following early ablation of a given brain area depends on the degree of maturation of the neural structures to which the lesioned area is connected. If these neural structures are still functionally immature (i.e., not engaged in the function) when the lesion is made, they may still be plastic enough to take over the functions of the ablated zone. If, on the contrary, the spared tissue is already engaged or is at least partially mature at the time of the lesion, its capacities for ensuring functional reorganization may be lost.

In more recent experiments Goldman and Galkin (1978) have made frontal lesions in monkeys at the fetal stage (102th to 109th day) that are subsequently replaced in utero until the day of natural birth. When tested at the age of 1 or 2 years, these monkeys showed no deficit in the delayed response or in the delayed alternated response tasks. Histological study of their brain revealed no degeneration in the thalamic dorsomedial nuclei, where projections to the prefrontal cortex normally originate. These results indicate that when an area is destroyed before its connections develop normally, a complete anatomical reorganization seems possible. In the case of prefrontal lesions the axons of the thalamic cells may reach structures other than their normal targets. Such a reorganization would explain the more complete functional sparing observed in these animals.

It is often difficult to evaluate the effects of early cortical lesions in humans comparatively, due to the lack of information about their extent, both on the cortical surface and in depth. There are exceptions, however, particularly in the case of surgical ablations. In the present chapter we deal with the effects of lesions acquired during the first years of life, on both language functions and visual perceptual abilities.

In the case of aphasia occurring in children as a consequence of left hemisphere lesions, a relatively fast recovery may be observed. This recovery raises the problem of the degree of specialization of a given brain-area, or equipotentiality of the two hemispheres, at least during a limited period of time. On the other hand, in the case of hemianopia due to early cortical ablations involving the visual cortex, remarkable residual visual abilities may be demonstrated. These abilities raise the problem of functional substitution by cortical or subcortical vicariate areas.

Acquired Aphasia in Children with Early Left-Hemisphere Lesions

As early as 1885, Bernhardt had insisted that aphasia is frequent in children and that the nature of the impairment is transient. These facts were confirmed in the systematic analysis of a series of cases by Guttman in 1942. Several other studies have been devoted to this problem (Alajouanine and Lhermitte, 1965; Basser, 1962; Branco-Lefèvre, 1950; Lenneberg, 1967). In 1976, Hécaen, in a study of 26 cases with cortical lesions, stressed the particular character of aphasia in children (frequent mutism, rare paraphasia, no logorrhea). In the same study, Hécaen showed that right hemisphere lesions do not produce more language disturbances in children than in adults (see also Krashen, 1973), a result in contradiction to some previous studies (Freud, 1897; Lenneberg, 1967). Finally, most of the cases in the Hécaen's series showed a relatively good functional recovery.

The current study is based on the 26 cases from the earlier study, to which 30 new cases have been added. Thus under consideration are 56 children aged $3\frac{1}{2}$–15 years, all with cortical lesions and all hospitalized at Hôpital Sainte-Anne in the units of neurosurgery or ster-

TABLE 1

Total Number of Cases with Aphasia

Handedness and lesion side	Adults			Children		
	N	Aphasic	%	*N*	Aphasic	%
Right handers						
Left-side lesions	366	232	63	34	25	74
Right-side lesions	239	1	0.4	7	1	14
Bilateral lesions	—	—	—	3	2	67
Left handers						
Left-side lesions	87	34	39	6	5	83
Right-side lesions	53	28	53	6	3	50

eotactic neurosurgery. Lesion lateralization was determined in most cases by surgical data or X-ray data (CT [computer tomography] scans for the new cases), or, in rare situations, clinical data (hemiplegia, hemianopia).

Of the 56 cases, 40 had left hemisphere lesions (34 of these in right-handers), 13 had right hemisphere lesions (7 of these in right-handers), and 3 had bilateral hemisphere lesions. All subjects were tested with a complete neuropsychological battery that was developed in our laboratory.

Initially we determined only the presence or absence of aphasia, regardless of type or severity. In Table 1, we see the frequency of aphasia in these children according to lesion lateralization or handedness. For purposes of comparison, Table 1 includes the frequency of aphasia in adults taken from our own series of right-handers with hemisphere lesions and from the series of left-handers with hemisphere lesions published earlier (Hécaen, Agostini, & Monzon-Montes, 1981).

Table 2 shows the frequency of aphasia in the 34 right-handed

TABLE 2

Cases with Aphasia, according to Age[a]

Age	*N*	Aphasic	%
$<$10 years	14	12	86
$\geq$10 years	20	13	65

[a]Left-side lesions in right-handed patients.

TABLE 3

Cases with Aphasia, according to Etiology[a]

Etiology	N	Aphasic	%
Tumors	15	8	53
Trauma	12	10	83
Hematoma (angioma)	6	6	100

[a]Left-side lesions in right-handed patients.

children with left-side lesions, grouped by age (up to or older than 10 years); Table 3 shows the same children, grouped by lesion type (tumor, trauma, hematoma due to ruptured angioma). Subsequently, we analyzed the frequency of specific types of language disorder (Table 4). These are studied by lesion localization (Table 5), age (Table 6), and lesion etiology (Table 7). Overall frequency of aphasia in the 34 right-handed children with left-side lesions was 74% (25 out of 34). In 4 of the 25 labeled as aphasic, only very mild disorders of oral or written expression were found. In the 7 right-handed children with right-side lesions, one case of very mild aphasia was found.

Satz and Bullard-Bates (1981) have emphasized the statistical bias represented by the small proportion of patients with right-side lesions in the series studied. The current series confirms their observation (34 patients with left-side versus 7 patients with right-side le-

TABLE 4

Overall Frequency of Aphasic Symptoms[a]

	Overall frequency		
Symptom	N	Cases (n)	%
Mutism	34	16	47
Articulatory disorders	34	18	53
Auditory comprehension disorders	34	12	35
Naming disorders	34	15	44
Paraphasias	34	3	9
Reading disorders	30	12	40
Writing disorders	30	19	63

[a]Left-side lesions in right-handed patients.

TABLE 5

Frequency of Aphasic Symptoms, according to Localization[a]

Symptom	Frequency by localization: Anterior lesions (frontal–rolandic) *N*	Cases (*n*)	%	Temporal lesions *N*	Cases (*n*)	%
Mutism*	11	7	63	10	1	10
Articulatory** disorders	11	9	81	10	2	20
Auditory comprehension disorders	11	5	45	10	3	30
Naming disorders	11	5	45	10	3	30
Paraphasias	11	1	9	10	1	10
Reading disorders	8	2	25	10	2	20
Writing disorders	8	5	62	10	5	50

[a]Left-hand lesions in right-handed patients.
*$p < .05$. **$p < .02$.

sions) and reemphasizes the rarity of aphasia in right-handers with right-side lesions.

Comparing overall frequency of aphasia in right-handed children with left-side lesions (74%) with that in right-handed adults (63%), we find more aphasia in the children, although the difference is not statistically significant. The frequency of aphasia in children is even greater in this series in the children under the age of 10 years (86%).

TABLE 6

Frequency of Aphasic Symptoms, according to Age[a]

Symptom	<10 yr *N*	Cases (*n*)	%	≥10 yr *N*	Cases (*n*)	%
Mutism	14	9	64	20	6	30
Articulatory disorders	14	9	64	20	9	45
Auditory comprehension disorders	14	6	43	20	6	30
Naming disorders	14	9	64	20	6	30
Paraphasias	14	3	21	20	0	0
Reading disorders	11	4	36	19	8	42
Writing disorders*	11	10	91	19	9	47

[a]Left-side lesions in right-handed patients.
*$p < .05$.

TABLE 7

Frequency of Aphasic Symptoms, according to Etiology[a]

Symptom	Frequency by etiology								
	Hematoma (angioma)			Trauma			Tumors abcess		
	N	Cases (n)	%	N	Cases (n)	%	N	Cases (n)	%
Mutism*	6	4	67	12	9	75	15	3	20
Articulatory disorders	6	4	67	12	8	67	15	6	40
Auditory comprehension disorders	6	3	50	12	6	50	15	3	20
Naming disorders	6	4	67	12	6	50	15	5	33
Paraphasias	6	2	33	12	0	0	15	1	7
Reading disorders	6	2	33	10	7	70	13	3	23
Writing disorders	6	6	100	10	8	80	13	5	38

[a]Left-hand lesions in right-handed patients.
*$p < .05$.

For the children 10 years of age or older, the frequency of aphasia is 65%—that is, nearly the same as that for the adults.

Clinical features of aphasia in these children are different from those in adults. The predominant clinical symptom, at least in the initial stage, is a suppression of spontaneous speech (mutism). At a later stage, aphasia in children is characterized by a higher frequency of anarthria or dysarthria, although paraphasia is rare and logorrhea is lacking.

Lesion localization and rapidity of lesion onset are two factors that seem to play a major role in symptom production. Anteriorly located lesions (frontal or rolandic) are associated with dysarthria in 81% of cases, whereas temporal lesions are associated with only 20% of dysarthria difficulties. In fact, all aspects of language, including auditory and visual verbal comprehension, are more disturbed following anterior than following temporal lesions.

As for rapidity of lesion onset, mutism is strikingly more frequent with rapid as compared with slow onset of illness. The same observation is true for writing disorders and, to a lesser degree, for difficulties with naming and with auditory comprehension.

In the seven right-handed children with right hemisphere lesions, we found only one case with language disability. This child had mainly articulatory problems, and recovery was rather quick. In this regard, Woods and Teuber (1978) commented that aphasia in children with right hemisphere lesions was found with relative frequency only in the period prior to the existence of antibiotics, and that, in fact, these cases probably reflected bilateral damage. Nevertheless, some cases of that period were due to brain tumors.

We were able to follow six of our right-handed aphasic children for periods of 1 to 8 years. Of these, four showed considerable improvement, two of whom retained only writing difficulties. A fifth child became more aphasic (his lesion was an astrocytoma, which progressed). The sixth child showed no change 5 years after a head injury.

Of the 13 cases that could only be followed for periods of 1½ to 3 months, 6 had apparently complete recovery. Considerable improvement was noted in the remaining 7, with writing difficulty being the major persisting language symptom. No apparent relation to etiology, age, or lesion localization could be discerned.

According to Woods and Carey (1979) any child over 1 year of age who received an aphasia-producing lesion in the left hemisphere would be likely to have permanently impaired performance on some verbal tests. One should be somewhat cautious, therefore, before concluding that complete recovery is to be expected in the childhood aphasias. Our own observations indicate that persistence of aphasic symptoms is linked to the size or bilaterality of the lesions. Current knowledge is insufficient to determine which factors are unequivocally favorable or unfavorable for recovery, a conclusion that was reached also by Satz and Bullard-Bates (1981).

Krashen (1973) and Hécaen (1976) provided evidence contradicting the model proposed by Lenneberg (1967) according to which the critical period for maturation of areas responsible for development of language extended to puberty. Krashen (1973) compared (1) the frequency of aphasia following right-side lesions in children younger and older than 5 years in several series of childhood aphasias with (2) the frequency of aphasia in adults with right-side lesions. They noted that the frequency of aphasia in the children 5 years and older was similar to that in adults. Even the limit of 5 years may be questioned, as is demonstrated in the reviews by Satz and Bullard-Bates (1981) and Carter, Hohenegger, and Satz (1982), which conclude that in right-handed children who have acquired language, the risk of aphasia exists virtually exclusively with left-side lesions. Such a conclusion, which rejects the notion of the equipotentiality of the two hemispheres for language during a critical period corresponding to maturation, is in accord with our current series. We found only one case of aphasia following a right-side lesion in a right-hander.

As for specific aspects of the language disorders among aphasic children, the current study generally confirms the results of earlier work. In aphasic children, we commonly find writing disorders and disturbances of oral expression, rarely find paraphasias and do not find logorrhea or jargonaphasia.

The important role played by intrahemispheric localization is clearly evident, because mutism and dysarthria are significantly more frequent following frontal–rolandic, as compared with temporal, lesions. There is a tendency for all aphasic symptoms in these children to be more common following anterior, as compared with posterior, lesions. One might speculate, on the basis of this evidence, that the anterior (frontal–rolandic) region of the left hemisphere is more engaged in diverse aspects of language in the child than in the adult, even though the specialization of this region is already fixed for verbal expression.

One could reasonably conclude, therefore, that studies of acquired aphasia in children support the notion of early cerebral lateralization and even of innate cerebral organization for the representation of language. Other evidence in favor of this position of "invariance" includes the characteristics of neuropsychological sequellae following neonatal unilateral hemispheric lesions, the verbal deficits and the recourse to novel cognitive strategies of subjects having received left hemispherectomies prior to language acquisition (Dennis, 1980; Dennis, Lovett, & Wiegel-Crump, 1981), the asymmetry of the *planum temporale* in the newborn and in the fetus (Wada, Clarke, & Hamm, 1975), and the electrophysiological demonstrations of perceptual asymmetries in the newborn (Molfese, 1977). We may thus consider the possibility that in the human species there exists a region of brain tissue specially evolved for the representation of language and present even before the appearance of language in the individual child.

Visual Functions following Early Visual-Cortex Damage

Visual functions following early damage of the visual cortex do not show a uniform degree of sparing or recovery. Complex perceptual activities such as recognition of mixed or hidden figures, spatial orientation in mazes, or route-finding tasks are impaired in children with early lesions, even when they are matched for mental age with normal controls (Rudel, Teuber, & Twitchell, 1974; Teuber & Rudel, 1962). When tested in adulthood, however, these patients may show impairments only in the most difficult spatial tasks. Kohn and Dennis (1974) have shown that in patients hemispherectomized for perinatal brain damage, either on the right or the left side, could reach near-maximum scores for complex pattern recognitions, although patients from the right-hemidecorticated group were more impaired than those from the left hemidecorticated group for spatial tasks, such as resolving a maze or orienting in a path drawn on a map.

Simpler visual functions such as detection of luminous flux or movement, spatial localization of objects, or simple pattern discrimination have not been studied systematically until the 1970s. Rudel *et al.* (1974) have found homonymous hemianopia in only 2 cases from a series of 63 children with early brain lesions who were tested for visual-field defects by the confrontation technique. Both cases corresponded to relatively late lesions (after the first year of life). This finding clearly raises the question of the relevance of the precocity of lesions to the recovery of visual-field defects. In fact even though occipital scotomata may remain unaltered for many years in certain patients, the age at time of injury can influence recovery at least during the initial stages. In a follow-up study of brain-wounded patients, Teuber (1975) observed that this holds true even within a restricted age range. Improvement in visual field (diminution in the number of affected quadrants) between the initial examination (up to 1 week after wounding) and the later ones several years after (up to 20 years) was better in patients who were wounded between 17 and 19 years of age (67%) than in those wounded between 20 and 25 years (43%) and those wounded after 26 years (14%). One could thus expect an even greater recovery following brain damage that occurred in infancy. But apart from studies like that of Rudel *et al.* (1974), concerning cases with more diffuse lesions the literature on this topic is quite limited. In fact, early brain lesions with a well-defined site are most often represented by congenital malformations such as large porencephalic cysts or cortical atrophies resulting from birth injuries, and for which an hemispherectomy is sometimes later performed. Evolution of visual capacities in such cases cannot be related to local reorganization due, for instance, to partial sparing of the striate cortex as can be the case in the previously mentioned studies. Instead we are faced here with the question of whether residual visual capacities could still be demonstrated within one hemifield when the whole occipital cortex or even all visual projections to the cortex have been excluded on one side in early life.

Anecdotal reports have been made on the visual capacities of this kind of patient. Marquis (1935) mentioned a case of an 11-year-old boy with a total absence of the left occipital lobe due to a porencephalic cyst (as observed during surgery) who had "only a slightly constricted defect of the right homonymous visual fields" (p. 813). In contrast, a total hemianopia has been found in most cases of hemispherectomy (e.g., Goodall, 1957; Laine & Gros, 1956; Obrador, 1964; Ueki, 1966; Wilson, 1970). The only exception is produced by Damasio, Lima, and Damasio (1975), who did not find a clear hemianopia in a patient hemidecorticated on the right side 13 years before examination: This subject could see moving or fixed targets in his left hemifield up to 20° from the fixation point. In fact, the possibility that some residual vision could remain within what appears to be a completely hemianopic field by perimetric standards has been raised by Williams and Gassel (1962). After dark adaptation their two hemispherectomized patients could detect bright targets and localize them by hand pointing. The authors, however, hypothesized that this effect could be related to the spread of light into the normal hemifield.

During the past 10 years the problem of residual vision in perimetrically blind fields has undergone important methodological improvement. The first results were obtained in adult patients with extensive, chronic lesions (such as occipital lobectomy or surgical interruption of the optic radiations). Provided they were forced to use a "guessing" mode of response irrespective of their perceptual awareness, they appeared to be able to localize targets within their scotoma either by orienting their gaze or by pointing at them with their hand (Perenin & Jeannerod, 1975; Poeppel, Held, & Frost, 1973; Weiskrantz, Warrington, Sanders, & Marshall, 1974).

In the late 1970s, we decided to reevaluate the visual capacities of patients who had undergone an hemispherectomy in early life by using this new method of testing (Perenin, 1978; Perenin & Jeannerod, 1978). The main purposes of this work were (1) to determine how visual functions are reorganized in such patients, (2) to compare this reorganization with that seen after lesions sustained in adulthood, and (3) to assess the functional role of the subcortical visual structures in extrastriate vision in man.

The 1978 study was carried out on a series of 6 subjects who had been operated on for intractable epilepsy with infantile hemiplegia as they were 6–9 years old in five cases and 17 years old in another case. The operation had been performed on the right side in four cases and on the left side in two cases. The elapsed time between operation and tests ranged from 3 to 13 years. Later we added to the hemidecorticated group two patients with porencephalic malformations that involved the whole left occipitoparietal region, as seen on CT scans. In both cases, hemianopia, their only neurological deficit, had been discovered following traffic accidents, at 16 and 18 years of age.

The 8 patients who are considered in the present study were tested in three different tasks; perimetry, spatial localization, and pattern discrimination. In the perimetry task the patients gave a response according to what they "saw," whereas in the two other tasks they made forced-choice responses irrespective of the subjective experience of presence or absence of a detectable visual target.

PERIMETRY

The visual field was mapped by conventional perimetry. Patients pressed a buzzer as soon as they could see a visual target in either part of their visual field. Both dynamic and static perimetry were performed using the Tubingen perimeter. All patients showed a dense hemianopia, even when they were presented with the brightest and biggest spot (318 candela per square meter [cd/m^2], 116′-diameter) of the perimeter on a mesopic background (3.18 cd/m^2). Thus we could not replicate the findings reported by Marquis (1935) and Damasio *et al.* (1975) of a large sparing of the visual field. A 1–5° area centered on the macula was always spared, however. In 3 patients in whom this was tested we could demonstrate a true macular sparing, that is, sparing not due to parafoveal or unstable fixation. These patients, when looking at the Haidinger brushes—an entoptic phenomenon only transmitted through the macular receptors—could see the whole figure turning around its center, whereas subjects with bitemporal hemianopia saw only half of the figure (Perenin & Vadot, 1981).

SPATIAL LOCALIZATION

The patients were tested for their ability to point by hand to visual targets flashed for a brief period of time in different parts of their visual field. The visual target (an 8°-wide vertical grating or a 2–4° spot) was projected randomly on a large, white, hemicylindrical screen from 15 to 75° from the midline along the horizontal meridian. At the onset of each trial, the patients were required to fixate a central mark on the screen; central fixation was monitored by means of a TV camera. Target exposure could be as short as 100 msec, that is, less than the oculomotor reaction time. Immediately after each target presentation the patients pointed rapidly toward the target location. This was easily performed on the normal side, where they could see the target. On the hemianopic side they were totally unaware of target location and had to give a forced-choice response, that is, had to point where they guessed the target had appeared.

This localization task was extensively studied in all patients by changing either the size or the duration of the targets from session to session. Although accuracy was not as high in the hemianopic as in the normal field, a clear statistical relation between pointing and target positions could still be found in all patients and in most sessions. Responses similar to those seen on Figure 1(a) were generally observed in the hemianopic field: The correlation was close to 1 for targets located up to 45°. The correlation was less clear for targets beyond 45° even though in most cases pointing-position values still increased with target eccentricity. The high level of correlation obtained for the overall sample of trials for all targets (between 15 and 75°) was not due only to the contribution of responses at targets within 30° of the midline. In fact there was still a highly significant correspondence between responses and target positions when the

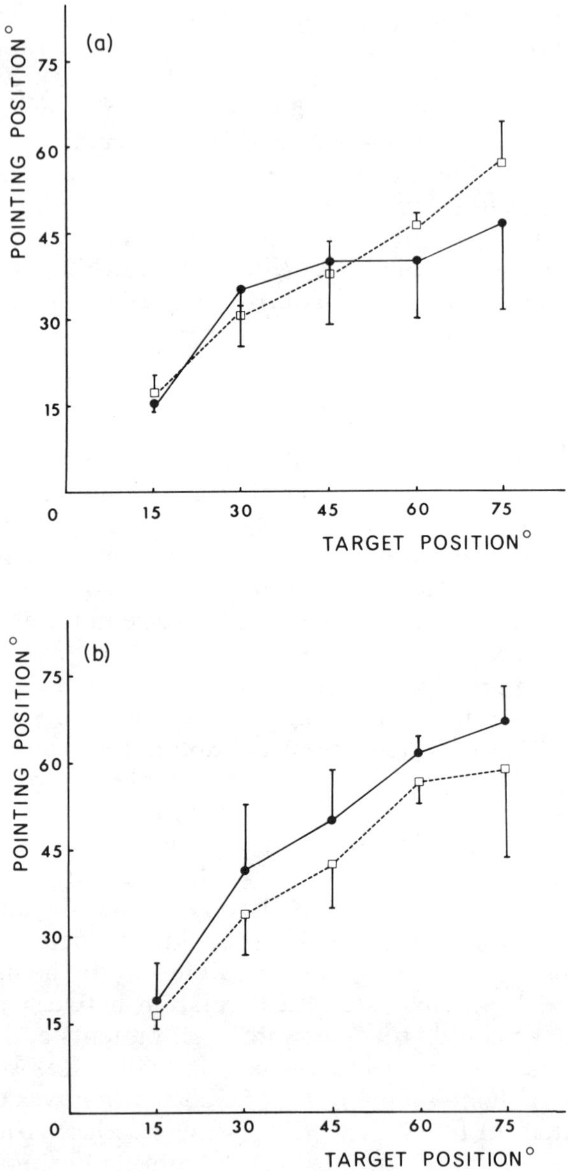

Figure 1. Hand-pointing responses in the hemianopic field of patients with (a) a left hemispherectomy and (b) a congenital porencephalic cyst of the left occipital lobe. The stimulus is an 8° grating, either stationary (dots) or moving (squares), with a 500 msec exposure time. Vertical bars represent one standard deviation.

data at and beyond 30° of eccentricity (or even 45°) were cumulated across all patients and all sessions. In 1 of the 2 patients with an occipital malformation, even better visual performances could be observed. In this patient, whose results appear in Figure 1(b), the correlation between pointing and target position remained within the whole extent of the hemianopic field. The greater sparing of visual function observed in this case could be related to the fact that part of the extrastriate visual cortex might be still functional.

For all 8 patients attempts were made to improve pointing accuracy either by increasing the duration (from 100 to 500 msec), or the size (from 2 to 8°) of the targets or by drifting the grating within the stimulated area. Each of these procedures was sometimes effective in reducing the scatter and the undershooting of the responses, but only in a few sessions and not in all patients.

PATTERN DISCRIMINATION

Pattern discrimination was investigated with pairs of large patterns (20°-wide triangles and circles) and pairs of horizontal and vertical lines, the stimuli of a given pair being equated for luminous flux or contour length. Each was flashed singly onto the hemianopic field. The patients were required to give a forced-choice response verbally or by showing on a card which one of two patterns had been presented.

In this kind of task, results were far less homogeneous than they were for target localization. In most cases scores were at chance level. However, when scores were cumulated across sessions, three patients performed above chance level (80, 72, and 52% correct responses). Their individual scores reached values as high as 87% correct responses for detection of line orientation and 82 and 97% for triangle versus circle discrimination, even though in the latter case the contrast was reversed: black patterns were flashed on a white background (Figure 2). Our findings suggest that differences in local luminous flux rather than in contour orientation are used for pattern discrimination in the hemianopic field: Nearly the same scores were observed with pairs of lines and pairs of dots.

INFLUENCE OF AGE AT THE TIME OF THE LESION

In both spatial localization and pattern discrimination tests, results differed from one patient to another. In fact, the three patients who were able to discriminate simple patterns within their hemi-

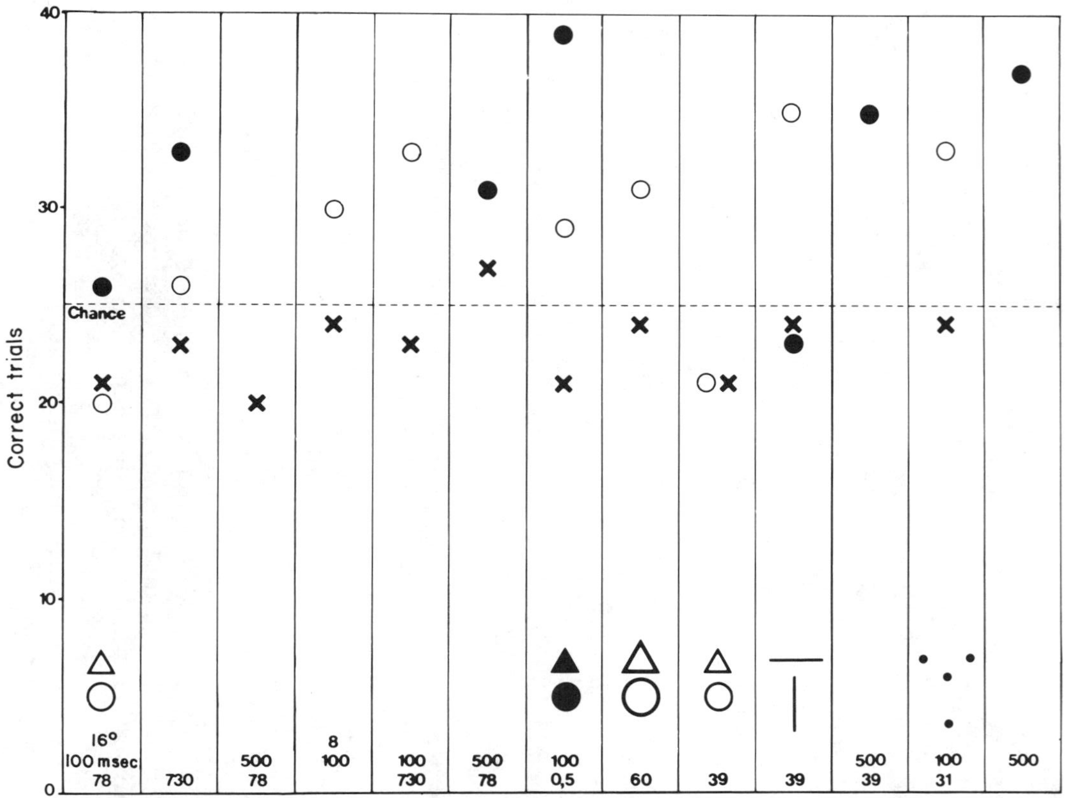

Figure 2. Pattern discrimination scores in the hemianopic field of two patients with hemispherectomy (open circles and exes) and one patient with occipital porencephalic cyst (darkened circles). Total percentage of correct responses (71.6, 52.2, and 80.0%, respectively) exceeds chance level in these three patients. In each vertical column, scores for each individual session have been represented, with stimulus characteristics (shape, eccentricity, exposure time, contrast) given at the bottom.

anopic field also performed best in pointing at targets. Neither the side of the lesion nor the time elapsed between lesion onset and tests could explain such discrepancies. The factor most likely to affect development of visual capacities in the hemianopic field is the age at the time of cortex injury. The best scores were indeed found in a subject with a congenital occipital cyst (although partial sparing of visual projections on the lesioned hemisphere might also have contributed to greater visual capacities in this subject). In three of the hemidecorticated patients the date of lesion, at least for the striate cortex, was found to coincide with the date of operation, since in these cases histological examination of the removed hemisphere showed a normal striate cortex. In two of these patients, who were operated on at the age of 7 years, a much greater amount of residual vision was observed than in the third patient, who was operated on at 17 years.

These results on early brain-damage patients tend to support the contention that those who have incurred early lesions have better residual vision than those with later injuries. One could expect an even-more-obvious age effect in comparisons of residual vision in cases of lesions sustained in early life with cases of lesions sustained in adulthood. Different amounts of residual vision have been reported in patients lesioned as adults. Performances observed by Weiskrantz *et al.* (1974), in their single case, seemed to be as good as (or even better than) the best of our early brain-damage patients. However, the cortical lesion in this patient was nearly restricted to area 17. In a previous study on six patients with larger occipital lesions sustained in adulthood, we found some abilities for locating bright flashes in the hemianopic field but no evidence for pattern discrimination (Perenin & Jeannerod, 1975).

A valid comparison of the effects of early and late brain damage should involve lesions of similar extent and also similar testing conditions. We recently pursued this ideal using exactly the same paradigm and apparatus as in our early brain-damage cases. We investigated six patients with occipital lesions that had occurred in adulthood. (These were as extensive as was available; hemidecortication is quite exceptional in adults.) These subjects had been operated on for angioma (four cases), hematoma (one case), or tumor (one case), which had necessitated resection of the occipital lobe, a large incision of the occipital cortex, or a ligature of the posterior cerebral artery. Following operation, all patients had a dense hemianopia with macular sparing. Our preliminary results on spatial localization in the hemianopic field show a significant correlation between pointing and

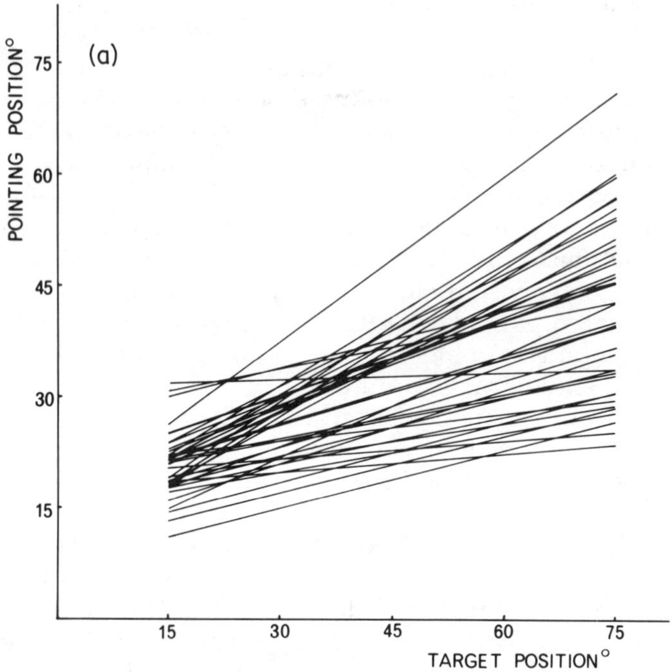
(a)
POINTING POSITION°
75
60
45
30
15
15
30
45
60
75
TARGET POSITION°

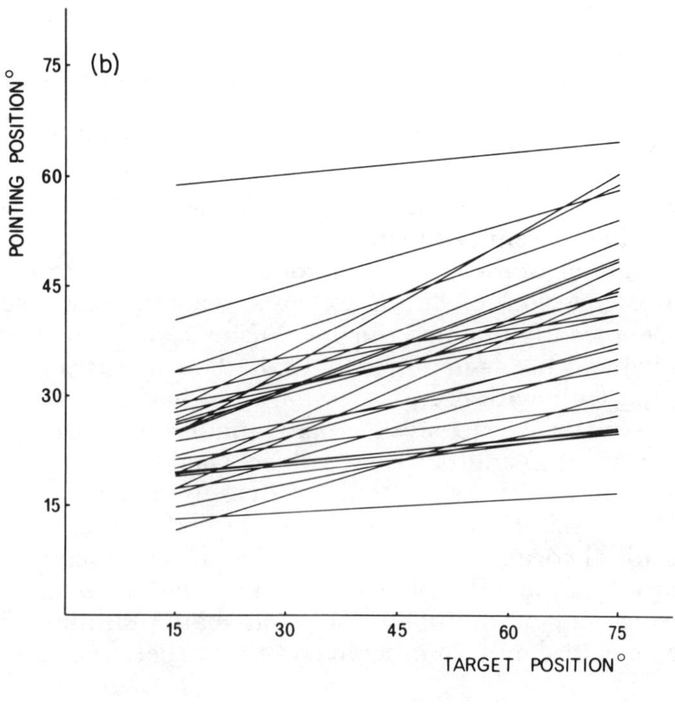
(b)
POINTING POSITION°
75
60
45
30
15
15
30
45
60
75
TARGET POSITION°

target position in 22 out of 28 sessions, which is less than in the early brain-damage group (35 out of 40). In addition, as illustrated by Figure 3, correlation was not as high in individual sessions. When comparing either the slopes of the regression lines or the values of *r* (Bravais–Pearson correlation coefficient), a significant difference ($p < .005$) was found between this group and the group of the early lesioned patients.

General Conclusion

A general conclusion can be drawn from these clinical observations that seems to apply to both recovery from language disorders and functional sparing of visual functions. In both cases the findings suggest the possibility of a lesser degree of localization of the anatomical substrate for functional representations in young children than in adult subjects.

Among patients suffering aphasia, a greater frequency of left-side lesions was found in children than in adults; this tendency was greater for the group of children under 10 years of age. It could be that in the earliest years of life the language areas in the left hemisphere are less limited than in adult brains. Consequently the probability of a left-side lesion producing aphasic symptoms would be higher in children. But this type of organization would also represent a great advantage for recovery, since such recovery would depend more on spared tissue adjacent to the lesion in the left hemisphere than on the tissue in a symmetrical area of the right hemisphere.

A remarkable sparing of visual functions can be observed in areas of the visual field that are no longer controlled by the cortex, provided the lesion has occurred neonatally or in early childhood. This finding implies that in early life, visual functions such as ability to locate objects or discriminate patterns are more widely distributed to subcortical structures than they are in adulthood. Anatomical structures such as the superior colliculus or the pretectal area could thus more easily become proficient in functions that, at a later stage, are effected almost exclusively by the visual cortex.

Figure 3. Regression lines obtained from all the sessions of hand pointing in the hemianopic field in (a) the group of patients lesioned early and (b) the group of patients lesioned in adulthood.

References

Alajouanine, T., & Lhermitte, F. (1965) Acquired aphasia in children. *Brain, 88,* 653–662.

Basser, L. S. (1962). Hemiplegia of early onset and the faculty of speech with special reference to the effects of hemispherectomy. *Brain, 85,* 427–460.

Branco-Lefèvre, A. F. (1950). Contribuicao para o estudo da psicopatología da afasia em cuancas. *Archivos de Neuropsichologia Sao Paulo, 8,* 345–393.

Carter, R. L., Hohenegger, M. K., & Satz, P. (1982). Aphasia and speech organization in children. *Science, 218,* 797–799.

Damasio, A., Lima, A., & Damasio, H. (1975). Nervous function after right hemispherectomy. *Neurology, 25,* 89–93.

Dennis, M. (1980). Capacity and strategy for syntactic comprehension after left or right hemidecortication. *Brain and Language, 10,* 287–317.

Dennis, M., Lovett, M., & Wiegel-Crump, C. A. (1981). Written language acquisition after left and right hemidecortication in infancy. *Brain and Language, 12,* 54–91.

Freud, S. (1897). Die infantile Cerebrallähmung. In *Specielle Pathologie und Therapie IV* Nothnagel. Wien: Holder.

Goldman, P. S. (1971). Functional development of the prefrontal cortex in early life and the problem of neuronal plasticity. *Experimental Neurology, 32,* 366–387.

Goldman, P. S., & Galkin, T. W. (1978). Prenatal removal of frontal association cortex in the fetal rhesus monkey: Anatomical and functional consequences in post-natal life. *Brain Research, 152,* 451–485.

Goldman, P. S., Rosvold, H. E., & Mishkin, M. (1970). Evidence for behavioral impairment following prefrontal lobectomy in the infant monkey. *Journal of Comparative and Physiological Psychology, 70,* 454–563.

Goodall, R. J. (1957). Cerebral hemispherectomy: Present status and clinical indications. *Neurology, 7,* 151–162.

Guttmann, E. (1942). Aphasia in children. *Brain, 65,* 205–219.

Harlow, H. F., Akert, K., & Schiltz, K. A. (1964). The effects of bilateral prefrontal lesions on learned behavior of neonate, infant and preadolescent monkeys. In J. M. Warren & K. Akert (Eds.), *The frontal granular cortex and behavior* (pp. 126–148). New York: McGraw-Hill.

Hécaen, H. (1976). Acquired aphasia in children and the ontogenesis of hemispheric functional specialization. *Brain and Language, 3,* 114–134.

Hécaen, H., De Agostini, M., & Monzon-Montes, A. (1981). Cerebral organization in left-handers. *Brain and Language, 12,* 261–284.

Jeannerod, M., & Hécaen, H. (1979). *Adaptation et restauration des fonctions nerveuses.* Lyon: Simep.

Kennard, M. A. (1936). Age and other factors in motor recovery from precentral lesions in monkeys. *American Journal of Physiology, 115,* 138–146.

Kennard, M. A. (1938). Reorganization of motor function in the cerebral cortex of monkeys deprived of motor and premotor areas in infancy. *Journal of Neurophysiology, 1,* 477–496.

Kohn, B., & Dennis, M. (1974). Selective impairments of visuo–spatial abilities in infantile hemiplegics after right cerebral hemidecortication. *Neuropsychologia, 12,* 505–512.

Krashen, S. (1973). Lateralization language learning and the critical period. Some new evidence. *Language Learning, 23,* 63–74.

Laine, E., & Gros, C. L. (1956). *L'hemispherectomie.* Paris: Masson.

Lawrence, D. G., & Hopkins, D. A. (1972). Development aspects of pyramidal control in the rhesus monkey. *Brain Research, 40,* 117–118.

Lenneberg, E. (1967). *Biological foundations of language.* New York: Wiley.

Marquis, D. G. (1935). Phylogenetic interpretation of the functions of the visual cortex. *Archives of Neurology and Psychiatry, 33,* 807–815.

Molfese, D. L. (1977). Infant cerebral asymmetry. In S. J. Segalowitz & F. A. Gruber (Eds.), *Language development and neurological theory* (pp. 21–35). New York: Academic Press.

Obrador, S. (1964). Nervous integration after hemispherectomy in man. In G. Schaltenbrand & C. N. Woolsey (Eds.), *Cerebral localization and organization.* Madison, WI: University of Wisconsin Press.

Passingham, R., Perry, H., & Wilkinson, F. (1978). Failure to develop a precision grip in monkeys with unilateral neocortical lesions made in infancy. *Brain Research, 145,* 410–414.

Perenin, M. T. (1978). Visual function within the hemianopic field following early cerebral hemidecortication in man. II. Pattern discrimination. *Neuropsychologia, 16,* 697–708.

Perenin, M. T., & Jeannerod, M. (1975). Residual vision in cortically blind hemifields. *Neuropsychologia, 13,* 1–7.

Perenin, M. T., & Jeannerod, M. (1978). Visual function within the hemianopic field following early cerebral hemidecortication in man. I Spatial localization. *Neuropsychologia* 16:1–13.

Perenin, M. T., & Vadot, E. (1981). Macular sparing investigated by means of Haidinger brushes. *British Journal of Ophthalmology, 65,* 429–435.

Poeppel, E., Held, R., & Frost, D. (1973). Residual visual function after brain wounds involving the central visual pathways in man. *Nature, 243,* 295–296.

Rudel, R. G., Teuber, H. L., & Twitchell, T. E. (1974). Levels of impairment of sensorimotor functions in children with early brain damage. *Neuropsychologia, 12,* 95–108.

Satz, P., & Bullard-Bates, C. (1981). Acquired aphasia in children. In M. T. Sarno (Ed.), *Acquired aphasia* (pp. 399–426). New York: Academic Press.

Teuber, H. L. (1975). Recovery of function after brain injury in man. In Ciba Foundation Symposium 34, *Outcome of severe damage to the central nervous system* (pp. 159–196). Amsterdam: Elsevier.

Teuber, H. L., & Rudel, R. G. (1962). Behavior after cerebral lesions in children and adults. *Developmental Medicine and Child Neurology, 4,* 3–20.

Ueki, K. (1966). Hemispherectomy in the human with special reference to the preservation of function. *Progress in Brain Research, 21,* 285–338.

Wada, J. A., Clarke, R., & Hamm, A. (1975). Cerebral hemispheric asymmetry in humans. Cortical speech zones in 100 adult and 100 infant brains. *Archives of Neurology, 32,* 239–246.

Weiskrantz, L., Warrington, E. K., Sanders, M. D., & Marshall, J. (1974). Visual capacity in the hemianopic field following a restricted occipital ablation. *Brain, 97,* 709–728.

Williams, D., & Gassel, M. M. (1962). Visual function in patients with homogeneous hemianopia. Part I: The visual fields. *Brain, 85,* 175–250.

Wilson, P. J. E. (1970). Cerebral hemispherectomy for infantile hemiplegia. *Brain, 93,* 147–180.

Woods, B. T., & Carey, S. (1979). Language deficits after apparent clinical recovery from childhood aphasia. *Annals of Neurology, 6,* 405–409.

Woods, B. T., & Teuber, H. L. (1978). Changing patterns of childhood aphasia. *Annals of Neurology, 3,* 273–280.

15

Early and Long-Term Recovery from Brain Damage in Children and Adults: Evolution of Concepts of Localization, Plasticity, and Recovery

Aaron Smith

Evolution of Current Concepts

Current concepts of recovery from brain insults in children and adults have evolved with accumulated findings in clinical studies of patients with diverse brain lesions supplemented by extrapolations from increasingly refined animal experiments. With the development of experimental techniques, there is a growing recognition (e.g., Finger, 1978; Laurence & Stein, 1978; Rosner, 1974); that the controversial findings and diverse hypotheses of the mechanisms of recovery reflect changing concepts of the localization, lateralization, and plasticity of cerebral functions. The concepts of plasticity and dominance of human hemispheric functions were first suggested by Dax in 1836.

Copyright © 1984 by Academic Press, Inc.
All rights of reproduction in any form reserved.
ISBN 0-12-052901-7

Dax noted that although sudden left hemisphere lesions resulted in aphasia, slowly developing lesions often did not (Finger, 1978). Broca initially localized speech in both frontal lobes (Broca, 1861), and it was not until 1865 that he specified only the third left frontal convolution as the seat of speech motor functions (Smith, 1966). Although he announced, "we speak with the left hemisphere," (Broca, 1865, p. 114) he also noted recovery of speech in adults and the development of normal speech in children with destruction of Broca's area, which he attributed to transfer of speech to the third right frontal convolution. Thus, Broca also indicated the plasticity of cerebral functions in children and adults.

The greater plasticity, sparing, and recovery of the young than of the old brain was clearly described in experimental studies of hemispherectomy by Vulpian.

> When one attempts an experiment of this sort in mammals, it is necessary whenever possible to make use of very young animals, for on the one hand, these support the operation well, and on the other, the functional relations between the different parts of the encephalon are not as yet narrowly circumscribed as they later become; to such effect that ablation from the brain has less influence on the action of other parts than in the adult animal. (Vulpian, 1866/1942, pp. 595).

In light of the sudden popularity of discrete localization of different functions, Kussmaul called attention to Vulpian's law of substitution—"The power of portions of the brain to act for other portions" (Kussmaul, 1877, p. 706). Consistent with Vulpian's earlier experimental studies, Bastian's findings in clinical studies strongly supported Vulpian's law of substitution and especially Vulpian's emphasis of age and the greater plasticity and recovery of language functions following earlier rather than later brain insults. Bastian concluded that "this plasticity is greatest in children though it continues to a diminished extent well on into adult life and is present still for varying periods even long beyond middle age" (Bastian, 1898, p. 342).

In a review of experimental studies of developmental plasticity, Goldman (1974) called attention to the marked morphological as well as functional differences between the immature and the adult brain. She also concluded that the full range of mechanisms underlying plasticity of cerebral functions had probably not yet been catalogued. Consistent with this, Wolf, Stricker, and Zigmond (1978) noted and described advances in biochemical and neuropharmacological techniques in elucidating the anatomy and functions of the central nervous system (CNS), as well as the processes in recovery from brain insult. However, other authors have rejected reports of recovery and have described the concept of greater plasticity and recovery from brain damage in children than in adults as a myth (see Smith, 1983).

Comparisons of lesion experiments with different species and clinical studies are obviously qualified by marked interspecies neuroanatomical and functional differences, as well as differences in the momentum (Finger, 1978) and the nature of clean and precisely designed, circumscribed surgical ablations in an intact animal brain versus the various types of slowly or rapidly evolving, naturally occurring amorphous lesions in humans. However, the interplay of experimental and clinical approaches in brain lesion research has been beautifully illustrated by Benton (1978). Although noting weaknesses and advantages of experimental and clinical approaches, Benton also illustrated their complementarity and integration in the cortical localization of visual functions in animals and humans.

Animal studies have contributed to the development of neurosurgery as well as to refinements of clinical diagnostic techniques. Experimental studies of hemispherectomy and commissurotomy for investigation of hemispheric functions provided developmental models that were later applied clinically in treatment of children and adults with malignant tumors or intractable seizures. Such conditions, in turn, provided unique opportunities to study the roles of each of the two human hemispheres in higher (cognitive) and lower (sensory and motor) cerebral functions. Similarly, experimental frontal lobe ablations prompted efforts to relieve chronic psychoses by psychosurgery, providing similarly unique opportunities to study the effects of carefully designed clean bilateral frontal lobe ablations in humans.

Emerging Sources of Ambiguity in Lesion Experiments

Despite these and other remarkable technical advances in experimental and clinical studies, the unresolved historical controversies and continual seemingly paradoxical and contradictory conclusions indicate that in both fields of study the findings are confounded by undefined sources of ambiguity. Reviewing the logic of the lesion experiment, Glassman (1978) called attention to various tacit or explicit assumptions in experimental and clinical studies. He also raised questions about the validity of inferences and interpretations of diverse findings cited as evidence of the localization of specific functions or of definitive brain structure–function relationships. For example, he described "the principle of double dissociation" as "an elegant answer to the 'where' question, which can distract us from the 'what'" (Glassman, 1978, p. 16). He indicated the principle of double dissociation was based on observations in animal experiments in which comparisons of effects of differently located ablations were reported to yield different behavioral deficits, either quantitatively or qualitatively. Thus if ablation of a circumscribed area (a) resulted in marked deficits in a specific function that was either absent or much lesser in degree following comparable ablation of another cortical area (b), the ablated area (a) producing the specific deficit was considered to play a special role in the specific function that was impaired.

The sudden proliferation of experimental studies focusing on recovery of functions (e.g., Eidelberg & Stein, 1974; Finger, 1978; Finger & Stein, 1982; Stein, Rosen, & Butters, 1974) represents more than concentration on efforts to elucidate the various anatomical and neurophysiological bases underlying the restitution of specific functions following carefully designed destruction of specific cortical areas. As Rosner (1974), Finger (1978), Laurence and Stein (1978), and others have noted, the sparing and partial or complete recovery of functions in such studies cannot be readily reconciled with traditional concepts of exclusive localization of discrete functions in the specific cortical areas destroyed. Thus, the findings in experimental and clinical studies of sparing and of recovery of functions following experimental or naturally occurring lesions in the young and the old brain have implications that extend far beyond the processes involved in recovery. A moment's consideration will show that such studies are essentially efforts to define the principles underlying not only the reorganization and recovery, but also the organization and development and the disorganization of brain functions following lesions incurred at different stages of cerebral maturation.

As noted above, the so-called principles of double dissociation were described by Glassman as an elegant answer to the *where* if not the *what* of localization of specific cerebral functions. In addition to the *where* and *what,* however, the *when* or, as described in the following, the condition of the residual brain as a whole at the time of observation, is one of the most important factors determining initial and later effects of experimental as well as naturally occurring lesions on its functions. Until more recent interest in the processes of recovery, studies of effects of specific lesions in animals were usually limited to 1 or 2 years.

Actually, however, the principle of double dissociation is really not a principle at all but an assumption. However seemingly logical, its validity is questionable, and conclusions about localization of specific functions based on such an assumption may often be unwarranted and misleading. For example, recovery of normal renal functional levels after removal of an entire kidney or recovery of hepatic functions after destruction of portions of the liver obviously cannot be interpreted as evidence that the removed kidney or destroyed portions of the liver had not previously participated significantly in renal or hepatic function. Unlike those cells in the liver and in the paired human organs, destroyed brain cells do not regenerate. However, the traditional and continuing focus in many lesion experiments on the specific areas destroyed in efforts to localize or study recovery of variously defined functions often does not take into account the immediate and later consequences of the lesion or the primary and secondary anatomical effects (Finger & Stein, 1982), including the later consequences on the already altered neuroanatomical economy and on the rapid or slow reorganization of cerebral mechanisms for partial or complete recovery of functions.

After a lifetime of experimental studies, Sherrington, the foremost physiologist of the twentieth century, noted the encephalization and specialization of functions unique to the human brain as the peak in the hierarchy of vertebrate forms. Yet, reinforcing Lashley's (1937, p. 386), similar criticism of claims of discrete localization (as quoted by Sherrington here), Sherrington concluded,

> Facts rebut the over-simplified conception such as ascribe to separate small pieces of the roof-brain, wedged together like a jig-saw puzzle, separate items of highly integrated behavior. A special place for comprehension of names, a special place for arithmetical calculation, a special place for musical appreciation, and so on . . . To suppose the roof-brain consists of point-to-point "centres" identified each with a particular item of intelligent concrete behavior is a scheme "over-simplified and to be abandoned." Rather . . . the contribution which the roof-brain in collaboration with the rest of the brain and spinal cord, makes toward integrated behavior will, when they are ultimately analyzed, resolve into components for which we at present have no names, having no conception of such processes . . . In localized disease or injury we . . . "must expect to find fractionings of behavior which cannot be expressed or understood in the current psychologic terminology." (Sherrington, 1941, p. 228)

As noted, the concepts of plasticity and recovery of functions were introduced to explain exceptional cases in which destruction of a specific brain area in which a discrete function was exclusively localized did not result in loss of the function. Thus, Lashley's initial concepts of equipotentiality and mass action were incompatible with the concepts of plasticity and recovery of brain function. After modifying his views to admit the possibility of regional localization and regional equipotentiality, Lashley abandoned his concept completely (Smith, 1962). Contemplating the continuing diverse findings in experimental and clinical studies of cerebral function in learning, Lashley observed,

> Direct control of all anatomic and behavioral variables is impossible, either in experimental studies or analyses of clinical material. The effects of interrupting transcortical associative connections can be estimated only by a study of a series of cases large enough to permit the partialling out of different factors contributing to deterioration through comparisons of the effects produced by various combinations and amounts of injury to different systems. (Lashley, 1944, p. 260)

More immediately relevant to clinical as well as to experimental studies of recovery and plasticity of cerebral functions following lesions was the comparative review of the myelogenetic cycles of regional maturations of the brain by Yakovlev and Lecours (1967). They reported that, contrary to prevailing views, myelination does not terminate after the first year of life and that the pattern of myelination of different cerebral regions varies from species to species.

> The myelination is an orderly process in which functionally allied systems of fibres are synchronized in an orderly sequence and in tempo of their myelination. The cycle of myelination of a fibre-system or region is an important parameter of regional maturation of the nervous system. The cycle reflects the position of a system or region in the hierarchy of functional organization of the brain as the organ of integration of motility experience. (Yakovlev & Lecours, 1967, p. 64)

In view of the different species used in experimental studies of recovery, their added observations have even greater heuristic implications for the design of future studies and afford bases for reconciling some of the seemingly paradoxical findings reported in experiments with different species.

> Myelination cycles of different fibre systems are highly species specific. Those systems with special functional importance to a given species appear earlier, but have longer cycles of myelination than those systems with more universal and less specific functions which differentiate later, but have shorter cycles of maturation (Yakovlev & Lecours, 1967, p. 67).

Although he attempted generalizations to human brain functions before abandoning his theories, Lashley preferred the clean, circumscribed ablations of experimental studies rather than investigations of clinical populations with diverse types of rapidly and slowly growing lesions in children and adults. Jackson (1915) once described neurological disease as an experiment on the brain performed by nature. However, as noted, in contrast to the lesion experiment, the occult processes underlying the onset, development, and specific boundaries of the various diseases and injuries of the human brain as well as of their dynamics, the changes in initial and later effects (which Jackson repeatedly emphasized) on adjacent cerebral structures and the brain as a whole, are reflected in continuing unresolved historical controversies on the localization, plasticity, and especially the complex processes underlying recovery of human functions. Thus Jackson also observed, "The tendency to appear exact by disregarding the complexity of factors is an old failing in our medical history" (Jackson, 1915, p. 112).

Some of the overlooked anatomical considerations in lesion experiments described by Woolsey (1978) suggest that Jackson's observation also applies to the seemingly more precise and "scientific" studies of the effects of clean, circumscribed ablations in animals. "With few exceptions, it is anatomically impossible to interfere with one functional group of neurons without inadvertently damaging portions of others" (p. 72). Although it was often overlooked, Woolsey also emphasized the critical importance of associated pathophysiological reactions including cerebrovascular and cerebrospinal fluid (CSF) circulation and other initial and later sequelae that affected cerebral structures variously remote from the lesion and the brain as a whole. "The lesson for the behaviorist is that a single lesion may have rather distant effects which should be considered in attempting to explain experimental results" (p. 79). And because of delayed neuroanatomical sequelae, these distance effects are clearly temporal as well as spatial.

Time and Other Interacting Factors

Riese observed, "One of the main reasons why the interpretation of brain lesions has been a mechanic rather than a dynamic one, has been the total neglect of one of the basic constituents of disease and the effects of injury, namely time" (Riese, 1960, p. 295).

The importance of time was dramatically illustrated in my first studies of initial and long-term effects of carefully designed bilateral frontal ablations in adult schizophrenics beginning in 1955. In contrast to the pattern of early recovery and later deterioration described later in this chapter, subsequent follow-up studies of children and adults with diverse lesions revealed different patterns in the rate and extent of deterioration or recovery.

These studies included populations with focal and diffuse traumatic brain injuries, malignant and benign neoplastic, toxic, anoxic, degenerative, vascular, and other types of cerebral lesions; hemispherectomy for tumor in adults and for infantile epileptogenic lesions; commissurotomy for intractable seizures in children and adults; and development of language, mental, motor and sensory functions in 279 hydrocephalics from 5 to 25 years of age with mild (normal CAT scans) to severe (CAT scans showing ventricular expansion occupying over 95% of the cranial cavity) hydrocephalus (Berker, Lorber, & Smith, 1983; Burklund & Smith, 1977; Campbell, Bogen, & Smith, 1981; Russell & Smith, 1961; Smith, 1966, 1971, 1972a, 1972b, 1975, 1978, 1979, 1981a, 1981b, 1983; Smith & Burklund, 1966; Smith & Sugar, 1975).

Economy precludes detailed considerations of the findings in individual studies. However, the consistency of certain findings supporting previously described principles of organization, disorganization, and reorganization of human cerebral functions has heuristic implications that may be further investigated in experimental as well as clinical studies.

Basing his observations on findings in clinical and experimental studies, Jackson (1874/1958a) noted underlying principles in the *evolution* (development from the general to the specific) of lower and higher level cerebral functions and of their *dissolution* (degeneration from the specific to the general). Citing consonant findings in animal experiments and his observations of neurological patients, Jackson's principles of *compensation* reflected his view that although various functions are specifically represented in particular areas of the brain, they are also variously re-represented in neighboring and distant structures (see *Selected Writings of John Hughlings Jackson,* Taylor, 1958, especially Vol. 1).

Consistent with Vulpian's, Jackson's, and Bastian's findings, von Monakow called attention to the reserve or overcapacity of brain structures that permitted early or later gradual compensation or recovery of functions by intact structures following brain insults. In documenting initial and later neuropathological and functional sequelae, he differentiated between early, frequently transient changes such as diaschisis and other temporary symptoms and later sequelae such as secondary degeneration and other residual symptoms. Thus, he too emphasized the critical importance of time and the condition of the entire brain in terms of the neuroanatomy underlying the development, recovery, or deterioration of the cerebral mechanisms.

Mechanisms of Recovery Indicated after Hemispherectomy and Commissurotomy

The subsequent development and partial or complete recovery of normal functions in children and adults with focal lateralized lesions may reflect the role of compensatory mechanisms in the damaged hemisphere (intrahemispheric compensation), of similar mechanisms in the undamaged, opposite hemisphere (interhemispheric compensation), or of both. The development of hemispherectomy for tumor in adults and for early epileptogenic lesions in infantile hemiplegics (Smith & Sugar, 1975) thus provided evidence of the interhemispheric compensatory capacities of children and adults following removal of a hemisphere damaged in early life as compared to excisions of one hemisphere in a brain that had matured normally until growth of a tumor in adulthood.

Neuropsychological studies of initial and long-term effects of right or left hemispherectomy for tumor in adults and for early epileptogenic lesions in infantile hemiplegics have provided the most dramatic confirmation of the suggestions of greater plasticity of the infant than the adult brain that were proposed in Vulpian's animal experiments and in the clinical studies by Bastian. Hemispherectory for tumor in adults has revealed a consistent pattern of reciprocal syndromes in all reported cases (Burklund, 1972; Burklund & Smith, 1977; Smith, 1966, 1969, 1972a, 1972b; Smith & Burklund, 1966). Right hemispherectomy results in a characteristic, enduring pattern of relatively intact language, verbal reasoning, and auditory memory, associated with severe, persisting impairment of nonverbal visual, ideational, spatial–constructional, and visual memory functions—with no evidence of recovery of nonverbal functions in cases tested 15 and 30 years postoperatively.

No cases of long-term survival have been reported after left hemispherectomy for tumor in adults. Early postoperative studies revealed very severe impairment of speech, reading, writing, and memory, less severe impairment of verbal comprehension, and relatively intact nonverbal visual, ideational, and spatial–constructional functions. However, in contrast to the severe, persisting nonlinguistic deficits in studies 15 and 30 years after right hemispherectomy, repeated studies during the 1st and 2nd year postoperatively of the 2 patients with longest survival after left hemispherectomy revealed gradual, continuous improvement of language functions until recurrence of the tumor resulted in deterioration and death (Burklund & Smith, 1977).

In contrast to the pattern of drastic selective impairment and sparing of either linguistic and verbal or nonverbal, visual, and ideational functions in adults with either right or left hemispherectomy for tumor, studies of initial and long-term effects of 36 infantile hemiplegics with left hemispherectomy and 28 with right hemispherectomy revealed no evidence of consistent or significant differences between hemispheres (Smith, 1972a, 1972b, 1981b, 1983a). Although the overall findings revealed that earlier damage to the *remaining* hemisphere limited subsequent developmental potentials in most of the patients, the remarkable capacities of the intact residual structures were demonstrated in long-term follow-up studies in two cases. At a 25-year follow-up; each had obtained a college degree and had enjoyed a successful career as an executive, following a right hemispherectomy in one case and left hemispherectomy in the other (Smith, 1983a). Thus, as Smith (1972a, 1972b) noted, the findings demonstrate that at birth each of the two cerebral hemispheres contains the neuroanatomical substrate necessary for the development of normal or even superior adult language and verbal and nonverbal cognitive functions.

The safety reserve factor apparently diminishes with increasing organization of cerebral structures and specialization of functions involving varying combinations of left and right hemisphere structures. However, in addition to studies of hemispherectomy, long-term studies of patients with commissurotomy for epilepsy resulting from early or later incurred lesions and other types of brain insult provide further evidence of inter- and intrahemispheric compensatory mechanisms. Administration of the same Michigan Neuropsychological Battery (Smith, 1975, 1981a, 1983b) in studies of a Los Angeles series of commissurotomy patients as that administered to hemispherectomy and other populations provided additional evidence of the critical role of the forebrain commissures in the reorganization of interhemispheric compensatory mechanisms following lateralized extracallosal lesions *before* commissurotomy.

As noted, following right or left hemispherectomy for early epileptogenic lesions, the remaining hemisphere and other intact residual structures can provide for the development of normal adult language, verbal and nonverbal reasoning, and memory. Continuous improvement of language functions until recurrence of the tumor in adults with left hemispherectomy indicates that although diminished, the plasticity of cerebral functions continues into the later decades of life.

Consistent with this, all reported intracarotid amobarbital studies have indicated the compensatory role of the right hemisphere in recovery of language functions following aphasiogenic left hemisphere lesions in older adults (Smith, 1981a). Goldstein (1948), Russell and Espir (1961), and Russell (1963) have suggested that the partial or complete recovery of language functions in such cases is accomplished by a reorganization of interhemispheric compensatory mechanisms in which the remaining viable structures in the damaged left hemisphere are linked to intact structures in the right hemisphere via the forebrain commissures.

Neuropsychological studies of 10 patients with complete and 2 with frontal commissurotomy (Campbell *et al.*, 1981) reported differences in the nature and severity of preoperative, initial, and long-term postoperative deficits in verbal and nonverbal cognitive, memory, and sensory–motor functions. Neurosurgical studies before and after commissurotomy revealed various types of extracallosal damage in all 12 patients, including 4 with gross structural lesions in the right hemisphere before surgery. Analyses of the data revealed that differences in the nature and severity of postoperative deficits varied according to the nature and laterality of associated extracallosal damage before as well as after operation. Following complete commissurotomy, in contrast to negligible changes in neuropsychological test performances by the remaining 6 patients with complete commissurotomy, all 4 patients with preoperative structural lesions in the right hemisphere revealed the unique pattern of marked selective impairment of nonverbal cognitive functions characteristic of adults with right hemispherectomy for tumor. The emergence of this pattern among the 10 patients in only the 4 patients who had right hemisphere structural lesions before complete commissurotomy indicates that the forebrain commissures had played a critical role in the reorganization of interhemispheric mechanisms.

The emergence of the profound selective impairments in nonverbal cognitive functions in all 4 patients (and in 1 of these, the emergence of a left-side somatosensory deficit that had not been present preoperatively) after complete commissurotomy indicates that sectioning of the forebrain commissures sundered the interhemispheric compensatory mechanisms that had been reorganized for restitution of these functions following right hemisphere structural lesions. In 2 of the 4 patients, the damage to the right hemisphere was incurred in adulthood. Since these 2 showed the same pattern of profound selective impairment of nonverbal cognitive functions as the remaining 2 with early right hemisphere damage after complete commissurotomy, the findings are consistent with those in follow-up studies of brain-wounded veterans that indicate recovery of nonverbal cognitive functions after right hemisphere missile wounds (Smith, 1981a).

The findings in other studies of patients with commissurotomy have been cited in support of remarkable generalizations on diverse functions of the two adult cerebral hemispheres, as is illustrated in controversies by Gazzaniga (1983a, 1983b), Levy (1983), and Zaidel (1983). For example, the right hemisphere has been described as "the mute, minor hemisphere . . . a passive, silent passenger who leaves the driving mainly to the left hemisphere" (Sperry, 1975 p. 11) and as "vastly inferior to the cognitive skills of a chimpanzee" (Gazzaniga, 1983a, p. 536); on the other hand "our sense of subjective awareness arises out of our dominant left hemisphere's relentless need to explain actions" (Gazzaniga, 1983a, p. 536) Perhaps even more remarkable is the suggestion of anthropomorphic criteria in comparisons of the two great cerebral hemispheres by Eccles. "I use the word person for a subject who is responsible for his actions, and the left hemisphere is a human person . . . whereas the right hemisphere is not" (Eccles, 1982, p. 164). Interestingly, the findings in studies of right and left hemispherectomy for early epileptogenic lesions fail to support these claims. Although this may reflect the greater plasticity of the younger than the older brain, the studies of adults with right or left hemispherectomy for tumor cited earlier also provide no support for these generalizations of the findings in studies of commissurotomy. In any case, the major findings in the follow-up studies of recovery of commissurotomy patients by Campbell *et al.* (1981) demonstrate that the forebrain commissures play a critical role in the reorganization of interhemispheric compensatory mechanisms following lateralized lesions in early and later life.

The remarkable plasticity of the infant brain has also been illustrated in long-term studies of overall cerebral development in 600 children with congenital hydrocephalus (Lorber 1965, 1977, 1980). Lorber reported the development of normal and even superior intelligence in 50% of those with even the most severe hydrocephalus (CAT scans showing ventricular expansion occupying 95% of the cranium). He also noted that one of this patients "gained a first-class honours (Sheffield University) degree in mathematics and is socially completely normal. And yet the boy has virtually no brain" (quoted by Lewin, 1980, p. 1232).

Consistent with the findings in numerous clinical and experimental studies reviewed by Finger and Stein (1982), our studies of 279 of these patients (Berker, Lorber, & Smith, 1983) and 125 normal children have also demonstrated that experiential, environmental, or extracranial factors may also play a significant role following early brain insults. Analyses of neuropsychological test performances of the 279 hydrocephalics and 125 controls revealed that, regardless of the severity of hydrocephalus (ventricular dilation indicated in CAT scans), cognitive development of hydrocephalics (as well as of normals) systematically increased with education and socioeconomic status of the parents.

As noted, clinical studies since the nineteenth century have abundantly documented partial or complete recovery from functional deficits resulting from brain insults in adults as well as children. However, as von Monakow (1914) emphasized, the initial and later effects and ultimate consequences of any cerebral lesion depend on the condition of the brain as a whole before as well as after any insult is incurred. Delayed consequences may not emerge for many years. One of the most common examples is the late development of neurological signs and progressive dementia in boxers—the punchdrunk syndrome. Neuropathological studies (Corsellis, 1976; Strich, 1978) have documented structural changes after the earlier accumulation of cerebral trauma in boxers who developed various symptoms long after retirement.

Early Recovery and Later Degeneration

The critical importance of time and consequently of long-term follow-up studies of the effects of brain insults is strikingly illustrated in studies of the effects of psychosurgery for relief of psychoses. Economy and focus preclude review of the history of lobotomy and subsequent psychosurgical procedures. However, we may note that, reflecting the interplay of experimental and clinical approaches, the study of bilateral frontal ablations in two chimpanzees by Jacobsen, Wolfe, and Jackson (1935) was prompted by Brickner's (1932) report of behavioral sequelae of bilateral frontal lobectomy in man. In turn, the report by Jacobson *et al.* of amelioration of experimental neurosis immediately after bilateral frontal ablations prompted the development of lobotomy by Moniz (1936). Who would dream that Jacobsen's studies of the two hapless chimpanzees, Becky and Lucy, would soon lead to psychosurgical ablations in over 50,000 patients?

With dissipation of the early enthusiasm and with the development of tranquilizers, the use of psychosurgery declined. Because of the apparently diverse and contradictory findings reported in clinical studies of the effects of lobotomy and other psychosurgical frontal ablations, and despite the continuing interest in experimental animal studies of the effects of various frontal lesions, the studies of effects of psychosurgical lesions have largely been ignored. However, three related projects marked a major advance in controlled clinical studies of frontal psychosurgical ablations—Lewis, Landis, and King (1956) and Mettler (1949, 1952). Increasingly refined research designs, including the introduction of a standardized surgical procedure with excisions of defined, smaller or larger portions of different frontal cortical areas; the use of equated controls, including simulated "mock" surgery; strict criteria in the selection of older and younger patients to evaluate possible differences of psychosurgical lesions as a function of age; and the use of standardized and objective mental tests at fixed preoperative and postoperative intervals, were also major advances in human brain research. But because the overall results for all such surgeries failed to reveal significant clinical benefits of the diverse surgical procedures, the operations were discontinued. However, the design of these three related studies most closely approximated or even exceeded the scientific criteria of most animal studies. The accumulated data in preoperative, initial, and later postoperative tests thus afforded unique data on initial and later effects on mental functions of clean, circumscribed bilateral ablations of varying amounts from different areas in the frontal lobes.

Comparisons of ablated and control groups revealed initial postoperative declines by all ablated groups followed by recovery after 1 year of preoperative levels that approximate those of the controls. Thus the drop-and-rise patterns were cited as evidence that regardless of patient age or site or amount of damage, bilateral excisions of homologous areas in both frontal lobes did not impair intellectual capacities. The drop-and-rise pattern was interpreted as evidence for recovery from what were considered to be temporary or transient early postoperative deficits.

Follow-up studies from 8 to 12 years postoperatively of 59 ablated and 35 control subjects from the three projects, however, revealed the emergence of significant intellectual deterioration—exceeding that of the early postoperative stages—among some of the ablated groups. The long-term deficits occurred in both younger and older patients with standardized posterior frontal ablations; they occurred in those with larger rather than smaller excisions, regardless of age and site.

By contrast, younger adults with standardized frontal (orbital) ablations showed no significant deterioration when compared to controls and to preoperative or 1-year postoperative levels (Smith, 1960, 1962, 1964; Smith & Kinder, 1959). Reexaminations 14 years postoperatively of patients with topectomy and controls from one of the three projects showed further mental deterioration by those with posterior frontal ablations, which suggested that the processes of progressive deterioration had been continuing (Hamlin, 1970).

Although often overlooked, these findings bear directly on the significance and interactions of the various factors that determine the consequences of focal cerebral damage. Differences in effects of standardized orbital and superior (approaching the convexity) ablations of homologous areas within the human frontal lobes between younger and older adults indicate that the age factor is a continuum. Differences in the initial and later postoperative sequelae as a function of site and quantity of tissue excised, as well as of time and of age, afford bases for reconciling many of the diverse findings reported in earlier studies. For example, the mental deterioration documented in long-term follow-up studies in patients with posterior or larger frontal ablations is strikingly consistent with the findings in neuropathological studies of lobotomized patients. In addition to the positive correlation between survival time and amount of secondary degeneration, Yakovlev (1953, 1954) reported marked and sometimes massive secondary degeneration following posterior cuts but little degeneration after anterior cuts of comparable size. Conversely, the recovery of preoperative mental capacities and the absence of later deterioration by younger adults with standardized, limited bilateral anterior (orbital) ablations is consistent with earlier reports of a critical mass beyond which bilateral lesions result in permanent intellectual deficits.

Studies of long-term effects of brain injuries have also documented the emergence of mental deterioration, memory and judgment disturbances, neuroses, psychoses, epilepsy, and other sequelae many years after cerebral trauma (Lishman, 1978). My own studies have shown that following recovery from closed head-injury, a relatively slight head injury that would result in only mild or transient symptoms in patients with no previous cerebral trauma may produce drastic, enduring deficits with far more limited recovery. This suggests that the compensatory capacities of the brain are limited; that the processes of recovery are accomplished by the recruitment of intact brain structures in the reorganization of compensatory mechanisms;

and that although functional recovery after severe trauma may be complete it is accomplished by expenditure of the reserve emergency capacities of the brain.

Long-Term Recovery or Development of Functions

In contrast to the emergence of deterioration of mental functions after bilateral frontal lesions demonstrated in the long term-follow-up studies just cited, continuing follow-up studies have demonstrated reciprocal processes of recovery or development of functions reflecting different temporal patterns in the reorganization of compensatory mechanisms in children and adults with focal lateralized and diffuse cerebral lesions. (Smith, 1981a). Conclusions based on single studies of children and adults reflect the tacit assumption that the functional deficits recorded at varying intervals after brain injuries are fixed, expecially in the later so-called chronic stages. Thus, the deficits recorded in children with pre-, peri-, or early postnatal brain insults and in adults with later incurred lesions are assumed to be permanent: Even though later follow-up studies may reflect continuing development with cerebral maturation, such development is assumed to stay at the same attenuated rate as indicated on initial observation. This assumption is predicated on the notion that the processes of reorganization in cases with chronic lesions have terminated at some unspecified time before examination. Follow-up studies may indeed show neither appreciable accelerated development at a catch-up rate in children nor significant recovery in adults. However, the varying rates and degrees of recovery documented in long-term follow-up studies next cited indicate that in most if not all such cases, the underlying brain insults not only destroyed specific neural structures that normally mediate the functions lost *but also compromised the structures necessary for reorganization of spontaneous compensatory mechanisms.*

As noted, the greater plasticity of the infant than the adult brain is illustrated in comparisons of effects of right or left hemispherectomy for infantile epileptogenic lesions and for tumor in adults, as well as in the development of normal and occasionally even superior intellectual capacities in adult hydrocephalics. Follow-up studies of hemispherectomy for infantile epileptogenic lesions and of children with subtotal agenesis of the right or left hemisphere have documented continuing intellectual development at an accelerated catch-up rate, with the gradual disappearance or diminution of long-persisting sensory or motor deficits (Smith, 1981a).

The persisting, severe selective deficits in language or nonverbal cognitive functions after left or right hemispherectomy for tumor in adults thus indicate the absence or limitations in the plasticity of these various functions that occur with cerebral maturation, or in Vulpian's terms, the establishment of more narrowly circumscribed functional relationships between different parts of the encephalon (within and between the two adult hemispheres). However, the importance of time and long-term follow-up studies is also dramatically illustrated in studies of adults after anterior left temporal lobectomy for epilepsy (Blakemore & Falconer, 1967). Serial postoperative tests showed persisting marked impairments and no appreciable improvement of difficulties in remembering or learning new spoken or written material, a cognitive deficit which did not occur after comparable right temporal lobectomy. Thus, the persisting deficits apparently support earlier, more limited postoperative studies reporting that the impairment was permanent.

Studies in the 4th or 5th postoperative years, however, revealed rapid improvement and recovery to normal preoperative levels, with diminution and disappearance of the patients' difficulties. We do not know whether children with comparable ablations would show more rapid recovery; that is, if the delay in recovery by adults might reflect the longer time necessary to reorganize the inter- or intrahemispheric compensatory mechanisms after the more narrowly circumscribed relationships of different parts of the encephalon for development of these functions had been established. However, it is important to note that in addition to the studies cited earlier indicating interhemispheric compensation of other language and nonlanguage functions after lateralized lesions in adults, this study also demonstrates that the processes of spontaneous reorganization and recovery and the plasticity of the brain continue into adulthood, as Bastian observed, and also that such processes may not become manifest for several years after persisting chronic defects.

Diaschisis

Reviewing the controversial findings in experimental and clinical studies of the effects of early and late brain lesions, Finger and Stein

(1982) called attention to the recondite diverse interactions in initial and later physiological and structural changes following experimentally designed as well as naturally occurring brain lesions. Their emphasis on the importance of diaschisis and other variously enduring early effects of brain lesions on recovery that had been previously described in earlier clinical studies illustrates a salutary and successful effort to integrate the diverse findings in experimental and clinical studies that characterize the literature as a whole.

Although economy precludes more detailed consideration, we may note that von Monakow, who introduced the term *diaschisis,* also emphasized that age was one of the most important factors determining the severity and duration of the "distance effects"—the suspension or reduction of functions of anatomically intact structures in both the damaged and undamaged hemispheres—resulting from lateralized lesions. As reported by von Monakow and Mourgue (1928), such effects increase with advancing age. Studies of the partial or complete recovery from aphasia in younger and older adults provide evidence not only of the role of the forebrain commissures and the right hemisphere in reorganization of compensatory intercerebral mechanisms, but also of the significance of diaschisis in the rate and extent of language recovery.

As noted by Finger and Stein, diaschisis is usually transient. However, in addition to increasing with advancing age, it may also be permanent. Studies of 255 young adult aphasics with brain missile wounds by Russell and Espir (1961) and Russell (1963) revealed remarkable recoveries in cases of even extensive lesions restricted to the left hemisphere. However, in cases with less extensive bilateral lesions or left hemisphere lesions involving the corpus callosum (and especially the splenium), such recoveries were rare. Thus the findings suggest that the failure to recover from aphasiogenic lesions in adults in many cases reflects the extent to which the brain damage produces specific functional deficits according to not only its specific site or extent but also the extent to which it has compromised the processes and potential reserve structures which in other cases would permit the establishment of compensatory cerebral mechanisms for recovery.

Von Monakow's observation that the inhibitory effects of diaschisis can be permanent suggests that the variable rates, limitations, or absence of recovery in cases with lateralized aphasiogenic lesions may reflect the persistence of diaschisis. Studies of 122 right-handed chronic aphasics (mean duration was 18 months) with reported vascular lesions restricted to the left hemisphere revealed *left-sided* sensory–motor defects in 70 (5.7%), indicating associated attenuation or inhibition of right hemisphere functions; 34 (49%) of these had constructional dyspraxia, also indicating right hemisphere dysfunction (Smith, 1974). Not surprisingly, objective tests revealed significantly greater persisting impairment in all language functions in the 70 (mean age was 53 years) when compared to the 52 (mean age was 44 years) without left-side sensory–motor deficits. Although the sample was restricted to cases with reported infarctions limited to the left hemisphere, how can we be sure that the signs of right hemisphere dysfunction were not simply reflections of associated, unsuspected right as well as left hemisphere lesions in older stroke patients with generalized arterial disease? We cannot. However, subsequent studies of over 300 similar cases, many with CAT scans indicating only left hemisphere lesions, have demonstrated the same patterns. Although language functions are unique to the human species, the significance of age as a factor determining the production, duration, and recovery of bilateral motor and sensory deficits can be investigated experimentally in infant, younger, and older adult animals with lateralized lesions.

Discharging Lesions: Epilepsy

In my studies of initial and long-term effects of hemispherectomy for infantile epileptogenic lesions and of other children and adults with diverse types of brain insult (Smith, 1981a), one of the significant factors limiting or even reversing the processes of recovery was the persistence or emergence of posttraumatic or postoperative epilepsy. The emergence of early and delayed seizures in children and adults with disease or injury of the brain as well as after neurosurgical intervention for nonepileptogenic resectable lesions has been abundantly reported. Incidence, onset, frequency, severity, and duration of seizures have been reported to vary according to specific site of the brain, age, and other factors. The pathogenesis of the damage to the brain resulting from seizures and superimposed upon the previously existing epileptogenic lesions has been reviewed by Corsellis and Meldrum (1976). The incidence of epilepsy following clean, frontal lobe surgical ablation is illustrated in Hamlin's (1970) report that over half of the patients with superior topectomy developed from 1 to over 50 postoperative seizures. Thus, prescription of anticonvulsants is common in efforts to prevent epilepsy as a side effect of neurosurgical resections of nonepileptogenic lesions. Baraitser (1982) reported that the threshold for seizure is lowest in early life and rises with cerebral maturation.

It is therefore intriguing to note the absence of reports of epilepsy in lesion experiments with animals and especially with infant animals. It is possible that as the brain of an organism ascends on the phyletic scale it is more vulnerable to seizure following ablation. Thus, seizures following cortical ablations in animals may not occur or become manifest before the animals are sacrificed, usually not long after postoperative observations have been made. In our experiences in follow-up studies of children and adults with hemispherectomy, commissurotomy, traumatic, vascular, and other focal or diffuse brain lesions, the presence of seizures has been consistently associated with more limited recovery and, in some cases, with progressive deterioration. Thus the diverse findings reported in clinical and experimental studies of recovery or development of cerebral functions following early or late brain lesions may reflect the pathophysiological effects of covert as well as overt electrophysiological abnormalities, which may emerge at various intervals after the lesion has been incurred.

Principles of Organization, Disorganization, and Reorganization

> In a lecture at the National Hospital, London, Riese once startled an audience by saying, "Facts are cheap" in developing his theme that principles alone must always direct the accumulation and assessment of facts; and that in the end those illuminating and inspiring syntheses and insights which the great figures in philosophy and science have derived from the unwieldy and often contradictory collections of facts can only be achieved by those few who are prepared to study their subject in its completeness, and not in its analytical fragments. (Gooddy, 1977, p. 10)

The rich interplay and complementarity of experimental and clinical approaches in efforts to elucidate principles underlying the development, disorganization, and reorganization of human brain functions following lesions at different stages of cerebral maturation is illustrated by Ferrier. After learning of the concepts and principles that Jackson based on his own extensive clinical pathological studies, Ferrier integrated his clinical and animal studies "to put to experimental proof the views entertained by Jackson" (quoted by Rioch, 1953, p. 123).

In addition to the principles of evolution, dissolution, and compensation of brain functions, Jackson's differentiation of discharging versus destroying lesions has conceivable implications and applications for lesion experiments as well as clinical studies. "That parts suffer more as they serve in voluntary and less as they serve in automatic operations is, I believe, the law of destroying lesions of the central nervous system" (Jackson, 1873/1958b, 1915, pp. 75–76); "the most voluntary or most special processes suffer first and most . . . in cerebral lesions" (Jackson, 1874/1958a, 1915, p. 87). Thus, according to Jackson, even though different functions are variously represented and re-represented in different parts of the brain in general, efferent (voluntary) functions are more vulnerable than afferent (automatic) functions to the effects of brain insults.

The bearing of my own studies on these and other principles have been reported elsewhere (Smith, 1975, 1981a, 1983a). These include documented long-term follow-up studies of children and adults with brain lesions that incurred either before or after the brain had matured normally (1981a). Repeated follow-up studies have also provided evidence confirming Head's principles of inconstancy. Comparisons of early and later neuropsychological test performances at different stages in the course of evolving and resolving lesions have consistently shown abnormal fluctuations in performance, reflecting marked changes in the efficiency of the specific cerebral mechanisms and functions involved. In repeated tests after brain insults, these fluctuations greatly exceed the quotidian variability of normals, the day-to-day or even hourly variations reflecting limited changes in the efficiency of different cerebral mechanisms. Such changes are more marked and frequent following brain insults and they generally increase in the later stages of evolving lesions and decrease in the later stages of resolving lesions. Repeated follow-up studies, however, also demonstrate that, barring the emergence of delayed posttraumatic complications, the processes of reorganization of compensatory mechanisms underlying the later development of functions in children and recovery in adults continue for many, many years.

Conclusions

It is clear that the results of any single study of the effects of lesions in experimental animals or of naturally occurring lesions in humans reflect the condition of the brain at a specific historical moment in the course of a complex dynamic process. Concurrent with the continuous processes of secondary degeneration and other variously progressive neuropathological changes, the early or later, partial or complete recovery in adults and development of functions in children reflects the versatility of the brain and its capacity for spontaneous reorganization in the recruitment of intact cerebral structures or the augmentation of the previously lesser role of undamaged portions of the brain for partial or complete restitution of function.

The systematic patterns of early sequential developmental milestones—the serially acquired abilities to sit up, stand, walk, understand speech, and then talk, at fixed stages in the early development of humans—clearly reflect principles underlying the organization, development, and integration of cerebral mechanisms with the gradual maturation of the human brain. The findings described in this chapter indicate that there are also principles underlying the disorganization of functions following insults to the brain at different stages in its cerebral maturation. These principles are both obscured by and reflected in the controversial findings in earlier clinical and experimental studies. Apart from secondary degeneration and other delayed complications following brain lesions, the potentials for subsequent development of recovery of functions following earlier or later incurred brain insults depend on the condition of the residual brain structures and the extent to which such insults may have compromised the access to and the integrity of residual, intact, specific structures in either or both hemispheres.

References

Baraitser, M. (1982). *The genetics of neurological disorders.* New York: Oxford.

Bastian, H. C. (1898). *A treatise on aphasia and other speech defects.* New York: Appleton.

Benton, A. L. (1978). The interplay of experimental and clinical approaches in brain lesion research. In S. Finger (Ed.), *Recovery from brain damage* (pp. 49–68). New York: Plenum.

Berker, E., Lorber, J., & Smith, A. (1983, February). Influences of extra-cerebral factors on cerebral development of 289 patients with varying degrees of hydrocephalus. *11th Annual Meeting, International Neuropsychological Society, Mexico City.*

Blakemore, C. B., & Falconer, M. A. (1967). Long term effects of anterior temporal lobectomy on certain cognitive functions. *Journal of Neurology, Neurosurgery & Psychiatry, 30,* 364–367.

Brickner, R. M. (1932). An interpretation of frontal lobe function based on the study of a case with partial bifrontal lobectomy. *Proceedings of the Association for Research of Nervous and Mental Disease, 13,* 259–352.

Broca, P. (1865). Sur la siège de la faculté du langage articulé. In H. Hécaen, & J. Dubois (Eds.), *La naissance de la neuropsychologie du langage* (1825–1865). Paris: Flammarion, 1969, p. 114. (Reprinted from *Bulletin Socièție de Anatomie Paris, 6,* 336–357.)

Burklund, C. W. (1972). Cerebral hemisphere function in man: Fact versus tradition. In W. L. Smith (Ed.), *Drugs, development and Cerebral function* (pp. 8–36). Springfield: IL: Thomas.

Burklund, C. W., & Smith, A. (1977). Language and the cerebral hemispheres: Observations of verbal and non-verbal responses during eighteen months following left ("dominant") hemispherectomy. *Neurology, 27,* 627–633.

Campbell, A. L., Jr., Bogen, J. E., & Smith, A. (1981). Disorganization and reorganization of cognitive and sensorimotor function in cerebral commissurotomy: Compensatory roles of the forebrain commissures and cerebral hemispheres in man. *Brain, 104,* 493–511.

Corsellis, J. A. N. (1976). Ageing and the dementias. In W. Blackwood & J. A. N. Corsellis (Eds.), *Greenfield's neuropathology.* Chicago, Year Book Publishers.

Corsellis, J. A. N., & Meldrum, B. S. (1976). Epilepsy. In W. Blackwood & J. A. N. Corsellis (Eds.), *Greenfield's neuropathology* (pp. 796–849). Chicago: Year Book Publishers.

Dax, M. (1865). Lésions de la moitié gauche de l'encéphale coincidait avec l'oubli des signes de la pensée - Lu au Congrès méridional tenu à Montpellier en 1836, par le docteur Mark Dax. *Gazette Hebdomadaire de Medicine et de Chirurgie, 35,* 259–262.

Eccles, J. (1982). Quoted (p. 164) in Gilling, D. & Brightwell, R. *The Human Brain.* New York: Facts on File Publications.

Eidelberg, E., & Stein, D. (1974). Functional recovery after lesions of the nervous system. *Neurosciences Research Progress Bulletin, 12*(2), 191–203.

Finger, S. (1978). Lesion momentum and behavior. In S. Finger (Ed.), *Recovery from brain damage* (pp. 135–164). New York: Plenum. Press.

Finger, S., & Stein, P. G. (1982). *Brain damage and recovery.* New York: Academic Press.

Gazzaniga, M. S. (1983a). Right hemisphere language in brain bisection. A 20-year perspective. *American Psychologist, 38,* 525–536.

Gazzaniga, M. S. (1983b). Reply to Levy and to Zaidel. *American Psychologist, 38,* 547–549.

Glassman, R. B. (1978). The logic of the lesion experiment and its role in the neural sciences. In S. Finger (Ed.), *Recovery from brain damage* (pp. 3–31). New York: Plenum.

Goldman, P. S. (1974). An alternative to developmental plasticity: Heterology of CNS structures in infants and adults. In P. G. Stein, J. J. Rosen, & N. Butters (Eds.), *Plasticity and recovery of function in the central nervous system* (pp. 149–174). New York: Academic Press.

Goldstein, K. (1948). *Language and language disturbances.* New York: Grune & Stratton.

Gooddy, W. (1977). In R. Hoops, Y. Lebrun, & E. Buyssens (Eds.), *Selected papers on the history of aphasia: Walter Riese* (p. 10). Amsterdam: Swets & Zeitlinger.

Hamlin, J. (1970). Intellectual function 14 years after frontal lobe surgery. *Cortex, 6,* 299–307.

Jackson, J. H. (1915). Epilepsy and epileptiform convulsions. *Brain 38,* 107–174. (Originally published 1863).

Jackson, J. H. (1958a). On the scientific and empirical investigation of epilepsies. In J. Taylor (Ed.), *Selected writings of John Hughlings Jackson.* London: Staples Press. (Original work published 1874)

Jackson, J. H. (1958b). On the anatomical and physiological localisation of movements in the brain. In J. Taylor (Ed.), *Selected writings of John Hughlings Jackson* (pp. 37–76). London: Staples Press. (Original work published 1873)

Jacobsen, C. F., Wolfe, J. B., & Jackson, T. A. (1935). An experimental analysis of the functions of the frontal association areas in animals. *Journal of Nervous and Mental Disease, 82,* 1–14.

Kussmaul, A. (1877). Die Storungen der Sprache. *Ziemssen's Handbuch der speciellen Pathologie und Therapie, XII,* Anhang, 1–300.

Lashley, K. S. (1937). Functional deteminants of cerebral localization, *Archives of Neurology and Psychiatry, 38,* 371–387.

Lashley, K. S. (1944). Studies of cerebral function in learning. *Journal of Comparative Neurology, 80,* 257–281.

Laurence, S., & Stein, D. G. (1978). Recovery after brain damage and the concept of localization of function. In S. Finger (Ed.), *Recovery from brain damage* (pp. 369–407). New York: Plenum.

Levy, J. (1983). Language, cognition and the right hemisphere. A response to Gazzaniga. *American Psychologist, 38,* 538–539.

Lewin, R. (1980). Is your brain really necessary? *Science, 210,* 1232–1234.

Lewis, N. D. C., Landis, C., & King, H. E. (Eds.) (1956). *Studies in topectomy.* New York: Grune & Stratton.

Lishman, W. A. (1978). *Organic psychiatry.* Oxford: Blackwell.

Lorber, J. (1965). Hydranencephaly with normal development. *Developmental Medicine and Child Neurology, 7,* 628–633.

Lorber, J. (1977). The medical treatment of hydrocephalus using isosorbide. *Modern Problems of Pediatrics, 18,* 178–180.

Lorber, J. (1980). Is Your Brain really necessary? *World Medicine,* May 3, 1980, pp. 21–24.

Mettler, F. A. (Ed.) (1949). *Selective partial ablations of the frontal cortex.* New York: Hoeber.

Mettler, F. A. (Ed.) (1952). *Psychosurgical problems.* Philadelphia: Blakiston.

Moniz, E. (1936). *Tentatives operatoires dans le traitment de certaines psychoses.* Paris: Masson.

Riese, W. (1960). Dynamics in brain lesions. *Journal of Nervous and Mental Disease, 131,* 291–301.

Rioch, D. M. (1953). Sir David Ferrier. In W. Haymaker (Ed.), *The founders of Neurology* (pp. 122–123). Springfield, IL: Thomas.

Rosner, B. S. (1974). Recovery of function and localization of function in historical perspective. In D. C. Stein, J. J. Rosen, & N. Butters (Eds.), *Plasticity and recovery of function in the central nervous system.* New York: Academic Press.

Russell, W. R. (1963). Some anatomical aspects of aphasia. *Lancet,* 1173–1177.

Russell, W. R., & Espir, M. L. E. (1961). *Traumatic aphasia.* London: Oxford University Press.

Russell, W. R., & Smith, A. (1961). Post-traumatic amnesia in closed head injury. *Archives of Neurology, 5,* 4–17.

Sherrington, C. S. (1941). *Man on his nature.* New York: Macmillan.

Smith, A. (1960). Changes in porteus maze scores of brain-operated schizophrenics after an eight-year interval. *Journal of Mental Science, 106*(444), 967–978.

Smith, A. (1962). Ambiguities in concepts and studies of 'brain damage' and 'organicity.' *Journal of Nervous and Mental Disease, 135,* 311–326.

Smith, A. (1964). Mental deterioration in chronic schizophrenia. *Journal of Nervous and Mental Disease, 139,* 479–487.

Smith, A. (1966). Certain hypothesized hemispheric differences in language and visual functions in human adults. *Cortex, 2,* 109–126.

Smith, A. (1969). Nondominant hemispherectomy. *Neurology, 19,* 442–445.

Smith, A. (1971). Objective indices of severity of chronic aphasia in stroke patients. *Journal of Speech and Hearing Disorders, 36,* 167–207.

Smith, A. (1972a). Dominant and nondominant hemispherectomy. In W. L. Smith, (Ed.), *Drugs, development and cerebral function* (pp. 37–68). Springfield, IL: Thomas.

Smith, A. (1972b). Hemispherectomy and the functional plasticity of the infant brain. *Proceedings of the XXth International Congress of Psychology, Tokyo,* p. 518.

Smith, A. (1974, February). Related findings in neuropsychologic studies of patients with hemispherectomy and of patients with chronic aphasia. *Presented at the Second Annual Meeting, International Neuropsychological Society, Boston.*

Smith, A. (1975). Neuropsychological testing in neurological disorders. In W. J. Friedlander (Ed.), *Advances in neurology* (Vol. 7, pp. 49–110). New York: Raven.

Smith, A. (1978). Lenneberg, Locke, Zangwill and the neuropsychology of language. In G. Miller & E. Lenneberg (Eds.), *Psychology and biology of language and thought: Essays in honor of Eric H. Lenneberg* (pp. 133–149). New York: Academic Press.

Smith, A. (1979). Practices and principles of clinical neuropsychology: Focusing on the hole rather than the doughnut. *International Journal of Neuroscience, 9,* 233–238.

Smith, A. (1981a). Principles underlying human brain functions in neuropsychological sequelae of different neuropathological processes. In S. Filskov & T. Boll (Eds.), *Handbook of clinical neuropsychology* (pp. 175–226). New York: Wiley.

Smith, A. (1981b). On the organization, disorganization and reorganization of language and other brain functions. In Y. Lebrun & O. Zangwill (Eds.), *Lateralisation of language in the child* (pp. 51–70). Lisse: Swets & Zeitlinger.

Smith, A. (1983a). Overview or underview? — Comment on Satz and Fletcher "Emergent trends in neuropsychology: An overview." *Journal of Consulting and Clinical Psychology, 51,* 768–775.

Smith, A. (1983b) Clinical psychological practice and principles of neuropsychological assessment. In C. E. Walker (Ed.), *Handbook of Clinical Psychology,* Homewood, IL: Dorsey Press, pp. 445–500.

Smith, A., & Burklund, C. W. (1966). Dominant hemispherectomy: Preliminary report on neuropsychological sequelae. *Science, 153,* 1280–1282.

Smith, A., & Kinder, E. F. (1959). Changes in psychological test performances of brain-operated schizophrenics after eight years. *Science, 129,* 149–150.

Smith, A., & Sugar, O. (1975). Development of above normal language and intelligence 21 years after left hemispherectomy. *Neurology, 25,* 813–818.

Sperry, R. W. (1975). Lateral specialization in the surgically separated hemispheres. In B. Milner (Ed.), *Hemispheric specialization and interaction* (pp. 5–19). Cambridge: MIT Press.

Stein, D. G., Rosen, J. J., & Butters, N. (Eds.), (1974). *Plasticity and recovery of function in the central nervous system.* New York: Academic Press.

Strich, S. J. (1976). Cerebral trauma. In W. Blackwood & J. A. N. Corsellis (Eds.), *Greenfield's Neuropathology.* Chicago: Year Book Publishers.

von Monakow, C. (1960). Localization of brain junctions. In G. von Bonin (Ed.), *Some papers on the cerebral cortex.* Springfield IL: Thomas. (Originally published 1911)

von Monakow, C., & Mourgue, R. (1928). *Introduction biologique a l'étude de la neurologie et de la psychopathologie.* Paris: Libraririe Felix Alcan.

von Monakow, C. (1914). *Die Lokalization im Grosshirn und der Abbau der Funktion durch kortikale Herde.* Wiesbaden: Bergmann.

Vulpian, A. (1942). Lecons sur la physiologie générale et comparée du système nerveux. [Lectures on general and comparative physiology of the nervous system] Quoted in M. A. Kennard & J. F. Fulton, (Eds.), Age and reorganization of the central nervous system. *Journal of Mount Sinai Hospital, 9,* 594–605. (Originally published 1866)

Wolf, G., Stricker, C. M., & Zigmond, M. F. (1978). Brain lesions: Induction, analysis and the problem of recovery of functions. In S. Finger (Ed.), *Revoery from brain damage* (pp. 91–112). New York: Plenum.

Woolsey, T. A. (1978). Lesion experiments: Some anatomical consideration. In S. Finger, (Ed.), *Recovery from brain damage* (pp. 71–89). New York: Plenum.

Yakovlev, P. I. (1953). Fronto-pontine bundle and associated projection fibers of the frontal lobe following frontal leucotomy. *Transactions of the American Neurological Association, 78,* 286–291.

Yakovlev, P. I. (1954). Anatomical studies in frontal leucotomies. *Transactions of the American Neurological Association, 79,* 53–56.

Yakovlev, P. I., & Lecours, A. R. (1967). The myelogenetic cycles of regional maturation of the brain. In A. Minkowski (Ed.), *Regional development of the brain in early life* (pp. 3–64). Philadelphia: Davis.

Zaidel, E. (1983). A response to Gazzaniga: Language in the right hemisphere. Convergent perspectives. *American Psychologist, 38,* 542–546.

16

Early Brain Injury and Cognitive Development

H. Gerry Taylor

Introduction

Each year, thousands of children suffer brain damage either congenitally or some time during their early childhood years. Cerebral palsy, seizure disorders, head trauma, and bacterial and viral infections of the brain and its surrounding tissue are among the most frequent conditions associated with early brain injury. Given the large number of children involved and the obvious risk that early brain damage would seem to pose for psychological development, it is both surprising and unfortunate that we are able to make so few predictions about long-term consequences. Even less is known concerning which children might most benefit from developmental intervention, or what kinds of intervention might be most helpful.

This inability to predict and to optimally treat the problems of the brain-injured child stems primarily from the diversity of effects of early brain injury on human development and the complexities of the

EARLY BRAIN DAMAGE, Volume 1
Research Orientations and Clinical Observations

Copyright © 1984 by Academic Press, Inc.
All rights of reproduction in any form reserved.
ISBN 0-12-052901-7

issues involved. Existing data on the effects of early brain lesions have been the subject of numerous speculations regarding functional plasticity, or sparing, and its neurological basis. The weight of evidence is against the child being either completely impervious to early brain lesions, on the one hand, or unalterably impaired by these lesions, on the other hand. Nevertheless, these two extreme views of the effects of early brain lesions each receives some support. The purpose of the present chapter is to discuss these two opposing views as points of departure for a more realistic formulation of the relationship between early lesions and later development. Although few researchers are likely to adopt either the early-plasticity or early-vulnerability view in its entirety, discussion of the strengths and weaknesses of each position serves to discourage all-or-none conceptions of functional sparing and to clarify research needs.

In addressing the topic of cognitive–behavioral sparing following early brain lesions, the present chapter intentionally avoids the issue of whether early lesions have greater or lesser effects than do later lesions. The disposition of the present chapter is that the effects of early brain injuries are difficult to compare with the effects of brain injuries occurring later in life. Meaningful comparisons are prevented by unavoidable complications due to differences in nature of the injury sustained, neural organization at the time of injury, time between injury and behavioral assessment, age at assessment, and intervening experiential influences (Johnson & Almli, 1978; Robinson, 1981). Whereas it may be of some interest to know whether brain damage in infancy or childhood compromises eventual functioning to the same degree as does brain damage in adulthood—or more specifically, if "it is better to have your brain lesion early" (Schneider, 1979, p. 557)—the most essential task is to determine the extent and nature of the effects of brain injury on subsequent development. The primary concern of this paper, therefore, is with the sequelae of brain injuries sustained previous to adulthood. Because the impact of early injury is gauged by the child's ability to maintain normal developmental progress, rather than by the preservation of or return to premorbid levels of ability, outcome is discussed more appropriately in terms of sparing than in terms of recovery.

Early Plasticity

Origins

The view that early brain injuries carry a better developmental prognosis than do later injuries comes close to what might be regarded as conventional wisdom (Geschwind, 1974; St. James-Roberts, 1979). The hypothesis advanced to account for the allegedly better functioning in early-lesioned as compared to later-lesioned individuals is that brain physiology and structure are more modifiable early in life. The most commonly cited findings in support of this hypothesis are those of Kennard (1936, 1938), who found that cortical ablations leading to motor impairment in adult monkeys and chimpanzees were much less devastating to younger members of these species. Subsequent investigators found similar early sparing with lesions in a number of sensory and association areas–for rats and cats as well as for monkeys (Hécaen & Albert, 1978).

Behavioral findings in many children with early central nervous system (CNS) insults are also consistent with the early-plasticity view. Among the more convincing of these findings is the rapid resolution of aphasia observed in many young children (Alajouanine & Lhermitte, 1965; Lenneberg, 1967) and the frequent absence of focal somatosensory deficits following early brain damage (Rudel, Teuber, & Twitchell, 1974). Case studies of individuals having achieved high IQs despite severe damage or dysgenesis of the brain early in life provide further confirmation for the plasticity position (Lewin, 1980; Smith & Sugar, 1975; Sperry, 1973). A final body of support is provided by those studies demonstrating sparing of function following early malnutrition or other pre- and perinatal risk events (St. James-Roberts, 1979). Although the evidence is mixed, pre- and perinatal complications (e.g., anoxia) frequently fail to precipitate any developmental problems. The transitory disturbances reported in some studies appear in many cases to wash out with time against the more potent influences of social and environmental factors (Sameroff & Chandler, 1975).

Limitations

On closer inspection the evidence in favor of early plasticity is of a rather limited nature. The sparing of functions that was initially observed in early-lesioned laboratory animals became less impressive as these animals matured (Kennard, 1942). According to more recent research, functional recovery is dependent on the specific focus of damage and the behavior assessed as well as on age at injury. Certain anatomical areas are more susceptible to permanent deficit than other areas; and some forms of learning are more affected than other forms (Hécaen & Albert, 1978; Johnson & Almli, 1978; Nonneman & Isaacson, 1973).

Findings have also been equivocal with respect to behavioral sparing in humans. Whereas it is clear that specific language and sensory–motor deficits are often absent in children who have recovered from aphasia, relevant studies have indicated that early lesions may indeed have a developmental impact. In their study of 32 cases of childhood aphasia, Alajouanine and Lhermitte (1965) studied 14 children who had returned to school after recovery from aphasia. These investigators found unsatisfactory progress in 12 of the 14. The majority either did not return to their previous level of schooling or did so with great difficulty. Vocabulary skills were normal or higher, but IQ fell below normal levels in two thirds of these patients. According to Alajouanine and Lhermitte, "in spite of a normal language—the children have great difficulty in learning lessons, understanding the general meaning of a course and in applying to a new problem a logical system which they have been taught. In short, they were able to regain what they had learned but were unable to acquire new data" (p. 661). Similar residual deficits in 10 other cases of childhood aphasia have been described by Byers and McLean (1962).

Survey of the literature on all forms of early brain damage—including head injuries, CNS infections, hemispherectomies and infantile hemiplegias, vascular diseases, seizure disorders, and prophylactic CNS irradiation for leukemia—suggests that later impairments in higher cognitive function may be more a rule than an exception (see reviews by Levin, Ewing-Cobbs, & Benton, in press; Rutter, 1981). In some cases earlier brain disease may be even more devastating to eventual cognitive status than is damage sustained later in life (Isaccson, 1975). Greater eventual impairment with early disease has been reported for head injury (Levin *et al.*, in press), meningitis (Taylor, Michaels, Mazur, Bauer, & Liden, in press; Wright, 1978), Reye's syndrome (Davidson, Willoughby, O'Tuama, Swisher, & Benjamins, 1978), prophylactic CNS treatment for cancer (Eiser, 1978), and seizure disorders (Dikmen, Matthews, & Harley, 1975; O'Leary, Seidenberg, Berent, & Boll, 1981). These more pessimistic findings with respect to early plasticity may beg the question of how some individuals with significant early brain damage can develop many normal or supernormal functions, but the myth that early injuries are generally of little consequence to development is clearly dispelled.

The significance of favorable outcomes following pre- and perinatal complications may also have been overstated. Pre- and perinatal risk events do not necessarily result in brain insults. Therefore, one cannot be sure of the extent to which children with early complications have been compromised neurologically. Behavioral outcomes have been more unequivocally negative in studies in which at least transient neurological abnormalities have followed the pre- or perinatal complications (Prechtl, 1960; Rubin & Balow, 1980). The impunity to these complications demonstrated in many follow-up studies may be better explained in terms of the absence of severe or chronic forms of brain damage than in terms of early plasticity.

Early Vulnerability

Hebb's Formulation

At the end of the spectrum opposite the early-plasticity position is the view that the psychological developmental of the child is particularly vulnerable to early brain injury. The early-vulnerability position has been less popular than the opposing early-plasticity view. Nevertheless, the hypothesis that development is particularly liable to disruption by early CNS insult accords with some of the facts discussed in the previous section and thus deserves consideration as an alternative to early plasticity.

Hebb's (1942) formulation of the differential effects of early versus late brain lesions on intelligence provides the most comprehensive statement of the early-vulnerability view. To support his argument for early vulnerability, Hebb (1942) summarized the specific effects of brain injury on adult intellectual functions. He noted that nonaphasic brain-damaged adults infrequently show impairment in vocabulary or in other verbal or practical reasoning skills; and that, conversely, aphasic adults infrequently manifest severe impairment on nonverbal tasks (e.g., block constructions). In contrast to this bimodal pattern of adult outcomes, Hebb observed that children with early injuries exhibited generalized mental impairment with some tendency for greater deficits in verbal than in nonverbal skills. His child data were based on the testing of a group of 32 cases of exogenous, or "brain-injured," retardates from a school for the brain-injured. The sample excluded children with severe retardation (Stanford-Binet IQ below 50) or with gross motor handicaps that would have interfered with testing. The absence in children of a parallel to the bimodal pattern of defits characteristic of brain-damage adults led Hebb to speculate that the brain mechanisms responsible for the development of intellectual functions were different from the mechanisms responsible for the retention of acquired intellectual functions in the audlt.

According to Hebb (1942) the development of intellectual abilities is dependent on "intellectual power," defined as the "capacity to develop a test ability in the absence of any previous relevant experience" (p. 287). Hebb described intellectual power, termed *intelligence* A, as the ability to engage in new mental constructions by "synthesis and invention" (p. 257). Tasks in which this type of intelligence is manifested include those measures most sensitive to adult brain-damage (e.g., tasks requiring visual route finding, abstract verbal reasoning, and speeded visual–spatial and constructional performance). In contrast to intelligence *A* is the operation of previously acquired mental functions, or *intelligence* B. Intelligence *B* has to do with the retention and use of intellectual products rather than with their original acquisition. As such, intelligence *B* results from the experiential accumulation of skills and is manifested in tasks that are insensitive to late-occurring brain disease, such as of vocabulary knowledge or verbal comprehension.

The distinction between intelligence *A* and intelligence *B* formed the basis for Hebb's conception of early vulnerability. In agreement with Lashley's (1938) equipotentiality position on recovery, intelligence *A* was conceived of as dependent on overall neural integrity. Damage to any part of the brain would diminish intelligence *A*. With intelligence *B*, however, came "stable changes in neural organization" (p. 286) that were less dependent on the integrity of the entire cerebrum. Hebb did not speculate on the exact neural basis of intelligence *B*, but he did imply a certain degree of localization of function. The distinction between the neural mechanisms subserving these two types of intelligence allowed prediction of the differential effects of early versus late brain insults. Consistent with Hebb's observations, early brain injury would be predicted to result in more generalized cognitive impairment than would insults to the brain later in development. Although early brain damage might not interfere with those intellectual products already formed, such damage would set limits on future intellectual products due to a lowering of intellectual power through the growth period.

The major advantage of Hebb's (1942) formulation is its compatibility with the lack of normal cognitive growth in groups of children who have sustained early CNS disease (Ernhart, Graham, Eichman, Marshall, & Thurston, 1963; Fitzhugh, Fitzhugh & Reitan, 1962; Reed & Fitzhugh, 1966; Reed, Reitan, & Klove, 1965; Rutter, 1981). Vocabulary and other verbal abilities are often as impaired as nonverbal skills, and tests of general mental abilities such as the Wechsler Intelligence Scale for children—Revised (WISC-R) are as sensitive to skill deficits as are neuropsychological test batteries (Reitan, 1974; Rutter, 1981). This pattern of findings is in marked contrast to the pattern observed in persons who have sustained brain damage as adults. As Hebb (1942) appropriately noted, brain injuries in adults often have little impact on well-practiced verbal and social skills, even when deficits in abstract reasoning and constructional abilities are clearly present.

Critique

Support for Hebb's (1942) early-vulnerability hypothesis is just as ambiguous as the evidence favoring early plasticity. One problem is that several of the favorable studies drew their samples from schools or training centers for brain-injured children. Although the admission criteria for these institutions are rarely reported, admission is likely based both on neurological abnormality and on mental or behavioral defect. The general mental subnormality observed in these groups, therefore, may not have been due as much to early brain injuries as to an overrepresentation of mentally impaired individuals in the samples studied. The tendency for mentally deficient children to manifest relatively greater impairments in verbal tests than in nonverbal tests (Kaufman, 1979) would in turn explain the somewhat greater verbal deficits reported for Hebb's (1942) brain-injured sample.

The fact that children with early brain lesions often show isolated forms of functional impairment is also problematic for the early vulnerability hypothesis. Brain-injured children of normal intelligence may display any one of a number of specific problems, including behavioral and psychiatric disturbances, deficiencies in constructional, visual–spatial, and visual–memory tasks, attention disorders, slowed psychomotor speed, motor incoordination, somatosensory deficits, specific learning disabilities, poor concept utilization, and difficulties in acquiring new skills (Benton, 1962; Birch & Bortner, 1967; Byers & Lord, 1943; Meyer & Byers, 1952; Rutter, 1981). As noted earlier, childhood aphasias are frequently accompanied by later disturbances in visual–motor skills, spatial conceptualization, and academic learning, even in cases where the aphasia resolves and where many verbal abilities develop normally (Alajouanine & Lhermitte, 1965; Byers & McLean, 1962). Although not widely recognized, this same tendency has been reported in many other studies as well, usually in terms of a superiority of verbal IQ over performance IQ on the Wechsler scales (Boll & Barth, 1981; Chadwick, Rutter, Shaffer, & Shrout, 1981; Dennis, Fitz, Netley, Sugar, Harwood-Nash, Hendrick, Hoffman, & Humphreys, 1981; Holroyd & Wright, 1965; Reed & Reitan, 1969; Taylor *et al.*, in press).

Hebb's (1942) distinction between intellectual power and intellectual products provides a manner in which to conceptualize the specific deficits of some children with early brain disease. If one assumes that early brain damage impairs intellectual power (intelligence *A*) more than intellectual products (intelligence *B*), and that selective impairments in performance areas are due to diminished intellectual power, then one would expect performance skills to be more affected than verbal skills. The major limitation of Hebb's model is that it does not allow for these differential effects when lesions are sustained *early* in life. Under these conditions and because the establishment of intellectual products is dependent on the operation over time of intellectual power, the development of intellectual products should be completely constrained by the level of intellectual power.

A final difficulty with Hebb's formulation stems from his conclusion that "The apparently generalized effect of infant lesions argues for some degree of equipotentiality of the cortex in development" (p. 290). By equipotentiality Hebb was referring to Lashley's (1938) concept of a dependence of some behaviors on mass action of the brain rather than on the functioning of restricted cortical areas. It is difficult to refute this statement outright, for there is clearly substantial support for a limited form of equipotentiality. Woods and Carey (1979), for example, tested persons who had sustained a left hemisphere injury either before or after their first birthday. These investigators found that the early-injury group was more linguistically intact than the group with somewhat later left hemisphere insults. In agreement with the Woods–Carey finding, Lansdell (1969) also discovered verbal abilities to vary as a function of the age of onset of left hemisphere disease. The earlier the onset of left hemisphere injury, the greater were the individual's verbal aptitudes. Additional evidence favoring some form of equipotentiality is provided by data summarized by Lenneberg (1967) and Annett (1973). These data showed a relatively high incidence of speech and language delays among children who had sustained early damage to either cerebral hemisphere. If one ignores the possibility that some of the right hemisphere-damaged cases may have involved bilateral damage (Woods & Teuber, 1978), the implication is that areas of the cortex other than those that eventually mediate language functions subserved those functions early in development.

The problem with Hebb's (1941) conclusion regarding equipotentiality of the brain early in life is that this concept can be easily overextended. Although Hebb did not specify the limits of equipotentiality, he implied that the growth of most normal functions, including verbal abilities, was based on "the integrity of the whole cerebrum" early in life (p. 290). Recent studies favor a more delimited form of equipotentiality. A series of studies by Dennis and her colleagues has shown disturbances in later developing linguistic abilities among patients with early left hemispherectomy, and disturbances in more complex and later developing visual–perceptual skills in cases of early right hemispherectomy (see Dennis & Whitaker, 1977). Investigations of other forms of early unilateral brain disease have yielded similar results (Kershner & King, 1974; Rudel *et al.*, 1974). Also somewhat damaging to the equipotentiality view is the fact that isolated left hemispheres can process high-level linguistic information, just as isolated right hemispheres can deal adequately with more complex visual–spatial tasks (Dennis & Kohn, 1975; Kohn & Dennis, 1974). Although there is reason to believe that some form of equipotentiality exists, such equipotentiality may be restricted to the earliest months of life. Equipotentiality may be further limited by the fact that specific cerebral regions are essential to the full acquisition of certain mental functions.

A Reformulation

Accounting for the Existing Facts

Clearly, neither the early-plasticity nor the early-vulnerability view adequately accommodates what is currently known about the effects of early brain lesions on cognitive development. On the one hand, the early-plasticity view underrates the frequency of stunted intellectual growth in children who have sustained early lesions. On the other hand, Hebb's (1942) early-vulnerability hypothesis cannot account for the frequent attainment of many normal functions despite pervasive early insults. Existing data imply a need for an alternative formulation of the developmental consequences of early brain lesions. This alternative should account for the following: (1) a limited form of either equipotentiality or vicarious neural functioning early in life in which undamaged tissue subserves behaviors normally mediated by the damaged areas; (2) the fact that sparing is more evident for some aspects of cognitive development than for other aspects; and (3) the tendency for damage sustained either congenitally or in early childhood to lead to mental subnormality. A nonpolarized view regarding the impact of early brain injury on cognitive development must strike a compromise between early plasticity and early vulnerability.

A good example of such an alternative view is provided by Goldman (1974). In her studies on developmental-sparing phenomena in rhesus monkeys, Goldman proposes an age-related commitment of specific CNS structures to specific behaviors. According to her model of CNS *heterology*, if a CNS structure is damaged early in life and before other less mature structures have become committed to certain behavioral functions, these uncommitted or prefunctional structures will be capable of assuming the functions of the damaged areas. However, if a CNS structure is damaged at a time when other structures have already become committed to their respective functions, there will be no sparing. Further, if a prefunctional area is itself damaged, the organism may escape immediate deficit, but it will then be subject to future impairments. The onset of these later impairments will depend on the time that would have been required for the prefunctional area to have otherwise matured, or to have taken over its normal functions.

Goldman's hypothesis of an age-related commitment of CNS structures to given functions receives support from recent histological studies of tissue regrowth following experimental brain ablations in young animals (Goldman & Lewis, 1978; Schneider, 1979). The possibility of neural reorganization following early brain lesions in children is less firmly grounded. One problem is that mechanisms in addition to neural reorganization undoubtedly contribute to the cognitive sparing observed in brain-injured children. The most obvious example is behavioral substitution, in which the child compensates for deficient skills by deploying alternative cognitive strategies (Geschwind, 1974). The extent to which behavioral substitution may contribute to instances of sparing following childhood lesions is difficult to ascertain and awaits the development of methods to appraise the *manner* in which children meet the demands of specific tasks. However, any explanation of sparing that relies on behavioral sutstitution alone fails to explain why earlier insults to the left hemisphere result in greater sparing of linguistic functions (Landsdell, 1969; Woods & Carey, 1979). It is also doubtful that sparing could be as complete as it is in certain instances (e.g., as when an entire hemisphere has been removed) without recourse to some form of CNS reorganization. The advantage of hypothesizing an age-dependent neural-recruitment mechanism is that it accounts for the sparing of some functions in children with congenital or very early brain injuries.

An additional advantage of Goldman's (1974) formulation is that it provides grounds for explaining the susceptibility of brain-injured children to specific deficits as well as to general mental subnormality. The implication of early recruitment of uncommitted neural structures is that sparing of certain functions will occur at the expense of other functions. Specifically, the behaviors mediated by recruited CNS structures should show some sparing, but at the expense of behaviors that would have been mediated by these structures had there been no brain damage. Assuming a preference for the development of certain verbal skills in early life—either on a genetic basis or due to environmental demands (Corballis & Morgan, 1978)—nonverbal skills would be expected to show least sparing as the child matures. Given that these nonverbal skills were essential to later stages of cognitive growth, general mental subnormality would also be predicted, depending on the extent to which neural structures either were themselves damaged or were sacrified to sparing.

Whether verbal functions in general show more sparing than nonverbal functions following early brain insults remains unclear. Even in cases of early removals of the left hemisphere, there are limits to which verbal sparing can occur. Dennis and Whitaker (1977), for example, report that persons who have sustained left hemispherectomies may develop adequate vocabulary knowledge, but they have difficulties on language tasks that require the processing of complex syntactical forms. As these results imply, extent of sparing may not fall cleanly along a verbal–performance continuum. Although the author is aware of no systematic investigations of this issue, a dimension that involves complexity of intellectual performance (defined, for example, in terms of the intricacy of rule systems followed) or perhaps something akin to Hebb's (1942) distinction between intellectual power and intellectual products may provide a better metric for the assessment of sparing than does the verbal–performance dichotomy (Lashley, 1938; Piercy, 1964; Teuber, 1970; Vygotsky, 1962). Perhaps those functions that place most demands on the integration of various neural systems are at greatest risk. A certain amount of "pre-wiring" may exist for certain behavioral functions, making these functions more dependent on the integrity of specific cortical sites. Other functions, on the other hand, may arise under the combined influences of wider cortical areas. In keeping with Lashley's

(1938) concept of equipotentiality, these latter functions may be less strictly preprogrammed for specific functions, but they may also be relatively more sensitive to diffuse forms of brain damage. For the present these possibilities remain a matter of speculation. The essential point is that, contrary to either the early-plasticity of early-vulnerability views, sparing is not an all-or-none process. Any sensible reformulation of the effects of early brain injury on cognitive development will need to attempt to describe the unevenness of sparing. The impact of this unevenness on the child's continued cognitive growth will also need to be taken into account in predicting eventual outcome.

Acknowledging Experiential Factors

In addition to their inability to account for the facts, the early-plasticity and early-vulnerability views fail to make any formal provision for the influences of early experience. Demonstration of the impact of environmental factors on sparing following early lesions is provided by both human and animal studies. With respect to children, several investigators have noted that recovery seems to be most substantial in cases in which acquisition of basic skills is directly emphasized (e.g., as with formal schooling), or in which environmental conditions are optimal (St. James-Roberts, 1981). The influence of premorbid cognitive and personality variables on the course of recovery following brain damage has also been documented (Finlayson, Johnson, & Reitan, 1977; Rutter, 1981). The adaptation of the child to the behavioral consequences of injury and the postinjury environment over time are of additional importance (Rutter, 1977).

Animal studies have been particularly helpful in even further broadening our appreciation for the complexities of environmental influences. Research on rhesus monkeys has demonstrated that behavioral impairment subsequent to orbital prefrontal cortical lesions in infancy can be greatly overcome given appropriate environmental stimulation (Goldman & Lewis, 1978). Comparable gains with stimulation are not seen in adults with similar lesions, nor are they observed with early lesions unless the stimulation occurs early in postoperative development. Early environmental enrichment or deprivation seems to have an especially potent effect on behavior at maturity. Early experience may serve not only to enhance the organism's capacity to compensate for behavioral dysfunctions induced by early brain injury, but may also be vital in guiding the neural reorganization of those functions (Wolff, 1981). For these several reasons, variations among brain-injured children in learning histories and in social and environmental circumstances deserve careful scrutiny. Assessment of these variables may improve predictions regarding cognitive and behavioral development subsequent to early brain injuries.

Expanding the Analysis of Behavior and Behavioral Change

A final problem with the early-plasticity and early-vulnerability positions is that these views discourage more refined analyses of behavioral sparing. Since these views tend to pit behavioral normality against behavioral impairment in an all-or-none fashion there is little incentive to study behavior in a more exacting fashion. If the sparing issue is to be reformulated in a manner that will encompass the possibility of selective sequelae, the study of behavior and behavioral change is critical. Data reviewed previously have shown that early lesions are more frequently associated with greater sparing of verbal IQ than of performance IQ. Tasks that require the learning of new material, spatial–constructional skills, motor and psychomotor efficiency, and developmentally more complex verbal and nonverbal skills may be especially sensitive to the effects of early brain lesions (Birch & Bortner, 1967; Dennis & Whitaker, 1977; Rudel *et al.*, 1974).

An illustration of this type of selective sparing is provided by the findings of a recently completed study by the author and his colleagues at the University of Pittsburgh (Taylor *et al.*, in press). In this study, 24 grade-school children who had sustained *Haemophilus influenzae* type b meningitis (age of onset, 3–36 months of age) were compared to their nearest school-age siblings. Comparisons were made on tests of intelligence, academic performance, and neuropsychological skills. In keeping with the previously noted trends, the postmeningitis group was deficient relative to the sibling group on WICS-R performance IQ and full-scale IQ. The postmeningitis group also obtained significantly lower age-corrected scores on neuropsychological tasks involving fine motor proficiency, gross motor and somatosensory skills, and verbal memory and learning. In contrast, the postmeningitis and sibling groups were closely comparable in age-adjusted standard scores across several academic measures; and although there was a tendency for verbal IQ to be lower in the postmeningitis group, the difference in verbal IQ was small and nonsignificant. Like the findings of several other neuropsychological investigations of brain-injured children, these results support the need to abandon all-or-none notions of sparing. Even more importantly, the outcome of this study underscores the advantages of more detailed analyses of cognitive skills.

Consideration of the burgeoning literature on neurological disorders and specific developmental disabilities suggests several requirements for improved behavioral analysis. As our study of meningitis indicates, one important requisite is that a wide range of abilities be assessed. In spite of a limited tendency for different skills to co-vary within individuals—the positive manifold, or *g*, factor—there is a long tradition of psychometric investigation that demonstrates the multifaceted nature of human intelligence (Guilford, 1967). Neuropsychological research in particular has been instrumental in bringing about an increased awareness of the limitations of traditional measures and in differentiating among types of intellectual skills (Kaufman, 1979; Rourke, 1976). This research has not revealed unitary patterns of dysfunction after early brain insults. Diverse skills may be affected, depending on the location and type of injury and the child's age at the time of testing. Hence it is critical that the scope of inquiry on the effects of early lesions be broadened beyond IQ tests alone (St. James-Roberts, 1979).

At the same time, it is essential that behavioral assessments not be expanded in a haphazard fashion. Although early lesions may lead to diverse sequelae (perhaps relating to the localization of the lesion and the commitment of the neural tissue in that area to a specific function), the pervasive developmental influences of some types of deficits and the tendency toward overall mental subnormality cannot be ignored (Isaccson, 1975). Judging from the tendency for performance IQ and other measures less dependent on previously acquired knowledge to be less spared than verbal IQ, distinctions like that Hebb (1942) proposed when he contrasted intellectual power (intelligence *A*) with intellectual products (intelligence *B*) may be important for understanding the effects of early brain injuries. The continued development of some higher level skills in individuals who have sustained substantial early injuries (e.g., the linguistic abilities of some patients with total right hemisphere removals in infancy) argues against Hebb's proposal for a close dependence of intellectual products on the integrity of the entire cerebrum in early life. Nevertheless, his insistence on a "capacity for achievement" that is distinct from achievement per se (Hebb & Morton, 1944, p. 221), is worth pursuing. A number of more recent theories of human abilities have promulgated a similar distinction (Guilford, 1967; Horn, 1968).

A second requirement is to expand behavioral analyses along the lines suggested by the methods of cognitive psychology. Contemporary theories of information processing provide potentially useful conceptual frameworks for exploring the nature of sparing subsequent to early lesions. Like Hebb (1942) theorists of information processing have proposed that intellectual behavior be construed as a reflection of both accumulated knowledge and current information-processing capacities (Estes, 1981; Hunt, 1980; Kail & Bisanz, 1982). Granting that the child's current information-processing capacities are less confounded by previous experience than are other cognitive achievements, the assessment of these capacities might prove particularly fruitful in evaluating the effects of early brain lesions. Awareness of these capacities may also be helpful in predicting future learning potential and in devising treatment methods (Estes, 1974). Although assessment of processing capacities may require extrapolation to clinical groups of experimentally based procedures, standardized and age-normed measures are becoming increasingly available (e.g., Kaufman & Kaufman, 1983).

A final element of improved behavioral analysis of cases of early brain injury should be the examination of developmental differences. A dysfunction at one point in development does not necessitate similar dysfunctions at other stages of life (Teuber & Rudel, 1962). Moreover, it is unsafe to assume that a given task will make demands on similar mental processes (or similar neural mechanisms) in persons of different ages (Ernhart *et al.*, 1963; Prechtl, 1981). For example, a vocabulary test that requires the child to express the meaning of a word (as opposed to, say, merely naming a pictured object) may draw heavily on the information-processing capacities of younger children. For adults, however, retrieval of stored information may be sufficient to perform this task. Because both knowledge ad information-processing capacities change with age (Kail & Bisanz, 1982), the manner in which children respond to task demands varies considerably in relation to their developmental status. For this reason the nature of developmental disabilities associated with early brain injuries is likely to change with age (Taylor, Fletcher & Satz, in press). Understanding the full implications of early lesions will be best achieved through longitudinal studies that allow assessment of both the changing status of the disability with age and the dependency of current problems on previous disabilities. If important information-processing capacities are compromised by early brain damage, the ability of the child to make use of learning experiences may be diminished and more general limitations in cognitive development may accrue over time. Due to the cumulative effects of earlier delays on later development and also to potential adaptations of the child to these delays, behavioral sparing (or its absence) must be studied "within the context of current theories of cognitive development" (Hutt, 1976, p. 636).

Conclusion

Survey of the relevant literature fails to provide support for any extreme position regarding the effects of early brain lesions on development. The complexities of cognitive development and the multiplicity of variables that influence outcome prevent any generalizations regarding cognitive sparing subsequent to early brain injury. To suppose that the nervous system is impervious to damage early in life is to ignore the evidence showing that brain-damage victims are prone both to specific deficits and to general mental subnormality. At the same time, to claim that the immature nervous system, when damaged, is particularly vulnerable to eventual cognitive dysfunction is to deny the fact that good behavioral outcomes can sometimes occur despite severe forms of early brain insult. The important task is not to decide whether sparing can occur, but to determine (1) the nature and extent of sparing and (2) the necessary and sufficient conditions that must exist in order for sparing to occur.

Research to date indicates that, at least for some groups of children, sparing may be fairly complete for many verbal and academic skills. More global assessments of cognitive status, however, suggest that sparing is incomplete, even for language. Performance IQ and other nonverbal measures, together with certain types of verbal tasks (e.g., those involving memory or abstraction), may be particularly sensitive to early CNS insult. Compromise of these latter skills may contribute to the propensity for groups of children with early brain lesions to manifest generalized mental subnormality. Nevertheless, no uniform pattern of deficits is present across individuals. Many children manifest difficulties in linguistic and nonlinguistic functions alike. Even among those groups of children that exhibit relatively delimited weaknesses on nonverbal tasks, the origins of these difficulties are poorly understood. More comprehensive analysis of the developmental sequelae of early brain injury awaits (1) an expanded repertoire of behavioral measures; (2) attempts to distinguish among types of mental abilities (e.g., task requiring application of already acquired knowledge versus those calling for deployment of information-processing capacities); and (3) longitudinal studies of behavioral change (Johnson & Almli, 1978; St. James-Roberts, 1979).

Progress in understanding the effects of early lesions will also require further analysis of the conditions that facilitate or impede behavioral sparing. There is reason to believe that diffuse brain damage may result in more serious developmental impairments than acute localized lesions (Finger & Stein, 1982; Levin, Benton, & Grossman, 1982), and that damage to specific areas of the brain may jeopardize some functions more than others (Dennis & Whitaker, 1977). In general, however, follow-up studies of children with early insults have rarely specified the extent or location of the brain damage. Other factors mediating outcome, including the age at injury and the types of experiences and interactions to which the child has been subject, are also poorly specified. Pending greater specification of both biological and environmental variables, the necessary conditions for sparing will probably remain elusive. Whether sparing, when it occurs, is achieved by virtue of behavioral substitution or of vicarious functioning of uncommitted neural areas would also seem indeterminant. Until more is known regarding both the nature of the behaviors spared and the biological and environmental correlates of such sparing, it will be difficult to formulate theories allowing prediction of consequences. Further progress toward this goal will require increased appreciation of the complexities of human development and of the manner in which biological and social variables impact on cognitive competence. Despite the difficulties of conducting research in this area, such studies are well worth the effort. They provide a unique opportunity to study the biological underpinnings of intellectual development and they hold promise for suggesting treatment alternatives. How some children learn to cope with their cognitive disabilities, or how functions once disabled may even be restored, may provide valuable insights. These insights, best gained by thoughtful evaluation and follow-up of children with early injuries, should suggest new avenues for preventing or at least reducing adverse developmental consequences (Chess, 1978).

Acknowledgments

The author wishes to express his appreciation to Arthur L. Benton and Jack M. Fletcher for their valuable feedback and constructive suggestions on the manuscript.

References

Alajouanine, T., & Lhermitte, F. (1965). Acquired aphasia in children. *Brain*, 1965, *88*, 653–662.

Annett, M. (1973). Laterality of childhood hemiplegia and growth of speech and intelligence. *Cortex*, *9*, 4–33.

Benton, A. L. (1962). Behavioral indices of brain injury in school children. *Child Development*, *33*, 199–208.

Birch, H. B., & Bortner, M. (1967). Stimulus competition and concept utilization in brain damaged children. *Developmental Medicine and Child Neurology*, *9*, 402–410.

Boll, T. J., & Barth, J. T. (1981). Neuropsychology of brain damage in children. In S. Filskov & T. J. Boll (Eds.), *Handbook of clinical neuropsychology*. New York: Wiley.

Byers, R. K., & Lord, E. E. (1943). Late effects of lead poisoning on mental development. *American Journal of Diseases of Children*, *66*, 471–494.

Byers, R. K., & McLean, W. T. (1962). Etiology and course of certain hemiplegias with aphasias in childhood. *Pediatrics*, *29*, 376–383.

Chadwick, O., Rutter, M., Shaffer, D., & Shrout, P. E. (1981). A prospective study of children with head injuries: IV. Specific cognitive deficits. *Journal of Clinical Neuropsychology*, *3*, 101–120.

Chess, S. (1978). The plasticity of human development: Alternative pathways. *Journal of Child Psychiatry*, *17*, 80–91.

Corballis, M. C., & Morgan M. J. (1978). On the biological basis of human laterality: I—Evidence for a maturational left–right gradient. *Behavioral and Brain Sciences*, *2*, 261–336.

Davidson, P. W., Wiloughby, R. H., O'Tuama, L. A., Swisher, C. N., & Benjamins, P. (1978). Neurological and intellectual sequelae of Reye's syndrome. *American Journal of Mental Deficiency*, *82*, 535–541.

Dennis, M., Fitz, C. R., Netley, C. T., Sugar, J., Harwood-Nash, D. C. F., Hendrick, E. B., Hoffman, H. J., & Humphreys, R. P. (1981). The intelligence of hydrocephalic children. *Archives of Neurology*, *38*, 607–615.

Dennis, M., & Kohn, B. (1975). Comprehension of syntax in infantile hemiplegics after cerebral hemidecortication: Left hemisphere superiority. *Brain and Language*, *2*, 472–482.

Dennis, M., & Whitaker, H. A. (1977). Hemispheric equipotentiality and language acquisition. In S. J. Segalowitz & F. A. Gruber (Eds.), *Language development and Neurological theory*. New York: Academic Press.

Dikman, S., Matthews, C. G., & Harley, J. P. (1975). The effect of early versus late onset of major motor epilepsy upon cognitive–intellectual performance. *Epilepsia*, *16*, 73–81.

Eiser, C. (1978). Intellectual abilities among survivors of childhood leukemia as a function of CNS irradiation. *Archives of Disease in Childhood*, *53*, 391–395.

Ernhart, C. B., Graham, F. K., Eichman, P. L., Marshall, J. M., & Thurston, D. (1963). Brain injury in the preschool child: Some developmental considerations (Vol. 2): Comparisons of brain-injured and normal children. *Psychological Monographs*, 1963, *77*,(Whole No. 573), 17–33.

Estes, W. K. (1974). Learning theory and intelligence. *American Psychologist*, *29*, 740–749.

Estes, W. K. (1981). Intelligence and learning. In M. P. Friedman, J. P. Das, N. O'Connor (Eds.), *Intelligence and learning*. New York: Plenum.

Finger, S., & Stein, D. G. (1982). *Brain damage and recovery: Research and clinical perspectives.* New York: Academic Press.

Finlayson, M. A. J., Johnson, K. A., & Reitan, R. M. (1977). Relationship of level of education to neuropsychological measures in brain-damaged and non-brain-damaged adults. *Journal of Consulting and Clinical Psychology, 45,* 536–542.

Fitzhugh, K. B., Fitzhugh, L. C., & Reitan, R. M. (1962). Weschler–Bellevue comparisons in groups with "chronic" and "current" lateralized and diffuse brain lesions. *Journal of Consulting and Clinical Psychology, 26,* 306–310.

Geschwind, N. (1974). Late changes in the nervous system: An overview. In D. G. Stein, J. J. Rosen, & N. Butlers (Eds.), *Plasticity and recovery of function in the central nervous system.* New York: Academic Press.

Goldman, P. S. (1974). An alternative to developmental plasticity: Heterology of CNS structures in infants and adults. In D. G. Stein, J. J. Rosen, & N. Butlers (Eds.), *Plasticity and recovery of function in the central nervous system.* New York: Academic Press.

Goldman, P. S., & Lewis, M. E. (1978). Develpmental biology of brain damage and experience. In C. W. Cotman (Ed.), *Neural plasticity.* New York: Raven.

Guilford, J. P. (1967). *The nature of human intelligence.* New York: McGraw-Hill.

Hebb, D. O. (1942). The effect of early and late brain injury upon test scores, and the nature of normal adult intelligence. *Proceedings of the American Philosophical Society, 85,* 265–292.

Hebb, D. O., & Morton, N. W. (1944). Note on the measurement of adult intelligence. *Journal of General Psychology, 30,* 217–223.

Hécaen, H. (1976). Acquired aphasia in children and the ontogenesis of hemispheric functional specialization. *Brain, 3,* 114–134.

Hécaen, H., & Albert, M. L. (1978). *Human neuropsychology.* New York: Wiley.

Holroyd, J., & Wright, F. (1965). Neurological implications of WISC verbal–performance discrepancies in a psychiatric setting. *Journal of Consulting Psychology, 29,* 206–212.

Horn, J. L. (1968). Organization of abilities and the development of intelligence. *Psychological Review, 75,* 242–259.

Hunt, E. (1980). Intelligence as an information-processing concept. *British Journal of Psychology, 71,* 449–474.

Hutt, S. J. (1976). Cognitive development and cerebral dysfunction. In V. Hamilton & M. D. Vernon (Eds.), *The development of cognitive processes.* London: Academic Press.

Isaacson, R. L. (1975). The myth of recovery from early brain damage. In N. E. Ellis (Ed.), *Aberrant development in infancy.* London: Wiley.

Johnson, D., & Almli, C. R. (1978). Age, brain damage, and performance. In S. Finger (Ed.), *Recovery from brain damage.* New York: Plenum.

Kail, R., & Bisanz, J. (1982). Information processing and cognitive development. In H. W. Reese (Ed.), *Advances in child development and behavior* (Vol. 17). New York: Academic Press.

Kaufman, A. S. (1979). Cerebral specialization and intelligence testing. *Journal of Research and Development in Education, 12,* 96–107.

Kaufman, A. S., & Kaufman, N. L. (1983). *Kaufman assessment battery for children, sampler manual.* Circle Pines, MN: American Guidance Service.

Kennard, M. A. (1936). Age and other factors in motor recovery from precentral lesions in monkeys. *American Journal of Physiology, 115,* 138–146.

Kennard, M. A. (1938). Reorganization of motor function in the cerebral cortex of monkeys deprived of motor and premotor areas in infancy. *Journal of Neurophysiology, 1*, 477–496.

Kennard, M. A. (1942). Cortical reorganization of motor function: Studies on a series of monkeys of various ages from infancy to maturity. *Archives of Neurology and Psychiatry, 47*, 227–240.

Kershner, J. R., & King, A. J. (1974). Laterality of cognitive functions in achieving hemiplegic children. *Perceptual and Motor Skills, 39*, 1283–1289.

Kohn, B., & Dennis, M. (1974). Selective impairments of visuo–spatial abilities in infantile hemiplegics after right cerebral hemidecortication. Neuropsychologia, 12, 505–512.

Landsell, H. (1969). Verbal and nonverbal factors in right-hemisphere speech: Relation to early neurological history. *Journal of Comparative and Physiological Psychology, 69*, 734–738.

Lashley, K. S. (1938). Factors limiting recovery after central nervous lesions. *Journal of Nervous and Mental Disease, 88*, 733–755.

Lenneberg, E. (1967). *Biological foundations of language.* New York: Wiley.

Levin, H. S., Benton, A. L., & Grossman, R. G. (1982). *Neurobehavioral consequences of closed head injury.* New York: Oxford University Press.

Levin, H. S., Ewing-Cobbs, L., & Benton, A. L. (in press). Age and recovery from brain damage: A review of clinical studies. In S. Scheff (Ed.), *Aging and recovery of function.* New York: Plenum.

Lewin, R. (1980). Is your brain really necessary? *Science, 210*, 1232–1234.

Meyer, E., & Byers, R. K. (1952). Measles encephalitis. *American Journal of Diseases of Childhood, 84*, 543–579.

Nonneman, A. J., & Isaacson, R. L. (1973). Task dependent recovery after early brain damage. *Behavioral Biology, 8*, 143–172.

O'Leary, D. S., Seidenberg, M., Berent, S., & Boll, T. J. (1981). Effects of age of onset of tonic–clonic seizure on neuropsychological performance in children. *Epilepsia, 22*, 197–204.

Piercy, M. (1964). The effects of cerebral lesions on intellectual function: A review of current research trends. *British Journal of Psychiatry, 110*, 310–322.

Prechtl, H. (1960). The long term value of the neurological examination of the newborn infant. *Developmental Medicine and Child Neurology, 2*, 69–74.

Prechtl, H. F. R. (1981). The study of neural development as a perspective of clinical problems. In K. J. Connolly & H. F. R. Prechtl (Eds.), *Maturation and development: Biological and psychological perspectives, Clinics in Developmental Medicine No. 77/78.* London: William Heinemann Medical Books.

Reed, H. B. C., & Fitzhugh, K. B. (1966). Patterns of deficits in relation to severity of cerebral dysfunction in children and adults. *Journal of Consulting Psychology, 30*, 98–102.

Reed, H. B. C., Jr., Reitan, R. M., & Klove, H. (1965). Influence of cerebral lesions on psychological test performances of older children. *Journal of Consulting Psychology, 29*, 247–251.

Reed, J. C., & Reitan, R. M. (1969). Verbal and performance differences among brain-injured children with lateralized motor deficits. *Perceptual and Motor Skills, 29*, 747–752.

Reitan, R. M. (1974). Psychological effects of cerebral lesions in children of early school age. In R. M. Reitan & L. A. Davison (Eds.), *Clinical neuropsychology: Current status and applications.* New York: Wiley.

Robinson, R. O. (1981). Equal recovery in child and adult brain? *Developmental Medicine and Child Neurology, 23*, 379–383.

Rourke, B. P. (1976). Issues in the neuropsychological assessment of children with learning disabilities. *Canadian Psychological Review, 17,* 89–102.

Rubin, R. A., & Balow, B. (1980). Infant neurological abnormalities as indicators of cognitive impairment. *Developmental Medicine and Child Neurology, 22,* 336–343.

Rudel, R. G., Teuber, H. L., & Twitchell, T. E. (1974). Levels of impairment of sensorimotor functions in children with early brain damage. *Neuropsychologia, 12,* 95–108.

Rutter, M. (1977). Brain damage syndromes in childhood: Concepts and findings. *Journal of Child Psychology and Psychiatry, 18,* 1–21.

Rutter, M. (1981). Psychological sequelae of brain damage in children. *American Journal of Psychiatry, 138,* 1533–1544.

St. James-Roberts, I. (1979). Neurological plasticity, recovery from brain insult, and child development. In H. W. Reese & L. P. Lipsitt (Eds.), *Advances in child development and behavior* (Vol. 14). New York: Academic Press.

St. James-Roberts, I. (1981). A reinterpretation of hemispherectomy data without functional plasticity of the brain (Vol. 1): Intellectual function. *Brain and Language, 13,* 31–53.

Sameroff, A. J., & Chandler, M. J. (1925). Reproductive risk and the continuum of caretaking casualty. In F. Horowitz (Ed.), *Review of child development research* (Vol. 4). Chicago: University of Chicago Press.

Schneider, G. E. (1979). Is it really better to have your brain lesion early? A revision of the "Kennard Principal." *Neuropsychologia, 17,* 557–583.

Smith, A., & Sugar, C. (1975). Development of above normal language and intelligence 21 years after left hemispherectomy. *Neurology, 25,* 813–818.

Sperry, R. W. (1973). Lateral specialization in the surgically separated hemispheres. In F. O. Schmitt & F. G. Worden (Eds.), *The neurosciences: Third study program.* Cambridge: MIT Press.

Taylor, H. G., Fletcher, J. M. & Satz, P. (in press). Neuropsychological assessment of children. In G. Goldstein & M. Hersen (Eds.), *Handbook of psychological assessment.* Pergamon.

Taylor, H. G., Michaels, R. H., Mazur, P. M., Bauer, R. E., & Liden, C. B. (in press). Cognitive, achievement, and behavioral outcomes six to eight years post-*H. influenzae* meningitis.

Teuber, H. L. (1970). Mental retardation after early trauma to the brain. Some issues in search of facts. In C. R. Angle & E. A. Bering, Jr. (Eds.), *Physical trauma as an etiological agent in mental retardation.* (Proceedings of a conference on the etiology of mental retardation.) Bethesda, MD: U.S. Department of Health, Education, and Welfare.

Teuber, H. L., & Rudel, R. G. (1962). Behavior after cerebral lesions in children and adults. *Developmental Medicine and Child Neurology, 4,* 3–20.

Vygotski, L. S. (1962). *Thought and language.* Cambridge, MA: MIT Press.

Wolff, P. H. (1981). Normal variation in human maturation. In K. T. Connolly & H. F. R. Prechtl (Eds.), *Maturation and development: Biological and psychological perspectives.* (Clinics in Developmental Medicine No. 77/78.) London: Heinemann Medical Books.

Woods, B. T., & Carey, S. (1979). Language deficits after apparent clinical recovery from childhood aphasia. *Annals of Neurology, 6,* 405–409.

Woods, B., & Teuber, H. L. (1978). Changing patterns of childhood aphasia. *Annals of Neurology, 3,* 273–280.

Wright, L. (1978). A method for predicting sequelae to meningitis. *American Psychologist,* 1037–1039.

Author Index

The numerals in italics indicate pages on which the complete references appear.

A

E

F

H

T

U

V

Subject Index